WIRELESS PHONES AND HEALTH

Scientific Progress

WIRELESS PHONES AND HEALTH

Scientific Progress

Edited by

George L. Carlo
Wireless Technology Research, L.L.C.

Associate Editors

Mary Supley
Susan E. Hersemann
Polly Thibodeau

Foreword by
George L. Carlo

KLUWER ACADEMIC PUBLISHERS
Boston / Dordrecht / London

Distributors for North, Central and South America:
Kluwer Academic Publishers
101 Philip Drive
Assinippi Park
Norwell, Massachusetts 02061 USA
Telephone (781) 871-6600
Fax (781) 871-6528
E-Mail <kluwer@wkap.com>

Distributors for all other countries:
Kluwer Academic Publishers Group
Distribution Centre
Post Office Box 322
3300 AH Dordrecht, THE NETHERLANDS
Telephone 31 78 6392 392
Fax 31 78 6546 474
E-Mail <services@wkap.nl>

 Electronic Services <http://www.wkap.nl>

Library of Congress Cataloging-in-Publication Data

Wireless phones and health : scientific progress / edited by George L.
    Carlo ; associate editors, Mary Supley, Susan E. Hersemann, Polly
    Thibodeau ; foreword by George L. Carlo.
        p. cm.
    Includes bibliographical references and index.
    ISBN 0-7923-8347-8 (alk. paper)
    1. Telephone, Wireless--Health aspects--Congresses.   2. Radio
frequency--Health aspects--Congresses.   I. Carlo, George Louis.
RA569.3.W55 1998
363.18'9--dc21   98-46064
                                                                      CIP

Printed on acid-free paper.

Printed in the United States of America

Contents

Section V: Non-biological Health Risks from Radio Frequency Radiation: Interference with Medical Devices

Appendices

State of the Science Colloquium
University "La Sapienza" of Rome
Rome, Italy
13-15 November 1995

viii

Foreword

Since questions about wireless phones and brain cancer were first raised in early 1993, numerous scientific studies and reviews have been conducted and published throughout the world with support from industry and government. The most comprehensive colloquium to date covering this science was co-sponsored by the International Committee on Wireless Communication Health Research and Wireless Technology Research, LLC, at the University "La Sapienza" of Rome in November 1995. Papers from that colloquium with appropriate updates form the foundation for the current volume. A follow-up to that colloquium is being planned for the spring of 1999 by the same group and the report of that colloquium will be the basis for Volume II of this series.

As the scientific story about wireless phones and health effects continues to unfold over the next several years, it is important to evaluate the work in a context that is beneficial to the enhancement of public health. Two themes are critical to an appropriate contextual understanding of this science.

First, no amount of science can ever prove that wireless phones are absolutely safe. While thoughtful and comprehensive batteries of in vitro and in vivo animal experiments can be predictive of both harm in humans and relative safety, and epidemiological studies can indicate what has happened in the human experience, assurance of the definite absence of harm is unattainable. For this reason, all the scientific work addressing wireless technology health questions that has been completed—much of it presented in this volume—or that which is underway (to be presented in future volumes), must necessarily be viewed in the context of post-market surveillance. Post-market surveillance is a search for problems following from the use of wireless technology so that interventions to solve those problems can be implemented. Timely intervention minimizes the adverse impact on the public of identified risks.

Second, wireless technology is perhaps the most rapidly evolving technology in our history. As such, it is nearly impossible to keep ahead of the technology evolution with our current tools of health risk evaluation and intervention. Within the two to three years it takes to complete a whole-life animal experiment or an epidemiological study, turnover in technology would have occurred to some degree. From a practical perspective, this suggests that scientific findings of today are variably relevant to today's technology and variably efficient at predicting tomorrow's risks. This dilemma further underscores the necessity of ongoing post-market surveillance, including both animal experiments and human epidemiology.

As you review the science presented in this and subsequent volumes of this scientific progress series, I urge you to think practically about what value each of these scientific findings has with regard to the protection of public health. That, after all, is why this work is being done.

G. L. Carlo

Acknowledgments

The papers included in this volume represent recent scientific progress in the study of potential health effects from wireless communication technology.

I would like to thank each of the presenters at the State of the Science Colloquium (Rome, Italy, 1995) for their contribution to both this volume and the scientific database on radio frequency radiation. Additionally, I would like to thank those individuals who chaired the colloquium sessions, as well as all who attended for their participation in this important scientific exchange.

The colloquium was co-sponsored by the International Committee on Wireless Communication Health Research, specifically Dr. Jorgen Bach Andersen, Dr. Paolo Bernardi, Dr. Guglielmo D'Inzeo, Gerd E. Friedrich, Dr. Zlatko Koren (deceased), Dr. Alastair F. McKinlay, Dr. Michael H. Repacholi, Dr. Paolo Vecchia, and Dr. Gary M. Williams. Dr. Guglielmo D'Inzeo graciously hosted and co-chaired the colloquium at the University "La Sapienza" of Rome, and was assisted in his efforts by Dr. Alessandro Palombo, Carlo Argiolas, Anna Bianchi, Sonia Bogliolo, Marina Breccia, Flavia Carmenini, Federica Censi, Stefano Cesare, Luca Ciminelli, Elena Cimino, Alessandro Ganci, Nora Grazioli, Federico Iori, Daniela Ippoliti, Luna Lazzarini, Fabio Mastrantonio, Stefano Pisao, and Aldo Vincenzi. Dr. Dina T. Simunic coordinated the participation of members of the COST 244 working group.

I would like to thank the staff of Wireless Technology Research (WTR), LLC responsible for organizing the colloquium: Mary Supley, Susan E. O'Donnell, and Patricia H. Carlo. The following WTR staff also provided support for the colloquium: Bryan W. Eddins, Michael Niemeyer, Jody Dosberg, Anita Sperling, Atticus Reaser, Claudine M. Valmonte, Elizabeth Estes Adams, Peter Sebeny, and Brian Jones.

I would like to thank the following individuals who served as rapporteurs for the colloquium: Kelly G. Sund, Martha Embrey, Gretchen K. Findlay, Dr. Graham H. Hook, Rebecca A. Steffens, Francesca Apollonio, Marta Cavagnaro, Andrea Donato, Mirka Zago, and Micaela Liberti. They were responsible for coordinating their respective sessions and the assembly of papers. Claudine M. Valmonte and Kathleen Kapetanovic provided additional assistance in assembling sections for this volume.

I would like to thank Mary Supley and Susan Hersemann for editing this volume. Polly Thibodeau and Sherry Farr also contributed to the editing process, and Eric Chrol and Jennifer Rumbaugh assisted in proofreading. This volume was formatted by Mary Supley and Polly Thibodeau, with the assistance of Jennifer Rumbaugh, Eric Chrol, Lisa Joson, Rebecca A. Steffens, Claudine M. Valmonte, and Marissa Gandee. Linda T. Solheim provided legal counsel on copyright and contractual issues related to this publication.

The wireless industry, through their financial support of WTR, provided support for the 1995 colloquium and this publication.

G. L. Carlo

I

DOSIMETRY AND MEASUREMENTS

Editor's Note:

The science of dosimetry as it pertains to radio frequency radiation health impact should be viewed in the context of assessing gradations in exposure to in vitro and in vivo test subjects as well as users of wireless instruments. Low-power radio frequency radiation from wireless communication instruments is difficult to accurately quantify and, where biological outcomes are of interest, must be carefully monitored for field uniformity and heating. The papers by Drs. Chou and Martens are directly applicable to this type of dosimetry and fairly represent the current state of scientific progress in that area.

Measurement of output from wireless communication instruments themselves is important in the context of product certification and regulatory compliance. Product certification is a voluntary program of the wireless industry aimed at standardizing and clarifying affirmations made to consumers about these products. Regulatory compliance is mandatory both in the US and around the world, and is dependent on specific criteria for measurements in different jurisdictions. The papers by Drs. Gabriel, Kuster and Gandhi address both regulatory compliance and product certification.

From the public health perspective, precise measurements of exposure in both experimental studies and epidemiology are necessary for scientific findings that can be relied upon for public health decisions. In effect, good public health decision making begins with good dosimetry.

Product certification and regulatory compliance are relevant to public health decision making, but only as regards the rigor of future post-marketing surveillance. A product specification regarding output of radio frequency radiation provides scientists with an upper bound on exposure to persons using wireless instruments. A history of regulatory compliance with a standard for emissions is also useful in quantifying an upper bound of exposure among the user population. Neither product certification nor regulatory compliance speak directly to safety or public health protection. These tools are only as good as the safety standard against which comparisons are made.

G. L. C.

1

STATE OF THE SCIENCE REGARDING IN VITRO AND IN VIVO EXPOSURE SYSTEMS FOR RF STUDIES

C.K. Chou

Abstract

To understand the biological effects of radiofrequency (RF) fields on humans, both in vitro and in vivo studies exposing cell cultures, isolated tissues, and animals have been conducted. Dosimetry of nonionizing radiation is far more complicated than that of ionizing radiation. Field frequency and polarization, tissue dielectric properties, object size and shape, and the presence of metallic stimulating and recording instruments can all affect energy absorption in exposed subjects, either in vitro or in vivo. In addition, temperature control in an exposure system can influence biological responses. Different exposure systems are reviewed in this paper. Relevance of the systems to wireless technology research is discussed.

Introduction

In this presentation, dosimetry was the first topic which included extrapolation from results with animals to humans and the use of specific absorption rate (SAR) for dosimetric quantification. Then, in vitro exposure systems were reviewed. Recording artifacts due to the electrodes and the importance of temperature control during in vitro experiments were emphasized. Some finite-difference time-domain (FD-TD) characterization results of an in vitro exposure system, which is supported by Wireless Technology Research (WTR), LLC, were presented. In vivo exposure systems, the third topic, dealt with whole-body and partial-body exposure systems. Progress of our WTR-supported, head-exposure system development was reported. Restrained and unrestrained exposure methods were compared. Finally, some conclusions were made on this subject.

Dosimetry

To study whether radio frequency (RF) electromagnetic exposure can cause effects on humans, one often conducts animal experiments then extrapolates the results to humans. However, the exposure intensities measured in the air by power survey meters do not tell us how much energy gets inside an animal or human. The reflection and absorption inside small laboratory animals and humans are vastly different. Therefore, incident power intensity cannot be used as a measure of exposure. Durney, Massoudi, and Iskander (1986) in their Dosimetry Handbook have shown that the rate of energy absorption in ellipsoidal human models is highly dependent on the orientation of the model versus the polarization of the incident fields. The maximum energy absorption occurs when the long axis of the body is parallel to the electrical field. There is a resonance curve for each size object. For an adult human (175 cm tall), the curve peaks at 70-80 MHz, which is near the frequency of TV Channel 5 in the United States. When smaller animals are exposed, the resonant curves shift to higher frequencies. For a laboratory rat 20 cm long, the maximum absorption occurs at 650 MHz; while for a mouse 7.5 cm long, the resonance peaks at 1500 MHz. For example, if a mouse is exposed to 10 mW/cm^2 2450 MHz fields (the most commonly used frequency in a laboratory due to availability of power source), the average rate of energy absorption is about 14 W/kg. At the same frequency and incident power density, the average absorption in an adult human is only 0.28 W/kg; it is 50 times lower than in a mouse.

Guy, Webb, and Sorensen (1976) investigated inhomogeneous energy depositions inside scaled man models exposed to high frequency electromagnetic fields (24-31 MHz). When a model was exposed to an electric field parallel to the body axis, more energy absorptions occurred at the neck, waist, knees and ankles, where current densities per cross-sectional areas were higher. If the magnetic field was perpendicular to the frontal plane of the body, energy absorption was primarily in the torso and more energy absorption occurred at the axilla and perineum, where the eddy current had to flow around sharp corners. The absorption patterns of the two exposure conditions are totally different.

The previous two examples, one on the average rate of energy absorption and the other on the spatial distribution of energy distribution, show the complexity of energy coupling in an exposed subject. External incident power density is not a suitable dosimetric parameter, and another quantification unit is needed, so that animal results can be extrapolated to human results. The National Council of Radiation Protection and Measurements (1981) gave a formal definition to the rate of energy absorption as SAR, which is defined as the time derivative of the incremental energy absorbed by an incremental mass contained in a volume element of a given density. In other words, SAR is the absorbed power density in tissue. The unit of SAR is watts per kilogram.

In Vivo Exposure Systems

Waveguide

Chou and Guy (1978) designed an S-band waveguide system for exposing isolated tissues to 2450 MHz microwaves. Since the tissues must remain in solution to be kept alive, a quarter-wavelength dielectric slab was inserted to match the impedance between the air-filled and solution-filled waveguide. Circulating ports were connected to a constant temperature circulator to minimize microwave thermal effects. Holes on the waveguide walls allowed the isolated tissues to be stretched either parallel or perpendicular to the electric field. This system was used to study pulsed and continuous microwave exposures on the nerve conduction and muscle contraction. At high SAR exposures (e.g., 1500 W/kg), the solution temperature inside the waveguide was raised by 1°C during circulation. The observed neuromuscular effects were reproducible by raising the solution temperature 1°C. No effect other than thermal was observed. In this study a 0.2 °C temperature rise caused a detectable latency shift in nerve action potential. Temperature control is extremely important in microwave bioeffect studies.

Galvin, Parks, and McRee (1980) modified the above system to expose two preparations in the same waveguide, using the one away from the dielectric matching slab as a control. At several penetration depths away, the energy absorption in the solution makes the exposure at that location negligible. This approach was adapted by Liu and Cleary (1988) to expose cells. To prevent cells from sinking to the bottom of the culture tubes, magnetic stirrers were used to keep the cells afloat. The magnetic stirrers were outside of the waveguide so they did not interfere with the fields inside the waveguide. Stirring also made the temperature fairly uniform inside the tube. However, since the test tube was 8.4 mm ID, it was difficult to keep the temperature constant, especially at high SAR levels. Lin (1976) used smaller pipettes for cell culture exposures to minimize the temperature rise. Field, Ginsburg, and Lin (1993) used the same waveguide design but with a separately perfused recording chamber to keep the tissue temperature constant. Snail neuron action potentials were recorded with 1 M KCl solution-filled microelectrodes. The concentration of the KCl solution was lower than the conventional 3 M solution, because high conductivity solutions can cause artifacts in the microwave field, especially in pulsed microwave fields. The pulsed field can push KCl solution out of the electrode and into cells, which can affect cellular function.

Joyner, Davis, Elson, Czerska, and Czerski (1989) described the design and dosimetry of an automated waveguide exposure system. Czerska, Elson, Davis, Swicord, and Czerski (1992) exposed human lymphocytes to continuous and pulsed 2450 MHz microwaves in this waveguide system to study the effects on spontaneous lymphoblastoid transformation. The temperature of the cell culture was not controlled. Liburdy and Magin (1985) used a tunable 2450 MHz waveguide to expose cell cultures. This device enables continuous control and monitoring of sample temperatures, sample mixing, and pO_2 conditioning. Tuning elements permit absorption of 99% of the forward power. This system was used to study microwave effects on cell membranes.

Stripline

Bawin, Kaczmarek, and Adey (1975) reported the calcium efflux effects using two large triangular aluminum plates (0.41 m^2) for exposing neonatal chick brains to amplitude modulated (0.5 to 35 Hz) 147 MHz fields. Wachtel, Seaman, and Joines (1975) exposed *Aplysia* ganglia to 1.5 GHz microwaves in a stripline to study the microwave effects on the neuron's firing rate. The preparation was placed inside the stripline between the center conductor and the ground plane. To avoid artifacts, due to high conductivity microelectrode fluid, they first filled the electrodes with a 2.5 M KCl solution, then removed all the solution except at the tips, after which they refilled the electrodes with a 0.5 M KCl solution. The temperature of the preparation was not controlled in this experiment.

Taylor and Ashleman (1975) used a parallel plate applicator to expose a cat's spinal cord, which was immersed in a reservoir with perfusing solution to keep the spinal cord temperature constant. The dorsal root was stimulated and the evoked responses were recorded at the ventral root, while exposed to 2450 MHz microwaves. Temperature of the spinal cord was measured with a thermistor or a thermocouple, while the microwave exposure was briefly turned off to avoid interference and perturbation. It was difficult to keep the temperature constant because the spinal cord is too large for thermal diffusion to work.

Transverse Electromagnetic Cell

Transverse electromagnetic (TEM) cells provide exposure conditions closest to a free-space environment and have been used by many investigators for cell culture exposures (e.g., Blackman et al., 1979; Dutta, Subramoniam, Ghosh, & Parshad, 1984; Sultan, Cain, & Tompkins, 1983). In these cells, the electric and magnetic fields are well characterized (Crawford, 1974). The example shown was used at the Environmental Protection Agency (EPA) for exposing chick forebrains to amplitude modulated RF fields at 50, 147, and 450 MHz in search of effects on the calcium efflux (Weil, Spiegel, & Joines, 1984). The TEM cell was placed vertically, and tissue samples were also exposed vertically. The temperature of the samples was controlled by a heater since the samples were exposed at 37°C instead of at room temperature.

During the Dosimetry Working Group meeting held on 2-3 December 1994 in Los Angeles, California, it was decided that the TEM cell is the most appropriate exposure system for in vitro studies. Under WTR support, Dr. Allen Taflove of Northwestern University is using the FD-TD method to characterize the SAR distributions in cell cultures exposed in TEM cells. Computations have been done with single and multiple flasks, with variable flask fluid levels, and with different flask locations and orientations. Preliminary data show a very nonuniform SAR distribution in the flasks, peaks at the edges of the flasks, and especially a very high peak at the leading edge of the flask. Temperature measurement in the middle of the flask cannot detect the high peak SAR as predicted by the FD-TD method. The dosimetry in the TEM cell is more complicated than was originally believed.

Coaxial Line

Guy (1977) designed a coaxial line system for exposing cells to broadband RF fields (0-100 MHz). The cells were placed inside a 5-ml stainless steel ring with a center conductor and an outer conductor and a Teflon bottom. The electric field orientation is between the inner and outer ring conductor. A Teflon cover kept the cells in a closed space. The culture cup was surrounded by a circulating mineral oil bath to keep the culture temperature constant. The temperature variation of the culture medium, which was monitored by a Vitek temperature sensor, was less than 0.2°C. This result indicated that the mineral oil circulation was able to keep the culture temperature constant.

In an unpublished experiment, Riley, Guy, Chou, Fitzmaurice, and Spackman (1979) used the coaxial line system to expose murine lymphoma cells to RF fields at 43°C. The exposed cells were then injected into mice to induce tumors. The tumor latency period was used as a measure for the RF exposure effect. Figure 1 shows the results using the system. The light bars, which are control data at 4°C, show that diluted cells have a longer latent period, as expected. When exposed to 43°C only (left dark bar), the latency was much longer, indicating some damaging effects to the tumor cells. The two dark bars to the right indicate that the higher the RF exposure, the more lively the tumor cells (shorter latent period). It appears that there was a protective effect from the RF field. This puzzling effect was resolved after a circulating pump was connected to the 5-ml cup to circulate and stir the cells so that they would not sink to the bottom of the cup. When cells stayed at the Teflon bottom, there was a thermal gradient due to the cooling of the bottom. With a higher intensity RF field, a cooler circulating temperature was needed to keep the culture at a constant temperature, and a higher thermal gradient was formed at the walls and the bottom. Figure 2 shows the results after the pump was in place. The protection effect disappeared. This experiment again signifies the importance of temperature control.

Horn Antenna

1)   Near Field.
Dhahi, Habash, and Al-Hafid (1982) exposed fungi cells in the near field of an applicator to a continuous wave of 8.7175 GHz. Because the magnetic stirrer was in the near field of the horn antenna, there were standing waves, and the field was severely disturbed. The resulting SARs were very complicated. However, since there were no demonstrated effects, further analysis is unnecessary.

Caddemi, Tamburello, Zanforlin, and Torregrossa (1986) placed an isolated chick heart in a petri dish, which was located in the near field of a rectangular slot in a

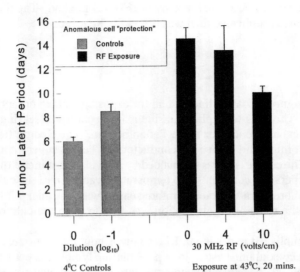

Figure 1. Apparent "protective" effect of 30 MHz RF exposure at 43°C upon tumor cells, as expressed by shorter latent periods in comparison with the latent periods of the thermal controls. The cell suspensions were stationary in the sample holders, with no cell circulation employed.

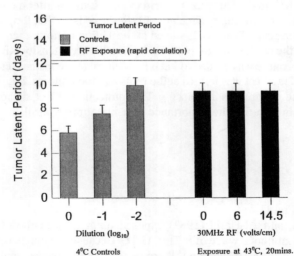

Figure 2. Lack of effect of 30 MHz RF exposure at 43°C tumor latent periods, in contrast to the thermal effect of 43°C. The cell suspensions were rapidly circulated in the sample holders, eliminating the anomalous effects depicted in Figure 1.

conductor plane and irradiated by an open-ended coaxial termination. The micropipets, filled with a low concentration (0.1 M) of NaCl solution, were used to record heart beats. The temperature of the bath was kept at 37°C. Due to the near-field configuration, accurate field distribution was difficult to obtain.

2)   Far Field.

To avoid the complicated near-field distribution, in vitro cell cultures were exposed in the far field of the antennas. Harrison, McCulloch, Balcer-Kubiczek, and Robinson (1985) placed a culture flask in a constant temperature bath, exposed at 20 wavelengths under a horn antenna. A quarter-wavelength matching window was placed at the surface of the bath to match the impedance. Field mapping shows that the incident power density was uniform to within 10% in the 25 cm x 25 cm region where the flask was located. With an SAR of 4.4 W/kg at the monolayer cells and at steady state, there was a 1.2 °C temperature rise in the flask. Brown and Marshall (1986) exposed murine erythroleukemia cells in cylindrical tubes parallel to the electric field in 1180 MHz far-field radiation. Temperature controlled air at 37.4°C was pumped through the exposed region to minimize temperature rise in the test tubes. Dardalhon, More, Averbeck, and Berteaud (1984) exposed Chinese hamster cells to 2450 MHz far-field microwaves. In addition to circulating cool air, they also rotated the samples to minimize field nonuniformity. Meltz, Eagan, Harris, and Erwin (1988) used a styrofoam float in a water bath to hold 10 flasks underneath and rotated it by water jets. The rotation also averaged the SARs produced by either 915 or 2450 MHz far-field exposure.

In Vivo Exposure System

Whole-body exposure

1)   Horn Antennas.

During the early years of RF bioeffect research, one example showed animals exposed in the laboratory with food and water ad lib in the cage. Another example showed rats tightly packed for RF exposure. No extra precaution was taken to adjust for the differences in ionizing and nonionizing radiation dosimetry. It took some time before more engineering inputs emerged to correct these situations.

    For small animals or objects, McRee, Hamrick, and Zinkl (1975) exposed fertilized Japanese quail eggs to 2450 MHz microwaves, in the far field, to study the teratogenic effects. The EPA had a 9 GHz X-band system for exposing mice from the top inside of an environmentally controlled chamber made of polystyrene foam (Liddle et al., 1980). Yang, Cain, Lockwood, and Tompkins (1983) exposed hamsters, from the top in an anechoic chamber, to 2450 MHz fields. An identical set-up was used for sham exposure except that no microwave horn was installed. Ray and Bahari (1990) used a 7.5 GHz horn to radiate rats inside a tapered microwave anechoic chamber, 3 hours daily for 60 days. Nine rats at a time were frontally exposed in individual cages. The power densities at the nine locations were measured with a dipole probe. The nonuniformity was due to both the distance from the horn and lateral position from the center beam. Using exposure from the bottom at far field, Galvin and McRee (1986) studied whether ventral exposure of rats to 2450 MHz fields can induce bradycardia. At the University of Utah, D'Andrea et al. (1986) used a monopole antenna system to expose 14 rats around the pole with the rat's long axis parallel to the electric field. There were two rooms; one for control and the other for exposure. The rats were exposed for 3 months before behavioral testing began.

For larger animals, Adair and Adams (1980) exposed monkeys to 2450 MHz microwaves in a partitioned room with sophisticated temperature and humidity control. A video monitor was used to watch the animal behavior. Lotz and Saxton (1987) also exposed monkeys in a microwave anechoic chamber to study the field effects of 225 MHz on behavior. Thermograms, taken of a live monkey and a bird carcass exposed to 2450 MHz microwaves inside a large anechoic chamber at the University of Washington, illustrated the complicated energy coupling of biological bodies with different shapes (Chou & Guy, 1985). The narrow cross sections of monkey ankles had high SARs, which is consistent with the scaled model mentioned before. For the bird, the neck and wing tips parallel to the electric field also had high SAR.

Using smaller exposure systems, Stern, Margolin, Weiss, Lu, and Michaelson (1979), in a refrigerated room, trained fur clipped rats to turn on an infrared lamp while under various intensities of 2450 MHz microwave exposure. The electric field was parallel to the long axis of the rat while the rat was pressing the control level. Guy, Kramar, Harris, and Chou (1980) dorsally exposed individual rabbits chronically in small chambers with microwave absorbers on the wall. Water was fed through a drip system to a cup. Water not drunk and urine were drained to the outside so that the fluid would not disturb the field inside the chamber. Thermograms showed high SAR values in the head and the back of the rabbit. This system was modified into a tapered miniature system for exposing mice, rats, and rabbits (Chou, Guy, Borneman, Kunz, and Kramar, 1983; Guy, 1979). Veyret et al. (1991) used a coaxial antenna coupled to a cylindrical reflector to generate a TM mode microwave propagation. Six mice were housed in a circular Plexiglas cage exposed to pulse-modulated or amplitude-modulated 9.4 GHz microwaves to study the effects on immune functions. SAR was estimated by referring to the Dosimetry Handbook (Durney et al., 1978).

2)   Cavity.

In the early 1970s, there was an American study showing that low-level microwave radiation caused significant behavior changes (Korbel, 1970). The exposure system, a cavity, was reproduced at the University of Washington (Guy & Korbel, 1972) to expose simulated rats (phantom muscle in plastic bottles). While the survey meter indicated a relatively low-level exposure, thermograms showed, when rats were drinking water with tails and feet touching metallic ground, that there were hot spots at the tongue and also at the parts in contact with the ground. The SARs were high enough to produce hyperthermia at these spots. This explains why the radiated rats had behavioral changes. The other example, a multimode cavity, was a modified 915 or

2450 MHz microwave oven used to expose rats for behavior studies (Justesen, Levinson, & Justesen, 1974). SAR was obtained calorimetrically from saline solution loads or from rectal temperature rise in anesthetized rats (Carrol, Levinson, Justesen, & Clarke, 1980).

3)   Waveguide.

Guy and Chou (1976) and Guy, Wallace, and McDougall (1979) designed 20.3 cm diameter circularly-polarized waveguides for chronically exposing rats to either 915 or 2450 MHz. The animals lived individually in a plastic cage with water and food ad lib. The animal absorption and the waveguide loss were measured by subtracting all transmitted and reflected power from the input power. To illustrate the sophistication of the design, details of the quarter-wavelength choke water bottle were shown as an example. This drinking bottle decouples RF current flow from the water to the rat to avoid the hot tongue effect shown before. Two thermograms, taken during anterior and transverse exposures, showed that the SAR patterns were different. Therefore, when the animal moved around inside the cage, the SAR pattern in the rat changed. Detailed dosimetry results measured with power meters, thermography, and calorimetry of the 2450 MHz circular waveguide system have been described (Chou, Guy, & Johnson, 1984). A lifetime exposure study was conducted for the Air Force (Chou et al., 1992). In this study, 200 rats were exposed for 21 hours per day for 25 months. This system was later modified to simultaneously expose four mice dorsally (Chou & Guy, 1982). Olsen, de Lorge, Forstall, and Ezell (1984) expanded the vertical circular waveguide to 76.2 cm diameter to expose 15 kg rhesus monkeys to 275 MHz fields.

When the rat body was exposed under a 915 MHz 13 cm x 13 cm applicator for a behavior study, the thermogram showed a very interesting pattern (Chou & Guy, 1985). Although the applicator was primarily located above the body, a very high peak SAR occurred at the base of the tail which was outside the applicator aperture. In this case, geometry of the tail played an important role in determining the SAR distribution.

4)   Transverse Electromagnetic Cell.

Marshall and Brown (1983) exposed mice in TEM cells at frequencies between 200 and 400 MHz. Since this is a closed system similar to the circular waveguides, whole-body averaged SAR can be determined from power meter measurements of incident, reflected, and transmitted powers. In a dosimetry study using calorimetry, SARs of live mice and cadavers were found to be twice as high as the prolate spheroid models, and when housed in Plexiglas cages, it was 2.5 times higher. Brooks Air Force Base has multifrequency TEM exposure systems (10-30 MHz, 40-400 MHz, 1-4 GHz) for animal studies (Rupp, Montet, & Frazer, 1975).

5)   Parallel Plates and Stripline.

At the Georgia Institute of Technology, a 435 MHz circular parallel plate waveguide system was designed to expose 100 rats at the same time on four plates (Bonasera, Toler, & Popovic, 1988). There were two identical rooms to house the exposed and control systems. A total of 200 rats were exposed and sham exposed. Gandhi (1975) placed rats in a stripline at different orientations and exposed them to RF fields ranging from 285 to 4000 MHz. The orientation effect on absorption and resonance effect were demonstrated using this system.

Before leaving the subject of whole-body exposure, Tables 2 and 3 of Chou, Guy, McDougall, and Lai (1985) showed the average whole-body, head, and tail SARs and the local SARs in a rat brain under seven exposure conditions: anterior and posterior exposure in a circular waveguide, in a near field with magnetic field parallel to the body, in a far field with electric field or with magnetic field parallel to the body, and inside a miniature chamber with electric field or with magnetic field parallel to the body. The SAR data vary considerably with system, orientation, and body parts.

Partial-body Exposure

1)   Torso.
Using a slot antenna on a cavity, applicators were designed to treat rat bladder cancer with 3.325 GHz microwave hyperthermia (Chou, See, Luk, & Chapman, 1987). Another example for partial-body exposure is the 27 MHz capacitive electrodes for heating the heart region of a pig. The heated heart pumps the warm blood to the other parts of the body. For a 60 kg pig, the rectal temperature was raised from 38° to 42°C within 30 minutes (Chou, McDougall, Chan, Vora, & Howard, 1993).

2)   Head Exposure.
Because of reports from Eastern European countries indicating that the nervous system is the most sensitive to microwave radiation, effects of microwave exposure on evoked responses of cats were studied in the early 1970s (Johnson & Guy, 1972). Anesthetized cats were stimulated with tactile or auditory stimuli and the evoked responses in brain were recorded. Effects on the amplitude and latency of the responses due to various intensities of 915 MHz microwave radiation of the head region were studied. The head exposure was to the back of the head. In a related topic, the choice of recording electrode was an issue. For conventional neurophysiological recordings, metallic electrodes are used. However, in RF electromagnetic fields, there are three problems associated with the metallic electrodes: electromagnetic interference, field intensification, and perturbation (Chan, Chou, McDougall, & Luk, 1988). For example, when a cat was exposed to 915 MHz fields, at 2.5 mW/cm², the peak SAR in the brain was 2.27 W/kg; after a 1 mm diameter metallic electrode was inserted for evoked response recording, the peak SAR at the tip of the electrode rose to 113 W/kg (Johnson & Guy, 1972). This large SAR increase makes it important not to use metallic sensors in microwave studies.

Sanders and Joines (1984) exposed rat heads in the near field of a 3 cm x 3 cm aperture antenna 3 cm above the head to 591 MHz fields to study rat brain physiology. The electric field was parallel to the midline. SAR was estimated from the Dosimetry Handbook and from temperature measurements. To study the inhibition of brain enzymes, Lenox, Gandhi, Meyerhoff, and Grove (1976) designed a high-power (3.5 kW) 2450 MHz applicator to heat the brain to inactivate brain enzymes. The exposure time necessary for a 325 g rat was 2.8 seconds. Guy and Chou (1982) used magnetic field coupling to heat the rat brain with 10 kW 915 MHz microwave energy. The heating was produced by the eddy currents induced by the magnetic field. Rats were stunned by a 28 kJ/kg energy pulse. The thermogram showed two heated regions, one in the brain and the other in the mouth. At 10 kW of power, a 98 msec pulse was able to raise the brain temperature by 13°C.

To expose one side of the head, Kramar, Emery, Guy, and Lin (1975) studied the microwave cataractogenesis in rabbits. A diathermy C director from a 2450 MHz diathermy machine was used to expose one rabbit eye. Thresholds for microwave-induced cataracts were established. It is an energy related phenomena. When the lens temperature was raised above 41°C, a cataract formed. The same experiment, including frontal exposure of both eyes, was conducted on monkeys. Only the eyebrow and the nose ridge were burned, but no cataracts were observed (Kramar, Harris, Emery, and Guy, 1976). The differences in eye and facial structures between rabbits and monkeys made the microwave energy coupling into monkey eyes difficult. Kues, Hirst, Lutty, D'Anna, and Dunkelberger (1985) also exposed monkey eyes to pulsed and continuous 2450 MHz microwaves in the near field of an aperture waveguide. They found corneal endothelial cell damages.

In a microwave auditory effect study, a human head exposure was conducted first to confirm the effect (Guy, Chou, Lin, & Christensen, 1975). Then the heads of guinea pigs and cats were exposed to pulsed 915 MHz fields inside a TE_{11} mode circular waveguide. Cochlear microphonics and brainstem-evoked responses were recorded (Chou, Guy, & Galambos, 1982). The only animal study which involved partial-brain exposure was the blood brain barrier study reported by Neilly and Lin (1986). A dielectrically loaded coaxial applicator was placed on one side of the rat head to deliver 3.15 GHz microwave energy for 15 minutes. Increased blood brain barrier permeability was associated with the temperature rise in the brain.

At the City of Hope clinic, a patient with a tumor under the left ear lobe was treated with 915 MHz microwave hyperthermia. The 15 cm x 15 cm applicator was in contact with the patient's head. In contrast to the 0.6 W of power used by a cellular telephone, up to 100 W of power was applied to heat the tumor to 43°C.

WTR Head Exposure System Development Update Conclusions

A research program intending to answer the concern of potential health effects produced by microwave energy radiating from a hand-held cellular telephone is being conducted by WTR. The above review indicates that most of the biological effect studies conducted in the past four decades were of acute whole-body exposure. Few involved only exposure to the head region. None of the studies simulated human exposure to cellular telephone fields. The results of these previous studies are irrelevant to the questions raised concerning cellular telephone safety. An appropriate animal exposure system is required for meaningful investigations that are relevant to in vivo biological research.

To simulate human exposure in animals for in vivo studies, one must first know the SAR distribution in humans. Both numerical and experimental dosimetry data have been available (Balzano, Garay, & Manning, 1995; Dimbylow & Mann, 1994; Gandhi, Chen, & Wu, 1994). The SAR is primarily at the side of the brain where the cellular phone was held. Biological parameters that need to be selected for the study include animal species, size, sex, and age. The rat has been chosen as the animal model. Strain and sex are to be determined by the biologists. Since these are head exposure investigations, the animal head size is the primary determining factor for microwave energy absorption. During growth, the rat head size changes considerably. Frequency, modulation, energy absorption level, and distribution are obvious engineering endpoints. Modulation and exposure time can be controlled at the power generator. As for the frequency, scaling was used for whole-body exposure. The frequency was scaled up to make the wavelengths in small laboratory animals equivalent to that in humans. Scaling is invalid if an effect is proven to be frequency-dependent. However, for cellular telephone exposure at 800-900 MHz in the human head, it is not necessary to scale the frequency as needed for a whole-body exposure study. As long as the SAR level and distribution patterns are similar, the same frequency can be used. The cellular telephone transmitting frequency of 837 MHz was chosen in this design. It is impossible to match the SAR patterns in human and rat brains. The head and brain shapes and the proportions of brain and muscle are different. Only approximations can be achieved. The FD-TD method was used to calculate SAR with an ellipsoidal model of a rat while models based on computed tomography images of a rat are developed. Dipole and loop antennas were evaluated. Thermographic techniques were used to verify the patterns.

Dipole antennas are inefficient and produce undesirable SAR distribution in the ellipsoidal phantom. The coupling is mostly due to the electric field. Various loop dimensions were tested. Appropriate SAR patterns were achievable when the loops were properly oriented. Loops primarily provide magnetic field coupling which is similar to the cellular telephone coupling as shown in human models. Thermographic tests on prototype loops show similar patterns as predicted by FD-TD calculations. However, loop loss was excessive due to impedance mismatch. The dielectric properties of the circuit board on which the loop is mounted also influence the impedance. Both transmission line and tuned circuit methods are being tested to match the impedance. Since cellular telephones, which have 0.6 W of maximum output, are being considered for feeding the antennas during the biological studies, maximum power transfer is critical.

Whether to use restrained or unrestrained animals is being discussed. To restrain an animal, the whole animal, especially the head, must be at a fixed location in a restraint. However, stress is the primary concern. Conditioning is necessary to reduce the stress. Unrestrained exposure can be achieved with at least two methods. One of them is having the rat eat and/or drink at a cone shaped location where the animal's head gets exposed. One of the problems is the difficulty of exposure time control. The other method is to mount the antenna on a helmet with the RF cable connected to a weight-balanced apparatus. This system has been used for many years in microdialysis and is commercially available. In terms of cost, the restrained method will be much cheaper. Considering the number of animals to be exposed (hundreds to more than a thousand rats), a compromised decision between biological endpoints and logistics must be made. The final product will be a duplicable system to expose a large population of animals to cellular telephone frequency fields.

Conclusions

In review of the in vitro and in vivo RF exposure systems, most of the exposures involved 915 or 2450 MHz microwaves. Most animal exposures were whole-body exposures. None of the biological studies simulate human exposure to cellular telephone fields. The dosimetry of various exposure systems indicate that SAR varies with many factors: 1) frequency, polarization, and phase of applied fields; 2) dielectric properties, geometry and size of tissue; 3) source configuration: near-field, type of antenna or applicator; 4) exposure conditions: free space, waveguide, cavity, ground plane, corner reflector, and metallic implant. Energy absorption in cells and animals vary greatly depending on the exposure systems. Cellular telephone frequency and SAR levels must be used for biological studies. To study the effects of cellular telephone exposure on humans, one must use suitably designed in vitro and in vivo exposure systems with well characterized SAR so extrapolating from animals to humans is possible. Close collaboration between engineers and biologists is essential for the success of this research program in providing answers to the safety of cellular telephones.

Editor's Update

The head exposure system described by Dr. Chou has now been completed and pilot tested. The WTR believes this exposure system to be the scientifically preferred exposure system for biological experiments of RF at this time. For more reference material on the exposure system, see the WTR web page located at http://www.wtrllc.com.

G. L. C.

References

Adair, A. R., & Adams, B. W. (1980). Microwaves modify thermoregulatory behavior in squirrel monkey. Bioelectromagnetics, 1, 1-20.

Balzano, Q., Garay, O., & Manning, Jr., T. J. (1995). Electromagnetic energy exposure of simulated users of portable cellular telephones. IEEE Transactions on Vehicular Technology, 44, 390-403.

Bawin, S. M., Kaczmarek, L. K., & Adey, W. R. (1975). Effects of modulated VHF fields on the central nervous system. In P. E. Tyler (Ed.), Annals of the New York Academy of Sciences:

16

Vol. 247. Biologic effects of nonionizing radiation (pp. 74-81). New York: New York Academy of Sciences.

Blackman, C. F., Elder, J. A., Weil, C. M., Benane, S. G., Eichinger, D. C., & House, D. E. (1979). Induction of calcium-ion efflux from brain tissue by radio-frequency radiation: Effects of modulation frequency and field strength. Radio Science, 14(6S), 93-98.

Bonasera, S., Toler, J. & Popovic, V. (1988). Long-term study of 435 MHz radiofrequency radiation on blood-borne end points in cannulated rats. Journal of Microwave Power, 23, 95-98.

Brown, R. F., & Marshall, S. V. (1986). Differentiation of murine erythroleukemic cells during exposure to microwave radiation. Radiation Research, 108, 12-22.

Caddemi, A., Tamburello, C. C., Zanforlin, L., & Torregrossa, M. V. (1986). Microwave effects on isolated chick embryo hearts. Bioelectromagnetics, 7, 359-367.

Carroll, D. R., Levinson, D. M., Justesen, D. R., & Clarke, R. L. (1980). Failure of rats to escape from a potentially lethal microwave field. Bioelectromagnetics, 1, 101-115.

Chan, K. W., Chou, C. K., McDougall, J. A., & Luk, K. H. (1988). Changes in heating patterns due to perturbations by thermometer probes at 915 and 434 MHz. International Journal of Hyperthermia, 4, 447-456.

Chou, C. K., Bassen, H., Osepchuk, J., Balzano, Q., Petersen, R., Meltz, M. , Cleveland, R., Lin, J. C. & Heynick, L. (1996). Radio frequency electromagnetic exposure: A tutorial review on experimental dosimetry. Bioelectromagnetics, 17, 195-208.

Chou, C. K., & Guy, A. W. (1978). Effects of electromagnetic fields on isolated nerve and muscle preparations. IEEE Transactions on Microwave Theory and Technique, 26, 141-147.

Chou, C. K., & Guy, A. W. (1982). Systems for exposing mice to 2450 MHz electromagnetic fields. Bioelectromagnetics, 3, 401-412.

Chou, C. K., & Guy, A. W. (1985). Research on non-ionizing radiation: Physical aspects in extrapolating infrahuman data to man. In J. C. Monahan & J. A. D'Andrea (Eds.), Behavioral effects of microwave radiation absorption (DHHS Publication No. 85-8238, pp.135-149). Washington, DC: U.S. Department of Health and Human Services.

Chou, C. K., Guy, A. W., Borneman, L. E., Kunz, L. L., & Kramar, P. (1983). Effects of chronic exposure of rabbits to 0.5 and 5 mW/cm² 2450 MHz CW microwave radiation. Bioelectromagnetics, 4, 63-77.

Chou, C. K., Guy, A. W., & Galambos, R. (1982). Auditory perception of radio-frequency electromagnetic fields. Journal of Acoustic Society of America, 80th review and tutorial paper, 71, 1321-1334.

Chou, C. K., Guy, A. W., & Johnson, R. B. (1984). SAR in rats exposed in 2450-MHz circularly polarized waveguide. Bioelectromagnetics, 5, 389-398.

Chou, C. K., Guy, A. W., Kunz, L. L., Johnson, R. B., Crowley, J., & Krupp, J. H. (1992). Long-term, low-level, microwave irradiation of rats. Bioelectromagnetics, 13, 469-496.

Chou, C. K., Guy, A. W., McDougall, J. A., & Lai, H. (1985). Specific absorption rate in rats exposed to 2,450-MHz microwaves under seven exposure conditions. Bioelectromagnetics, 6, 73-88.

Chou, C. K., McDougall, J. A., Chan, K. W., Vora, N., & Howard, H. (1993). Whole body hyperthermia with an RF electric field system. Proceedings 15th Annual International Conference of the IEEE Engineering in Medicine and Biology Society, Part 3, 1461-1462.

Chou, C. K., See, W. A., Luk, K. H., & Chapman, W. H. (1987). Microwave hyperthermia system for treating bladder carcinoma in rats. Endocurietherapy and Hyperthermia Oncology, 3, 147-152.

Crawford, M. L. (1974). Generation of standard EM fields using TEM transmission cells. IEEE Transactions on Electromagnetic Compatibility, 16, 189-195.

Czerska, E. M., Elson, E. C., Davis, C. C., Swicord, M. L., & Czerski, P. (1992). Effects of continuous and pulsed 2450-MHz radiation on spontaneous lymphoblastoid transformation of human lymphocytes in vitro. Bioelectromagnetics, 13, 247-259.

D'Andrea, J. A., DeWitt, J. R., Gandhi, O. P., Stensaas, S., Lords, J. L., & Nielson H. C. (1986). Behavioral and physiological effects of chronic 2,450-MHz microwave irradiation of the rat at 0.5 mW/cm^2. Bioelectromagnetics, 7, 45-56.

Dardalhon, M., More, C., Averbeck, D., & Berteaud, A. J. (1984). Thermal action of 2.45-GHz microwaves on the cytoplasm of Chinese hamster cells. Bioelectromagnetics, 5, 247-261.

Dhahi, S. J., Habash, W. Y., & Al-Hafid, H. T. (1982). Lack of mutagenic effects on conidia of aspergillus amstelodami irradiated by 8.7175-GHz CW microwaves. Journal of Microwave Power, 17, 345- 351.

Dimbylow, P. J., & Mann, S. M. (1994). SAR calculations in an anatomically realistic model of the head for mobile communication transceivers at 900 MHz and 1.8 GHz. Physics in Medicine and Biology, 39, 1537-1553.

Durney, C. H., Johnson, C. C., Barber, P. W., Massoudi, H., Iskander, M. F., & Lords, J. L. (1978). Radiofrequency radiation dosimetry handbook (2nd ed.; Rep. SAR-TR-78-22). Brooks Air Force Base, TX: USAF School of Aerospace Medicine.

Durney, C. H., Massoudi, H., & Iskander, M. F. (1986). Radiofrequency radiation dosimetry handbook (4th ed.; Rep. USARSAM-TR-85-73). Brooks Air Force Base, TX: USAF School of Aerospace Medicine.

Dutta, S. K., Subramoniam, A., Ghosh, B., & Parshad, R. (1984). Microwave radiation-induced calcium ion efflux from human neuroblastoma cells in culture. Bioelectromagnetics, 5, 71-78.

Field, A. S., Ginsburg, K., & Lin, J. C. (1993). The effect of pulsed microwaves on passive electrical properties and interspike intervals of snail neurons. Bioelectromagnetics, 14, 503-520.

Galvin, M. J., & McRee, D. I. (1986). Cardiovascular, hematologic and biochemical effects of acute ventral exposure of conscious rats to 2450-MHz (CW) microwave radiation. Bioelectromagnetics, 7, 223-233.

Galvin, M. J., Parks, D. L., & McRee, D. I. (1980). Microwave irradiation and in vitro release of enzymes from hepatic lysosomes. Radiation and Environmental Biophysics, 18, 129-136.

Gandhi, O. P. (1975). Discussion paper: Strong dependence of whole animal absorption on polarization and frequency of radio-frequency energy. In P. E. Tyler (Ed.), Annals of the New York Academy of Sciences: Vol. 247. Biologic Effects of Nonionizing Radiation (pp. 532-538). New York: New York Academy of Sciences.

Gandhi, O. P., Chen, J. Y., & Wu, D. (1994, September). Electromagnetic absorption in the human head for mobile telephones at 835 and 1900 MHz. Paper presented at the International Symposium on Electromagnetic Compatibility, Rome, Italy.

Guy, A. W. (1977). A method for exposing cell cultures to electromagnetic fields under conditions of controlled temperature and field strength. Radio Science, 12(6S), 87-96.

Guy, A. W. (1979). Miniature anechoic chamber for chronic exposure of small animals to plane-wave microwave field. Journal of Microwave Power, 14, 328-338.

Guy, A. W., & Chou, C. K. (1976). System for quantitative chronic exposure of a population of rodents to UHF fields. In C.C. Johnson & M.L. Shore (Eds.), Biological effects of electromagnetic waves: Selected Papers of the USNC/YRSU Annual Meeting, Boulder, CO, Vol. II (HEW Publication No. (FDA) 77-8011, pp. 389-410). Washington, DC: U.S. Department of Health, Education, and Welfare.

Guy, A. W., & Chou, C. K.. (1982). Effects of high-intensity microwave pulse exposure on rat brain. Radio Science, 17(5S), 169S-178S.

Guy, A. W., Chou, C. K., Lin, J. C., & Christensen, D. (1975). Microwave induced acoustic effects in mammalian auditory systems and physical materials. In P.E. Tyler (Ed.), Annals of the New York Academy of Sciences: Vol. 247. Biologic Effects of Nonionizing Radiation (pp. 194-218). New York: New York Academy of Sciences.

Guy, A. W., & Korbel, S. F. (1972, May). Dosimetry studies on UHF cavity exposure chamber for rodents. Summaries of papers presented at the 1972 Power Symposium, Ottawa, Canada.

Guy, A. W., Kramar, P. O., Harris, C. A., & Chou, C. K. (1980). Long term 2450 MHz CW microwave irradiation of rabbits: Methodology & evaluation of ocular and physiologic effects. Journal of Microwave Power, 15, 37-44.

Guy, A. W., Wallace, J., & McDougall, J. A. (1979). Circularly polarized 2450-MHz waveguide system for chronic exposure of small animals to microwaves. Radio Science, 14, 63-74.

Guy, A. W., Webb, M. D., & Sorensen, C. C. (1976). Determination of power absorption in man exposed to high frequency electromagnetic fields by thermographic measurements on scale models. IEEE Transactions on Biomedical Engineering, 23, 361-371.

Harrison, G. H., McCulloch, D., Balcer-Kubiczek, E. K., & Robinson, J. E. (1985). Far-field 2.45 GHz irradiation system for cellular monolayers in vitro. Journal of Microwave Power, 20, 145-151.

Johnson, C. C., & Guy, A. W. (1972). Nonionizing electromagnetic wave effects in biological materials and systems. Proceedings of the IEEE, 60, 692-718.

Joyner, K. H., Davis, C. C., Elson, E. C., Czerska, E. M., & Czerski, P. (1989). An automated dosimetry system for microwave and thermal exposure of biological samples in vitro. Health Physics, 56, 303-307.

Justesen, D. R., Levinson, D. M., & Justesen, L. R. (1974). Psychogenic stressors are potent mediators of the thermal response to microwave irradiation. In Biological Effects and Health Hazards of Microwave Radiation (pp. 134-140). Warsaw, Poland: Polish Medical Publisher.

Korbel, S. F. (1970). Behavioral effects of low intensity UHF radiation. In S.F. Cleary (Ed.), Symposium proceedings of biological effects and health implications of microwave radiation. BRH/DBE (pp. 180-184).

Kramar, P. O., Emery, A. F., Guy, A. W., & Lin, J. C. (1975). The ocular effects of microwaves on hypothermic rabbits: A study of microwave cataractogenic mechanisms. In P. E. Tyler (Ed.), Annals of the New York Academy of Sciences: Vol. 247. Biologic Effects of Nonionizing Radiation (pp. 155-165). New York: New York Academy of Sciences.

Kramar, P. O., Harris, C., Emery, A. F., & Guy, A. W. (1976). Acute microwave irradiation and cataract formation in rabbits and monkeys. Journal of Microwave Power, 13, 239-249.

Kues, H. A., Hirst, L. W., Lutty, G. A., D'Anna, S. A., & Dunkelberger, G. R. (1985). Effects of GHz microwaves on primate corneal endothelium. Bioelectromagnetics, 6, 177-188.

Lenox, R. H., Gandhi, O. P., Meyerhoff, J. L., & Grove, H. M. (1976). A microwave applicator for in vivo rapid inactivation of enzymes in the central nervous system. IEEE Transactions on Microwave Theory and Technique, 24, 58-61.

Liburdy, R. P., & Magin, R. L. (1985). Microwave-stimulated drug release from liposomes. Radiation Research, 103, 266-274.

Liddle, C. G., Putnam, J. P., Ali, J. S., Lewis, J. Y., Bell, B., & West, M. W. (1980). Alteration of circulating antibody response of mice exposed to 9-GHz pulsed microwaves. Bioelectromagnetics, 1, 397-404.

Lin, J. C. (1976). A new system for investigating nonthermal effect of microwaves on cells. In C.C. Johnson & M.L. Shore (Eds.), Biological effects of electromagnetic waves: Selected Papers of the USNC/YRSU Annual Meeting, Boulder, CO, Vol II. (HEW Publication No. (FDA) 77-8011, pp. 350-355). Washington, DC: U.S. Department of Health, Education, and Welfare.

Liu, L.-M., & Cleary, S. F. (1988). Effects of 2.45-GHz microwave and 100-MHz radiofrequency radiation on liposome permeability at the phase transition temperature. Bioelectromagnetics, 9, 249-257.

Lotz, W. G., & Saxton, J. L. (1987). Metabolic and vasomotor responses of rhesus monkeys exposed to 225-MHz radiofrequency energy. Bioelectromagnetics, 8, 73-89.

20

Marshall, S. V., & Brown, R. F. (1983). Experimental determination of whole body average specific absorption rate (SAR) of mice exposed to 200-400 MHz CW. Bioelectromagnetics, 4, 267-279.

McRee, D. I., Hamrick, P. E. & Zinkl, J. (1975). Some effects of microwave of the Japanese quail embryo to 2.45-GHz microwave radiation. In P. E. Tyler (Ed.), Annals of the New York Academy of Sciences: Vol. 247. Biologic Effects of Nonionizing Radiation (pp. 378-390). New York: New York Academy of Sciences.

Meltz, M. L., Eagan, P., Harris, C. R., & Erwin, D. N. (1988). Dosimetry considerations in far field microwave exposure of mammalian cells. Physiological Chemistry and Physics and Medical NMR, 20, 23-30.

National Council on Radiation Protection and Measurements. (1981). Radiofrequency electromagnetic fields: Properties, quantities and units, biophysical interaction, and measurements (NCRP Rep. No. 67). Bethesda, MD: National Council on Radiation Protection and Measurements.

Neilly, J. P. & Lin, J. C. (1986). Interaction of ethanol and microwaves on the blood-brain barrier of rats. Bioelectromagnetics, 7, 405-414.

Olsen, R. G., de Lorge, J. O., Forstall, J. R., & Ezell, C. S. (1984). A circular waveguide irradiation system for nonhuman primates: Design and dosimetry. Bioelectromagnetics, 5, 79-88.

Ray, S., & Behari, J. (1990). Physiological changes in rats after exposure to low levels of microwaves. Radiation Research, 123, 199-202.

Riley, V., Guy, A. W., Chou, C. K., Fitzmaurice, M. A., & Spackman, D. H. (1979, June). RF radiation effect on neoplastic cells (USAF/SAM Contract No. F33615-77-C-0617). Seattle, Washington: University of Washington School of Medicine, Department of Rehabilitation Medicine, Bioelectromagnetics Research Laboratory.

Rupp, T., Montet, J., & Frazer, J. W. (1975). A comparison of thermal and radio-frequency exposure effects on trace metal content of blood plasma and liver cell fractions of rodents. In P. E. Tyler (Ed.), Annals of the New York Academy of Sciences: Vol. 247. Biologic Effects of Nonionizing Radiation (pp. 282-291). New York: New York Academy of Sciences.

Sanders, A. P., & Joines, W. T. (1984). The effects of hyperthermia and hyperthermia plus microwaves on rat brain energy metabolism. Bioelectromagnetics, 5, 63-70.

Schwartz, J. L., & Mealing, G. A. R. (1993). Calcium-ion movement and contractility in atrial strips of frog heart are not affected by low-frequency-modulated, 1 GHz electromagnetic radiation. Bioelectromagnetics, 14, 521-533.

Stern, S., Margolin, L., Weiss, B., Lu, S. T., & Michaelson, S. M. (1979). Microwaves: Effect on thermoregulatory behavior in rats. Science, 206, 1198-1201.

Sultan, M. F., Cain, C. A., & Tompkins, W. A. F. (1983). Immunological effects of amplitude-modulated radio frequency radiation: B lymphocyte capping. Bioelectromagnetics, 4, 157-165.

Taylor, E. M., & Ashleman, B. T. (1975). Some effects of electromagnetic radiation on the brain and spinal cord of cats. In P. E. Tyler (Ed.), P.E. Annals of the New York Academy of Sciences: Vol. 247. Biologic Effects of Nonionizing Radiation (pp. 63-73). New York: New York Academy of Sciences

Veyret, B., Bouthet, C., Deschaux, P., de Seze, R., Geffard, M., & Joussot-Dubien, J. (1991). Antibody responses of mice exposed to low-power microwaves under combined, pulse-and-amplitude modulation. Bioelectromagnetics, 12, 47-56.

Wachtel, H., Seaman, R., & Joines, W. (1975). Effects of low-intensity microwaves on isolated neurons. In P. E. Tyler (Ed.), Annals of the New York Academy of Sciences: Vol. 247. Biologic Effects of Nonionizing Radiation (pp. 46-62). New York: New York Academy of Sciences

Weil, C. M., Spiegel, R. J., & Joines, W. T. (1984). Internal field strength measurements in chick forebrains at 50, 147, and 450 MHz. Bioelectromagnetics, 5, 293-304.

Yang, H. K., Cain, C. A., Lockwood, J., & Tompkins, W. A. F. (1983). Effects of microwave exposure on the hamster immune system. I. Natural killer cell activity. Bioelectromagnetics, 4, 123-139.

2

MODELING AND EXPERIMENTAL CHARACTERIZATION OF EXPOSURE SYSTEMS

Luc Martens

Abstract

This paper will give an overview of the key issues in the design of exposure systems. A design procedure will be proposed and applied to the design of generally used transverse electromagnetic (TEM) cells. The difference between cell and animal exposure is briefly discussed.

Introduction

Experiments with exposure systems can benefit from modeling and characterization for several reasons. First, modeling and characterization are used to determine the fields that are incident on the exposed biological structure under test (BSUT—animal or cell suspension) and that are present in the absence of the BSUT. This characterization is used in the first step of the design of the exposure system. Second, the incident fields are influenced by the presence of the BSUT. The change in the fields can be determined by electromagnetic modeling. Finally, knowledge of the electromagnetic fields and the specific absorption rate (SAR) in the BSUT determined by calculation allows a quantitative interpretation of the biological results.

The design of an exposure system depends on its specifications, which again depend on the type of experiments. For biological cell experiments, a known uniform electric field or SAR should be produced in the cell culture under study. An example of an exposure system producing a uniform field is a transverse electromagnetic (TEM) cell, which will be illustrated further. However, the fields in the exposure system will only be uniform without an exposed structure. Another point that should be addressed is the fact that the field distribution in the BSUT is dependent on the live cell complex concentration in a cell culture. Detailed modeling should take that into account. This was investigated in Steffensen, Raskmark, and Pederson (1995). In this paper, however, we will assume that the BSUT is a uniform structure described by its

24

macroscopic parameters (relative permittivity ε_r and conductivity σ). For animal studies, a realistic near-field environment should be simulated if biological effects of wireless mobile telephone antennas are under study.

It should be noted that designing and characterizing the exposure system is the first step in a well-defined biological experiment. It should be complemented with a detailed report on experiment conditions. In Valberg (1995), a list of 18 key exposure parameters to be reported for an unambiguous interpretation of the biological results is described. With these remarks in mind, we now describe the procedure for designing exposure systems based on electromagnetic calculations and measurements. We will further apply it to a TEM cell exposure system. Finally, we will comment on animal exposure systems.

Steps in the Design and Characterization

In Figure 1, the subsequent steps in the design of exposure systems are shown. The design starts with the choice of system, such as a TEM cell, a resonant cavity, or a waveguide system. As already mentioned, the choice of the system depends on the nature of the experiments. Together with the choice of the exposure system, the excitation signal must be defined (e.g., continuous wave or modulated signal with a specific duty cycle, power level, central frequency, and frequency bandwidth).

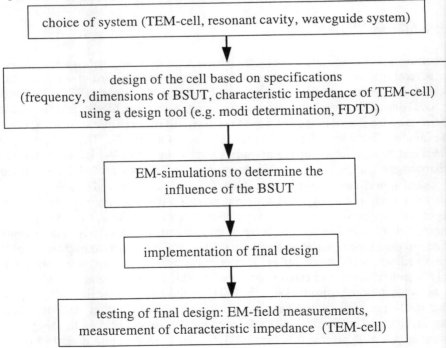

Figure 1. Subsequent steps in the design of an exposure system

Once the best choice is made, the specific design can be started. The dimensions of the system are determined by electrical specifications such as the frequency, the dimensions of the BSUT, and desired characteristic impedance of a transmission line system (e.g., TEM cell). The dimensions can be determined based on an electromagnetic simulation tool which calculates the fields inside the transmission line or cavity as a function of the dimensions. The electromagnetic calculations can also be used to determine the influence of discontinuities and transitions on the field distribution in the exposure system.

Electromagnetic simulations, such as the finite-difference time-domain (FD-TD) method are further used to determine the influence of the BSUT (i.e., calculation of the scattering of the incident field and the SAR distribution in the BSUT). In this phase of the design, the position and dimensions of the BSUT can be optimized in order to improve the uniformity of the fields in the BSUT.

Once the exposure system has been designed, the electrical design is converted to a mechanical design in a CAM-system and the exposure system is constructed following the mechanical specifications. The electrical specifications are further tested, for example, using field measurements with a nonperturbing probe to determine the field uniformity without BSUT and using the time domain reflectometry (TDR) technique in the case of a TEM cell to determine the impedance through the transmission line system. Field measurements can also be performed in the BSUT if the probes are small enough and nonperturbing. Though subsequent steps are now explained for the TEM cell, this does not mean that this is the best choice of an exposure system.

Application of the Design Procedure to a TEM Cell System for Cell Exposure

A popular exposure system, especially for lower frequencies (< 1 GHz), is the TEM cell. In the TEM cell a nearly uniform field is generated between the inner conductor (septum) and the outer conductor. Therefore the cell is suitable for biological cell experiments. Figure 2 shows a top view, a side view, and the cross section of such an exposure system. In what follows, the height and width (W) of the cell is 12 cm. The width (b) of the septum is 9.8 cm and its thickness (t) is 2 mm. Because power is delivered through a coaxial cable and connector and because termination of the cell at the other side can only be done at the coaxial connector level, two transitions from coaxial connectors to the main section of the TEM cell are provided. These transitions must be accurately designed because they can cause reflections and hence resonances, which disturb the field pattern as explained in Steffensen et al., (1995).

In a first step, the cross section is designed in such a way that the reflections in the TEM cell are minimized. To this end, the electrical parameters of the TEM transmission line such as the characteristic impedance were simulated using a 2D electromagnetic software tool (Olyslager, Faché, & De Zutter, 1991). The size of the cross section of the TEM cell determines the cut-off frequency of the first higher-order mode, the TE_{01}-mode. Since we want to study biological effects at the GSM carrier frequency of 900 MHz, we have chosen a 12 cm x 12 cm size corresponding with

26

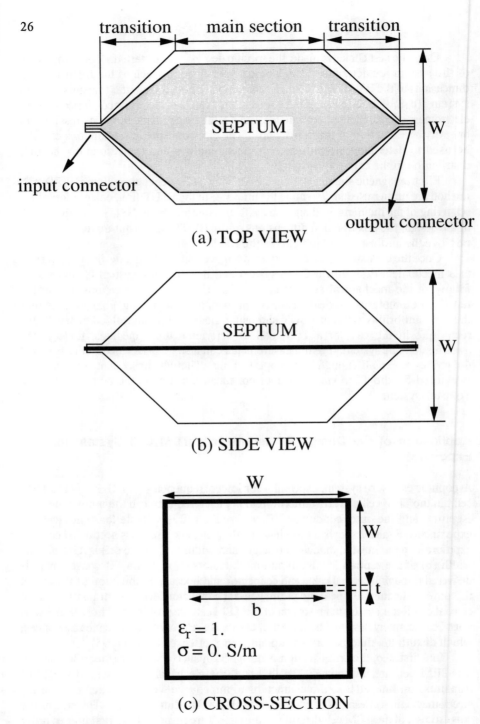

(a) TOP VIEW

(b) SIDE VIEW

(c) CROSS-SECTION

Figure 2. Top view (a), side view (b), and cross section (c) of a TEM cell

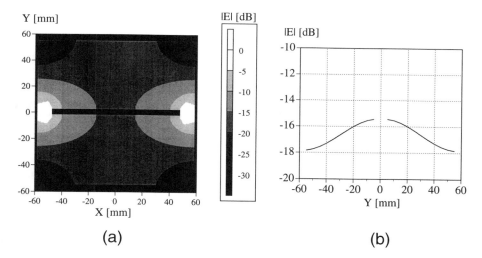

Figure 3. Electric field distribution of the TEM-mode in the cross section of the TEM cell (a), variation of the electric field of the TEM-mode along the x=0 axis (b)

1050 MHz for the TE_{01}-cut-off frequency. The width of the septum was then further adapted to obtain a 50 Ω characteristic impedance for the transmission line structure. Figure 3 shows the dimensions of the designed TEM cell and the electric field distribution of the lowest TEM-mode. As can be derived from the figure, the electric field is largest at the edges of the septum, which can be explained by the fact that the corners of the perfectly conducting septum act as singularities for the electromagnetic field resulting in very high levels for the fields. Cell suspensions that are placed near the edge will be irradiated with higher field levels than suspensions in the center of the septum. This should be kept in mind if a matrix of Petri dishes is placed on the septum. Also shown in this figure is the amplitude of the E-field along the x=0 axis. We observe a variation of 2.5 dB from the septum to the top or bottom of the TEM cell. Hence, it should be kept in mind that even in the empty cell, the electric field is not completely uniform above the septum.

However, the design of the empty cell does not suffice for a biological experiment. For a good interpretation of the biological results, we must quantify how much the insertion of the cell culture disturbs the incident field. This can be done using the FD-TD method (Burkhardt, Pokovic, Gnos, Schmid, & Kuster, 1995; Steffensen et al., 1995; Martens et al., 1993; Valberg, 1995; Van Hese et al., 1992). We investigated the field perturbation near and the field distribution inside a blood cell suspension which was placed in the center of the TEM cell on the septum. Figure 4 shows the blood cell suspension placed in the TEM cell with indication of dimensions. Dielectric parameters for blood at 900 MHz were found in the literature ($\varepsilon_r = 51$ and $\sigma = 1.28$ S/m). The transitions were not modeled in the calculations. For the FD-TD method, a cubic grid was used with elementary grid dimension of 2.5 mm. Figure 5

Cross section of the TEM-cell (with sample)

Longitudinal view of the TEM-cell

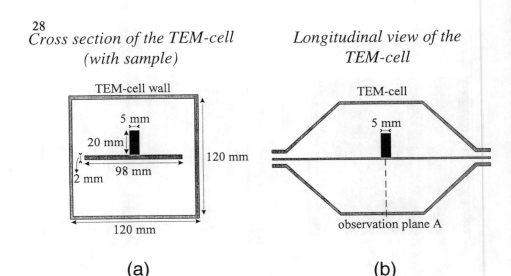

(a)

(b)

Figure 4. Blood cell suspension placed in the TEM cell: side view (a), cross section in observation plane A (b)

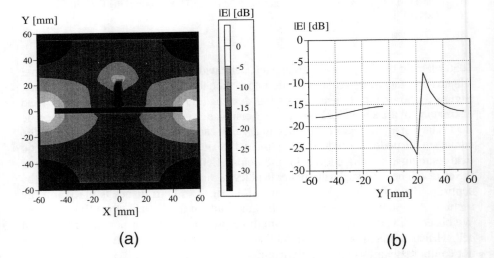

(a)

(b)

Figure 5. Electric field distribution in observation plane A indicated on figure 4 (a), variation of the electric field along the x=0 axis in this cross section (b)

shows the electric field distribution for 900 MHz in the cross section corresponding to the observation plane A. As can be noted, the electric fields are much lower in the cell suspension in comparison to the levels around it. This is also confirmed by the curve of Figure 5 (b) which again shows the amplitude of the electric field along the x=0 axis in this cross section. Note the jumps in the electric field at the bottom and the top of the cell suspension. This is due to the discontinuity of the normal component of the electric field at these surfaces. The electric field varies about 5 dB in the cell suspension, in spite of its small dimensions. It is clear that this is a bad positioning of the cell suspension. A better uniformity is achieved by placing the largest side of the suspension on the septum.

After these design and electromagnetic calculations, the TEM cell has been characterized. The TDR technique has been used to determine the reflections throughout the TEM cell. By using a time-domain input step signal (rise time 35 ps and voltage amplitude 200 mV over a 50 Ω load) and by measuring the voltage levels at the input with an oscilloscope, the reflections at the different discontinuities in the TEM cell are displayed on the screen of the oscilloscope. The TDR picture determines the quality of the impedance control (50 Ω) through the transmission line structure. The TDR picture for the realized TEM cell is shown in Figure 6. Only slight variations in the voltage level are measured at the position of the transitions. The deviation from 200 mV is always less than 10%. Hence, the cross section and the transitions are well designed, which is important to avoid standing waves, even when the TEM cell is terminated with a 50 Ω load.

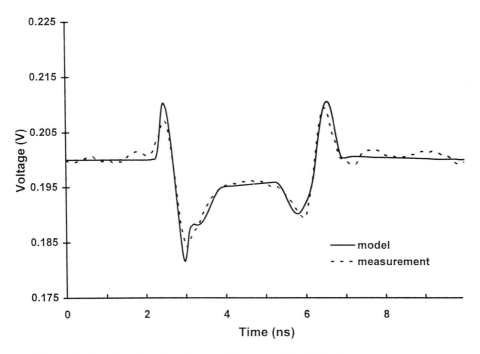

Figure 6. Time-domain voltage levels at the input of the TEM cell when an excitation of a time-domain step signal (rise time 35 ps and voltage amplitude 200 mV over a 50 Ω load) is used

Exposure Systems for Animal Studies

For animal studies, a commercially available near-field exposure set-up does not exist. The near-field exposure system used in Burkhardt and Kuster (1995), in which rats are exposed to the near field of a wire antenna, requires detailed knowledge of the fields inside the head of the animal. To that end, very good electromagnetic models of the antenna and the animal are required. Designing and quantifying the fields of such systems are fully dependent on the accuracy of the simulations. As was done in Burkhardt and Kuster, the detail of the model should be investigated before satisfactory accuracy is obtained. Calculated SAR distributions can be further verified through a comparison with invasive measurements using non-perturbing probes, such as an optical temperature sensor. Initial prediction of the inhomogeneity of the SAR distribution can also be done using an animal phantom (Thuroczy, Bakos, & Szabo, 1995). In animal exposure, other factors such as movement of the animals can strongly influence the SAR distributions. These factors must be taken into account.

Conclusion

In this paper, we discussed the subsequent steps in a good design of an exposure system. For a quantitative interpretation of the biological experiment, a complete electromagnetic characterization of the exposure system and the biological structure under test is a prerequisite. A final message is that the design and application of the exposure system should also be done by an engineer in close cooperation with the biologist performing the biological experiment.

Acknowledgment

The author would like to thank Dr. S. Criel for the simulations and Eng. K. Haelvoet for the design of and measurements on the TEM cell.

References

Burkhardt, M., & Kuster, N. (1995, September). Dosimetric analysis of a near field exposure system used for RF animal studies [abstract]. Proceedings of Latsis symposium on computational electromagnetics, Zurich, Switzerland, 234.

Burkhardt, M., Pokovic, K., Gnos, M., Schmid, T., & Kuster, N. (1996). Numerical and experimental dosimetry of petri dish exposure setups. Bioelectromagnetics, 17(6), 483-493.

Martens, L., Van Hese, J., De Zutter, D., De Wagter, C., Malmgren, L., & Persson, B. R. R. (1993). Electromagnetic field calculations used for exposure experiments on small animals. Journal of Bioelectrochemistry and Bioenergetics, 30, 73-81.

Olyslager, F., Faché, N., & De Zutter, D. (1991). New fast and accurate line parameter calculation of multi-conductor transmission lines in multilayered media. IEEE Transactions on Microwave Theory and Technique, 39(4), 673-681.

Steffensen, K. V., Raskmark, P., & Pederson, G. F. (1995). FDTD calculations of the EM-field distribution in a microtiter suspension well. In D. Simunic (Ed.), Proceedings of COST 244 Kuopio Workshop.

Thuroczy, G., Bakos, J., & Szabo, L. D. (1995). Practical considerations in bioelectromagnetics dosimetry: SAR measurements of RF and microwave exposure in animal phantoms related to mobile phones. In D. Simunic (Ed.), Proceedings of COST-244 Athens Meeting.

Valberg, P. A. (1995). Designing EMF experiments: What is required to characterize "exposure"? Bioelectromagnetics, 16(6), 396-401.

Van Hese, J., Martens, L., De Zutter, D., De Wagter, C., Malmgren, L., Persson, B. R. R., & Salford, L.G. (1992). Simulation of the effect of inhomogeneities in TEM transmission cells using the FDTD-method. IEEE Transactions on Electromagnetic Compatibility, 34(3), 292-298.

3
DIELECTRIC SPECTROSCOPY OF BIOLOGICAL MATERIALS: ITS ROLE IN DOSIMETRY
Camelia Gabriel

Dielectric spectroscopy is the study of the frequency dependence of the passive electrical properties of matter as a function of frequency. In the case of biological materials, the electrical properties (relative permittivity $\acute{\varepsilon}$ and total conductivity σ) are highly frequency-dependent from hertz to gigahertz which indicates strong electrical interactions. The interaction of magnetic fields with biological materials is much less eventful and is described in terms of their magnetic permeability. The magnetic permeability of most biological materials is largely frequency-independent, not different from that of a vacuum. This indicates little, if any, specific interactions.

A consequence of the dielectric properties of biological material is that an external electric field will induce a different internal field within it. This field, known as an average or macroscopic field, is itself due to interactions at all levels of organization within the material and the presence of local microscopic fields. The quantification of these fields is the scope of dosimetry.

Two main categories of electrical interaction can be observed in biological materials. These are (i) charge displacement, which subsides on the removal of the field, and (ii) charge drift. The former causes electrical polarization while the latter leads to charge conduction and the establishment of ionic currents. In biological tissue, different types of polarization occur at the cellular and molecular levels. The time constants associated with such mechanisms vary from picoseconds for the polarization of water and small organic molecules, to nanoseconds for large organic configurations, and milliseconds for the cellular structures. Dielectric spectroscopy is an important tool in the study of such mechanisms.

This paper will concentrate, albeit briefly, on two aspects of this science that impact dosimetry. First, the dielectric properties of tissues, which are essential input parameters in dosimetry, will be discussed in light of recent measurements, as well as a literature review of the subject. Second, it will be shown that dielectric studies can be used to quantify concepts such as microwave energy at the molecular level.

The Dielectric Properties of Tissues: Current State-of-Knowledge

Recent advances in dielectric measuring techniques (Gabriel, Chan, & Grant, 1994; Gabriel, Lau, & Gabriel, 1996a, Gabriel, Lau, & Gabriel, 1996b) made it possible to obtain dielectric data for tissues over more than ten decades. Examples of such measurements are given in Figures 1 and 2 (see appendix of this paper), which show the measured values of the relative permittivity and the conductivity of liver and kidney as a function of frequency in the range of 10 Hz to 20 GHz. Three experimental techniques were used with overlapping frequency coverage. When measurements are made on the same sample throughout, the agreement between data sets is particularly good.

Experimental data, such as those reported in Figures 1 and 2, fall well within corresponding dielectric data collated from the literature as shown in Figures 3 and 4 (see appendix of this paper). The data follow the well-known frequency dependence and fill in the gaps due to the scarcity of information in the literature.

In practice, people are often exposed to more than one frequency, continuous monochromatic sources being the exception rather than the rule. Quantitative assessment of exposure to pulsed or multiple frequency devices requires knowledge of the dielectric properties at all the frequencies involved. To facilitate the incorporation of these values in the numerical solutions invoked, the frequency dependence of dielectric properties is expressed as a parametric function. The spectrum is characterized by three or four dispersion regions that may be fitted to the following expression:

$$\varepsilon(\omega) = \varepsilon_\infty + \sum_{m=1}^{m=4} \frac{\Delta\varepsilon_m}{1 + (j\omega\tau_m)^{(1-\alpha_m)}} + \sigma_i/j\omega\varepsilon_0$$

This expression is known as the 4 Cole-Cole model. The first term is a real number; its value depends on water content of the sample and generally falls between two and five for dry and high water content tissues. ε_∞ represents the permittivity in the terahertz frequency range. The second term is the summation of 4 Cole-Cole expressions corresponding to the main features of the spectrum. Each dispersion is characterized by its amplitude: $\Delta\varepsilon$ corresponding to the observed change in permittivity in the frequency range corresponding to $\omega\tau \gg 1$ and $\omega\tau \ll 1$, τ being the main relaxation time, ω the angular frequency of the field, and α is the Cole-Cole parameter, which signifies a distribution of relaxation times and is therefore equivalent to a Cole-Cole dispersion with $\alpha = 0$. The last term in the 4 Cole-Cole model represents the contribution of the ionic currents in which σ_i is known as the ionic conductivity at the limit of low frequencies; ε_0 is the permittivity of free. The SI unit of conductivity is siemens per meter (Sm^{-1}), which presumes that in this term, ε_0 is expressed in farad per meter ($F\ m^{-1}$) and ω, the angular frequency, in radians per second.

Figures 5 and 6 (see appendix of this paper) show the 4 Cole-Cole model with parameters adjusted to give a good fit to the experimental data presented in Figures 1 and 2. The corresponding literature data identified in Figures 3 and 4 are also shown. The model adequately describes the frequency dependence of the dielectric properties in the frequency range from Hz to GHz. It can be used with confidence for frequencies above 1 MHz, where it is supported by the body of literature data. At lower frequencies, where the literature values are scarce and have larger than average uncertainties, the model should be used with caution in the understanding that it provides a "best estimate" based on present knowledge.

This treatment has been extended to the main tissues. The results for two types of bone, cortical and cancellous, are given in Figures 7 and 8 (see appendix of this paper); a more comprehensive account of the study will be published elsewhere (Gabriel, Gabriel, & Courthout, 1996; Gabriel, Lau, & Gabriel, 1996a; Gabriel, Lau, & Gabriel, 1996b).

Microwave Energy Absorption

The absorption of microwave energy in biological material is intrinsically linked to water content and the nature of the water in the vicinity of organic molecules. Pure water presents a Debye type dispersion of amplitude $\Delta\varepsilon \approx 75$ and relaxation time $\tau \approx 9ps$ at $20°C$. At $37°C$ the dielectric parameters are 69 and 6 ps respectively. The relaxation time of organic macromolecules is on the order of nanoseconds. For each substance, the rate of energy absorbed due to dielectric dispersion is maximum when $\omega\tau = 1$. A substance with a relaxation time of 70 or 80 ps will absorb energy most efficiently at about 2 GHz.

Dielectric studies have shown that a number of organic solutes lengthen the relaxation time of water, and some increase the amplitude of its principle dispersion (Bateman, Gabriel, & Grant, 1990). This observation is fairly general; it applies to a greater or lesser extent to aqueous solutions, cellular cultures, and biological tissues. Table 1 gives the dielectric parameters of water dispersion in some high- and low-water-content tissues; the corresponding parameters for water are given for comparison purposes. The lengthening of the relaxation time is clearly demonstrated together with an increase in the distribution parameter. These data reinforce the observation that the relaxation time increases with solute concentration and may reach values up to an order of magnitude higher (Bateman et al., 1990).

The practical consequences of this effect are that in the frequency range of 900 MHz to 2 GHz the rate of heating modified water will exceed that of unmodified water and greatly exceed that in the solute. The microwave energy is unevenly absorbed at the molecular level. Concepts such as these need to be expanded and incorporated in the calculation of temperature distribution in biological systems, including tissues.

Conclusions

Parametric expressions of the frequency dependence of the dielectric properties of tissues provide adequate data for the study of human exposure to electromagnetic fields. The availability of such data will remove an important source of differences between dosimetric studies.

Tissue	ϵ		τ (ps)		α	
Water	74.1		6.2		0.0	
Aqueous Humor	74.2	(0.3)	6.18	(0.08)	0.01	(0.01)
Retina	67.3	(0.4)	7.25	(0.08)	0.05	(0.01)
Tongue	57.7	(0.3)	9.12	(0.21)	0.08	(0.01)
Brain (Grey matter)	55.5	(0.5)	7.76	(0.15)	0.12	(0.02)
Cornea	53.0	(0.4)	8.72	(0.17)	0.13	(0.01)
Lens (Cortex)	52.1	(0.3)	9.18	(0.16)	0.11	(0.01)
Cerebellum	50.2	(0.4)	8.52	(0.21)	0.09	(0.02)
Dura	49.2	(0.5)	9.63	(0.28)	0.14	(0.02)
Cartilage	43.6	(0.6)	12.8	(0.58)	0.27	(0.02)
Bone (Cancellous)	22.1	(0.2)	14.4	(0.33)	0.22	(0.01)
Bone (Cortical)	14.9	(0.2)	13.8	(0.48)	0.26	(0.01)

The first column is equivalent to $\Delta\epsilon+\epsilon_\infty$, the number in brackets is the 95% confidence limit on the parameters. Pure water has a Debye type dispersion and hence $\alpha = 0$.
Table: Cole-Cole Parameters of Tissue Water at 37°C

An insight into microwave energy absorption by biological material revealed uneven distribution at the molecular level. This understanding points to the importance and the relevance of extending dosimetric studies to include thermal modeling. This approach is particularly suited to the assessment of exposures intended to study biological effects, since the biological response is more directly related to temperature rise rather than instantaneous energy absorption.

Acknowledgment

The work reported in this paper was supported by the U.S. Air Force under contract F49620-93-1-0561.

References

Bateman, J. B., Gabriel, C., & Grant, E. H. (1990). Permittivity at 70 GHz of water in aqueous solutions of some amino acids and related compounds. Journal of the Chemical Society Faraday Transactions 2, 86, 3577-3583.

Gabriel, C., Chan, T. Y. A., & Grant, E. H. (1994). Admittance models for open ended coaxial probes and their place in dielectric spectroscopy. Physics in Medicine and Biology, 39(12), 2183-2200.

Gabriel, C., Gabriel S., & Courthourt, E. (1996). The dielectric properties of biological tissues: 1. Literature survey. Physics in Medicine and Biology, 41 (11), 2231-2250.

Gabriel, S., Lau, R. W., & Gabriel, C. (1996). The dielectric properties of biological tissues: 2. Measurements in the frequency range 10 Hz to 20 GHz. Physics in Medicine and Biology, 41 (11), 2251-2269.

Gabriel, S., Lau, R. W., & Gabriel, C. (1996). The dielectric properties of biological tissues: 3. Parametric models for the dielectric spectrum of tissues. Physics in Medicine and Biology, 41 (11), 2271-2293.

References to literature on dielectric properties are not given explicitly but are mentioned in Gabriel, Gabriel, & Courthourt, 1996.

38

Appendix

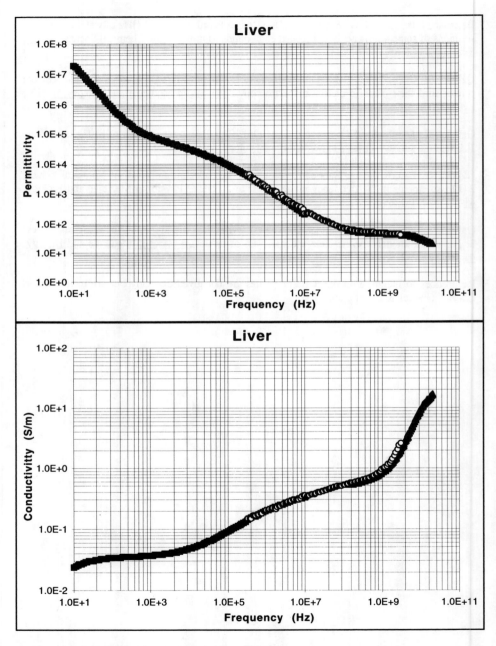

Figure 1. Permittivity and conductivity of ovine liver tissue at 37°C

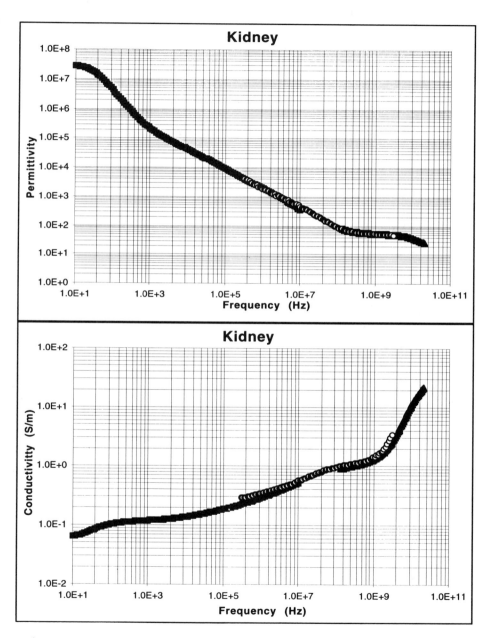

<u>Figure 2.</u> Permittivity and conductivity of ovine cortical kidney tissue at 37°C

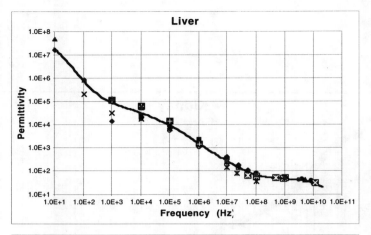

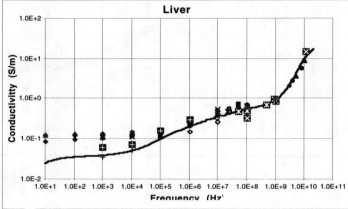

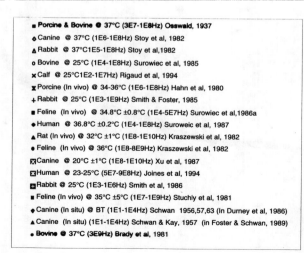

Figure 3. Experimental data from Figure 1 shown as a continuous line and corresponding literature data identified in the legend to follow

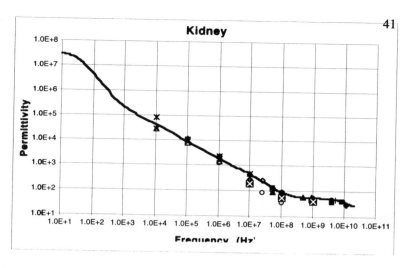

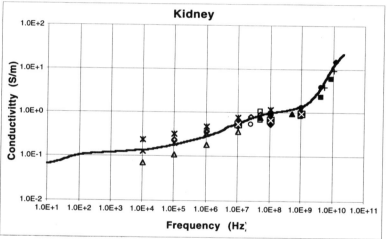

□ Porcine & Bovine @ 37°C (5E7Hz) Osswald, 1937 (in Stoy et al, 1982)

◆ Canine @ 37°C (1E5-1E8Hz) Stoy et al,1982

▲ Bovine @ 25°C (1E4-1E8Hz) Surowiec etal, 1985

○ Porcine (In vivo) @ 34-36°C (1E6-1E8Hz) Hahn et al, 1980

✕ Feline (In vivo) @ 34.7°C+/-0.9°C (1E4-1E8Hz) Suroweic et al, 1986

✕ Human @ 36.5°C (1E4-1E8Hz) Suroweic et al, 1987

+ Rat (In vivo) @ 32°C +/-1°C (1E8-1E10Hz) Kraszewski et al, 1982

■ Feline (In vivo) @ 36°C +/-2°C (1E8-8E9Hz) Kraszewski et al, 1982

◆ Canine @ 20 °C+/-1°C (1E8-1E10Hz) Xu et al, 1987

▲ Human @ 23-25°C (5E7-9E8Hz) Joines et al, 1994

● Canine (In vivo) (1E8-4E9Hz) Burdette et al, 1980

⊠ Feline (In vivo) @ 35 °C+/-1°C (1E7-1E9Hz) Stuchly et al, 1981

Figure 4. Experimental data from Figure 2 shown as a continuous line and corresponding literature data identified in the legend to follow

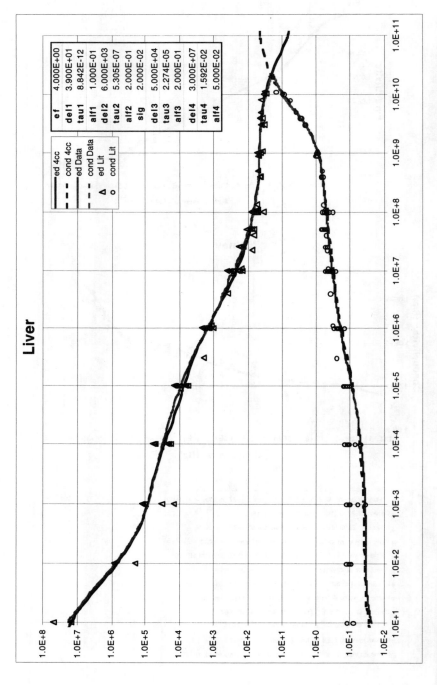

Figure 5. The 4 Cole-Cole model applied to liver tissue. The corresponding parameters are shown in a self-explanatory manner.

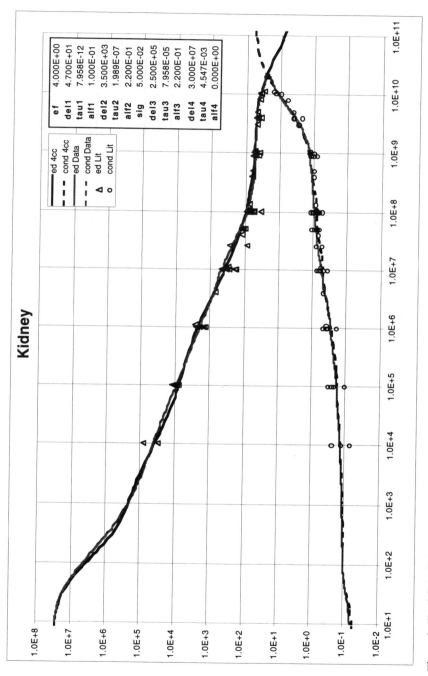

<u>Figure 6.</u> The 4 Cole-Cole model applied to kidney tissue. The corresponding parameters are shown in a self-explanatory manner.

44

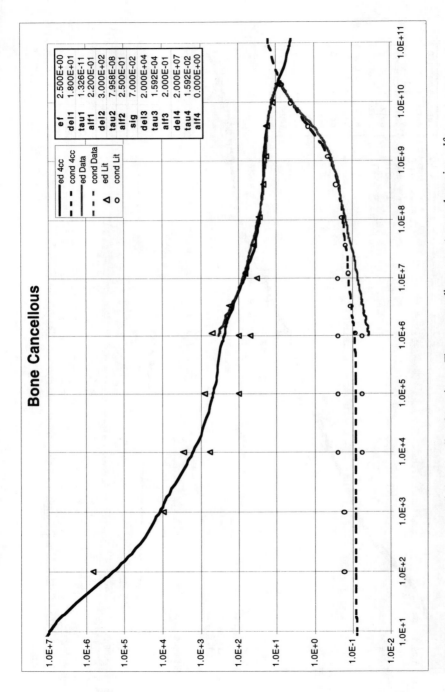

Figure 7. The 4 Cole-Cole model applied to cancellous bone tissue. The corresponding parameters are shown in a self-explanatory manner.

45

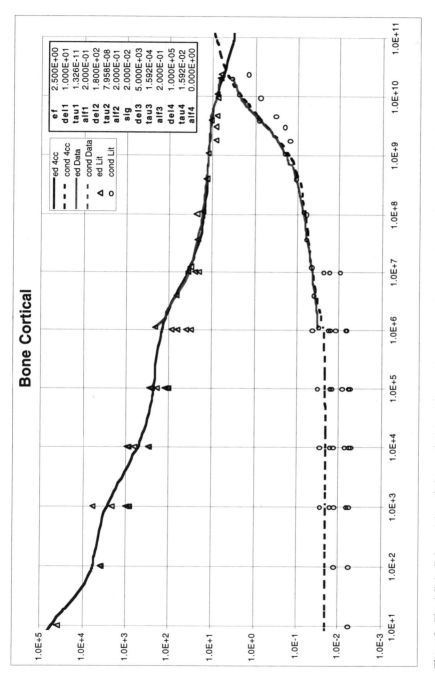

Figure 8. The 4 Cole-Cole model applied to cortical bone tissue. The corresponding parameters are shown in a self-explanatory manner.

4

COMPLIANCE TESTING OF HANDHELD MOBILE COMMUNICATIONS EQUIPMENT

Niels Kuster

Abstract

A scientifically sound procedure for certification of mobile telecommunications equipment (MTE) must satisfy a number of requirements: 1) assessment of the spatial peak SAR values defined in safety standards; 2) a reliable procedure to determine the uncertainty of the assessed values; 3) a simple but reliable test to validate proper functioning of the setup; 4) high reproducibility of all test results; 5) the ability to test randomly selected devices; 6) credibility in the eyes of both experts and consumers; 7) ease of use, without the need of highly specialized experts; 8) time efficiency; 9) availability for manufacturers during the product design process. Commercially available dosimetric scanners have been proven to satisfy all these requirements. Further arguments for dosimetric scanners are: 1) the actual MTE is tested and certified as it leaves the production line; 2) the measurement error of dosimetric assessments within homogeneous phantoms can be kept below ±20%; 3) homogeneous phantoms not only accurately simulate absorption in the heads of MTE users but also considerably reduce the number of tests required to ensure compliance with safety limits for a reasonable cross-section of users.

Requirements

A scientifically sound procedure for testing the compliance of handheld mobile telecommunications equipment (MTE) with safety standards—as has been called for by health agencies—is becoming a pressing need for industry, in order to maintain customer credibility and ward off the risk of potentially damaging liability suits. Two factors make the development of a compliance test difficult. 1) Current cellular phones induce spatial peak SAR close to or above the current safety limits (Meier, Egger, Schmid, & Kuster, 1995). 2) Small shifts in the position with respect to the head may significantly alter absorption, depending on the design of the device. The latter is crucial, since users have numerous habitual ways of holding MTE devices. This issue has recently been addressed by a working group of CENELEC (WGMTE of CENELEC TC211/B, 1997), which has drafted the range of operational conditions to be tested within a certification procedure.

48

A sound procedure should, therefore, ideally demonstrate compliance for all users and the numerous operating conditions with a minimum of measurements and simulations. Further requirements are:

- accurate assessment of the spatial peak SAR values defined in the safety standard;
- a reliable procedure to determine the total uncertainty of the assessment;
- a simple but reliable test to validate the correct functioning of the setup;
- high reproducibility of all test results;
- a very reliable setup;
- the ability to test randomly selected devices;
- time efficiency;
- ease of use, so that the tests do not need to be performed by very specialized experts;
- availability for manufacturers during the design process of their products;
- credibility in the eyes of experts and consumers.

Demonstration of compliance for handheld MTE is generally possible either by measurements or by numerical computations. Both approaches are currently being investigated by several groups worldwide. The approach which will finally succeed will be the one which best fulfills the above requirements. Minimal total uncertainty is seen as especially critical, in view of the small margins current cellular handsets have with respect to current safety levels (Kuster, Balzano, & Lin, 1997). In the following, the overall uncertainty of measurement setups such as the one developed at

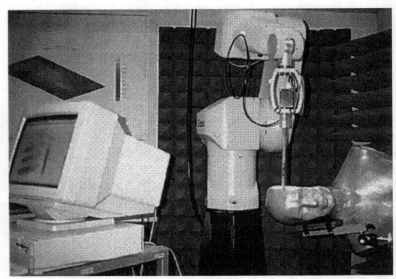

Figure 1. The dosimetric assessment system DASY2 (six-axis robot, isotropic E-field probe, data acquisition electronics, and PC) and the anatomically shaped shell phantom (corresponds to the third experimental phantom).

the ETH (Figure 1) is briefly discussed. In general, the total uncertainty is comprised of all uncertainties arising from the modeling of the handsets and the representation of the human head using shell phantoms as well as from the measurement system.

Uncertainties in Modeling the Mobile Phone

The object to certify is the MTE as it leaves the production line. A procedure which requires modifications or modeling of the test object is therefore critical per se. This is all the more true, since the spatial peak SAR has proven to be highly dependent upon the actual design of the MTE (e.g., see Figure 2). The physical explanation is that the SAR is predominately induced by induction, i.e., it is proportional to the square of the current distribution and inversely proportional to the square of the distances between those currents and the surface of the body (Kuster & Balzano, 1992). Therefore, minor details, even internal structures, can affect the spatial peak SAR considerably. Consequently, small modeling errors can result in SAR errors of several dBs. As long as procedures to reliably assess the uncertainty of a particular modeling are not available, certification by simulations or measurement techniques requiring modification of the device is of doubtful value or would demand large safety margins.

However, if the sensitivity of a measurement setup allows testing of the actual MTE as it leaves the production line, the uncertainty of modeling the device is zero, i.e., the total uncertainty of the procedure is independent of the device and is comprised of those of the setup only. This is seen as the reason for the superiority of measurement approaches, since the total uncertainty of the setup only needs to be determined once and not for each modeling of the MTE, i.e., for each dosimetric assessment.

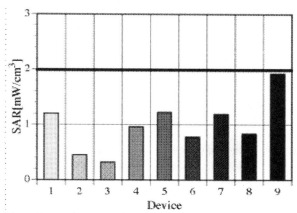

Figure 2. Maximum spatial peak SAR of nine GSM devices (nominal time averaged P_{in}: 250 mW) averaged over 10 cm³, measured according to the test conditions described in the WGMTE draft (1997).

Uncertainties in Modeling the Human Body

Currently available fully automated systems are limited to assessments made in tissue simulating liquids, which requires that compliance tests be conducted in homogeneous phantoms. This immediately poses the question of whether such phantoms are suitable for simulating absorption in the head of a mobile phone user. This question was very recently addressed by investigating the dependence of the induced spatial peak SAR at 900 MHz and 1800 MHz on 1) the outer shape of the head, 2) the distribution of the different tissues within the head, and 3) the dielectric properties of these tissues (Hombach, Meier, Burkhardt, Kühn, & Kuster, 1996; Meier, Kästle, Hombach, Tay, & Kuster, 1997). This study was performed using a finite integration technique (FIT; which is related to the FD-TD approach) and experimental techniques (Schmid, Egger & Kuster, 1996). Four different MRI-based numerical phantoms and three different experimental phantoms were used:

- The most complex experimental phantom was constructed with four tissue types: skull, muscle, skin, and eyes. The fifth tissue, brain, was simulated using a sugar-water-salt solution with the electrical parameters of the mean value between gray and white matter. This head was considerably smaller than that of an average adult. In addition, the skin-skull layer in the area above the ear was thicker (15.5 mm) than for an average person.

- The second experimental phantom was an exact copy of the outer shape of the above mentioned complex phantom. The shell was made of polyester with a thickness of approximately 3 mm.

- The third experimental phantom was a head-torso model of a human being. The shell was anatomically correctly-shaped and made of 3 mm thick fibreglass. The shape and size of this phantom differed from the shell copy of the complex phantom. It was considerably larger (4 liters instead of 2.5). This phantom is currently used for dosimetric characterizations of MTE in several laboratories in Europe and the United States.

- The first numerical phantom had a volume of 4.4 dm^3 and a resolution of 1 mm^3. Thirteen tissue types were simulated. The brain region was segmented very carefully.

- The second numerical phantom had a volume of 3.4 dm^3 and a resolution of 1.08 mm^3. It was developed for the training of medical students and distinguished among 120 tissue types. For the EM analysis the number of tissues was reduced to 13, the number for which dielectric parameters were available.

- The third numerical phantom had approximately the same volume as the first phantom but a resolution of only 10.5 mm^3 (voxel size of 1.875 mm x 1.875 mm x 3 mm). Although the original model did not identify the skin, it was added in this study. The brain region was homogeneous and assigned only one tissue type. Twelve tissue types were simulated. Compared to the other phantoms, the skull was considerably thicker.

• The fourth numerical phantom corresponded to the most complex experimental phantom described above. It was derived from MRI and CT cross sections taken every 2 mm.

Simple dipole excitations were chosen in order to avoid the uncertainties involved in modeling actual handsets. Dipoles of 0.45 λ length were positioned at a distance of 15 mm from the head and placed parallel to the body's axis.

The dependence of the spatial peak absorption on the size, shape, and internal anatomical composition of the head were assessed by comparing the results of the various phantoms using the same excitation. In addition, the tissue parameters were varied. The findings were verified by spherical phantoms of similar layer structures as derived from MRI scans.

Interestingly, the SAR values measured using the homogeneous phantoms were only slightly higher than those of the MRI-based phantoms. With the homogeneous phantoms, the spatial peak SAR averaged over a volume of 10 cm^3 overestimated the largest value obtained for the nonhomogeneous phantom by a factor of less than 10%. The overestimation of the spatial peak SAR averaged over 1 g, though greater, was still less than 25%. Since the homogeneous approach was only compared to four different human heads, the overestimation might even be considerably smaller if all users are considered.

These findings basically confirm the conclusions of Kuster and Balzano (1992), that the spatial peak SAR is scarcely affected by the size and shape of the human head for electromagnetic sources in very close proximity. In contrast to effects caused by other factors, such as the distance of the source from the head and the design of the devices, the effects caused by complex anatomy are minor if volume-averaged values are of interest.

An important advantage of using simple, homogeneous phantoms is that the number of tests can be reduced, since small shifts of the source parallel to the surface result in almost no change in the spatial peak SAR values. Strongly inhomogeneous phantoms might result in artificially low SAR values for some positions of the device with respect to the head. Hence, a large number of tests would need to be conducted to certify the device.

Uncertainties of SAR Assessments in Shell Phantoms

Dosimetric measurement setups providing the sensitivity needed to test actual mobile phones are all based on isotropic E-field probes of small dimensions (Balzano, Garay, & Manning, 1995; Schmid et al., 1996), whereby E-field distributions induced in shell phantoms filled with brain simulating liquids are scanned by robots. The uncertainty analysis for the spatial peak SAR has been analyzed for the system described in Schmid et al. (1996) considering:

- E-field probe errors, which include: 1) the pick-up of other signals as secondary modes of reception, 2) errors in isotropy, 3) errors due to limited spatial resolution, and 4) interaction with the measured field;

- probe calibration errors, which include: 1) temperature probe errors, 2) heat distribution effects, and 3) numerical simulation errors (if used as a basis for the calibration);

- probe positioning errors;

- data acquisition errors and data evaluation errors;

- long-term stability;

- errors in assessing the correct parameters for the tissue-simulating solution.

This analysis has been performed for the system described in Schmid et al. (1996), resulting in an overall uncertainty of less than ±20% at 900 MHz. This was achieved with the aid of two breakthroughs: 1) a novel E-field probe design with improved isotropy, immunity to ELF and RF fields, and a greater frequency and dynamic range; 2) an accurate broad band calibration procedure (Meier, Burkhardt, Schmid, & Kuster, 1996). The long-term stability and the proper functioning of the system can be checked with an easy-to-use validation kit. The check has a reproducibility of better than ±5%.

Conclusions

Accurate dosimetric assessments within shell phantoms filled with tissue-simulating liquids are achievable with E-field scanners. Time efficient and user-friendly setups are possible with robot-based systems. The uncertainty of measurements can be kept within 20%. The correct performance of the system can be monitored by easy-to-use system validation kits.

Homogeneous shell phantoms have been proven to be suitable for use in compliance tests for handheld MTE operating in the frequency band between 300-2500 MHz. Homogeneous phantoms not only accurately simulate the absorption in the head of the MTE user but also considerably reduce the number of tests required to ensure compliance with safety limits.

The most persuasive argument for a certification procedure based on measurements is that the actual MTE can be tested and certified as it leaves the production line. A dosimetric assessment testing any kind of configuration or position can be completed within approximately 15 minutes.

Acknowledgments

The author gratefully acknowledges the research teams at ETH, Motorola, German Telekom, Nokia, Ericsson and CSELT for their excellent cooperation and invaluable advice.

Update

The absorption studies using MRI-based head phantoms of different adult persons have recently been complemented by a study including head phantoms of a three-year-old child and seven-year-old child. The results showed no significant differences in the absorption of electromagnetic energy in the near field of sources between adults and children. The same was shown to be true for various linearly-scaled adult phantoms (Schönborn, Burkhardt, & Kuster, 1998).

The relatively minor dependence of the absorption on internal anatomy allowed the development of a generic phantom that does not underestimate real-world exposure for at least 90% of MTE users for any defined position of the phone with respect to the head (Kuster, Kästle, & Schmid, 1997). However, very precise positioning of the device is essential in order to provide a high degree of repeatability of the evaluations, since the position defines the distances of the various parts of the phone with respect to the surface of the phantom. In order to meet this requirement, a special device was developed allowing highly precise positioning of the phones in accordance with the CENELEC guidelines (Kuster, Kästle & Schmid, 1997), i.e., achieving a repeatability of the dosimetric assessments that is better that ±5%. This completes the scientific and technical basis to conduct reliable and sound compliance testing with known precision.

Ongoing research studies are being performed with the objective of further reducing the uncertainty of the evaluation, which involves the development of probes with better spatial resolution (Poković, Schmid, & Kuster, 1997a), as well as improved isotropy (Poković, Schmid, & Kuster, 1996), and improved and traceable calibration procedures (Poković, Schmid & Kuster, 1997b).

References

Balzano, Q., Garay, O., & Manning, T. J. (1995). Electromagnetic energy exposure of simulated users of portable cellular telephones. IEEE Transactions on Vehicular Technology, 44, (3), 390-403.

Hombach, V., Meier, K., Burkhardt, M., Kühn, E., & Kuster, N. (1996). The dependence of EM energy absorption upon human head modeling at 900 MHz. IEEE Transactions on Microwave Theory and Technique, 44(10), 1865-1873.

Kuster, N., & Balzano, Q. (1992). Energy absorption mechanism by biological bodies in the near field of dipole antennas above 300 MHz. IEEE Transactions on Vehicular Technology, 41(1), 17-23.

Kuster, N., Balzano, Q., & Lin, J. C. (Eds.). (1997). Mobile communications safety. London: Chapman & Hall.

Kuster, N., Kästle, R., & Schmid, T. (1997). Dosimetric evaluation of mobile communications equipment with known precision. IEICE Transactions on Communications, E80-B. (5), 645-652.

Meier, K., Kästle, R., Hombach, V., Tay, R., & Kuster, N. (1997). The dependence of electromagnetic energy absorption upon human-head modeling at 1800 MHz. IEEE Transactions on Microwave Theory and Technique, 44(11), 2058-2062.

Meier, K., Burkhardt, M., Schmid, T., & Kuster, N. (1996). Broadband calibration of E-field probes in lossy media. IEEE Transactions on Microwave Theory and Technique, 44(10), 1954-1962.

Meier, K., Egger, O., Schmid, T., & Kuster, N. (1995, March). Dosimetric laboratory for mobile communications. In Proceedings of the 11th Symposium on Electromagnetic Compatibility, (pp. 297-300). Zurich, Switzerland.

Poković, K., Schmid, T., & Kuster, N. (1996, June). E-field probe with improved isotropy in brain simulating liquids. In Proceedings of the ELMAR, (pp. 172-175). Zadar, Croatia.

Poković, K., Schmid, T., & Kuster, N. (1997, June). Specialized E-field probe for RF exposure evaluation of in vivo and in vitro experiments [abstract]. In The Second World Congress for Electricity and Magnetism in Biology and Medicine, (pp. 117). Bologna, Italy.

Poković, K., Schmid, T., & Kuster, N. (1997, October). Robust setup for precise calibration of e-field probes in tissue simulating liquids at mobile communications frequencies. In ICECOM87, (pp. 120-124). Dubrovnik, Croatia.

Schmid, T., Egger, O., & Kuster, N. (1996). Automated E-field scanning system for dosimetric assessments. IEEE Transactions on Microwave Theory and Technique, 44, 105-113.

Schönborn, F., Burkhardt, M., & Kuster, N. (1998). Differences in energy absorption between heads of adults and children in the near field of sources. Health Physics, 74(2), 160-168.

WGMTE of CENELEC TC211/B. (1997). Final Draft: Considerations for human exposure to electromagnetic fields from mobile telecommunication equipment (MTE) in the frequency range 30 MHZ-6 Ghz. Brussels, Belgium: CENELEC.

5

STATE OF THE SCIENCE REGARDING RF DOSIMETRY, MEASUREMENT, AND CERTIFICATION

Om P. Gandhi

Introduction

Cellular telephones and wireless personal communication systems (PCS) are being introduced into society at a very rapid rate. Whereas the present-day cellular telephones in the United States operate at midband transmission frequencies of about 835 MHz (about 900 MHz in Europe), higher frequencies on the order of 1900 MHz (1800 MHz in Europe) are to be used for the PCS systems, including mobile telephones, wireless local area networks, pagers, personal health monitoring systems, global positioning systems, etc. This has resulted in public concern about the health hazards of radiofrequency (RF) electromagnetic fields that are emitted by these devices. To allay public concerns, the Federal Communications Commission (FCC) in the United States has decided to require compliance with the ANSI/IEEE RF safety guidelines (American National Standards Institute/Institute of Electrical and Electronics Engineers [ANSI/IEEE], 1992) for uncontrolled environments for all personal wireless devices that use more than 100 mW of time-averaged input power to the antenna. According to ANSI/IEEE safety guidelines for uncontrolled environments (ANSI/IEEE, 1992), the mass-normalized rate of electromagnetic energy absorption (specific absorption rate or SAR) in any 1 gram of tissue should not exceed 1.6 W/kg except for the hands, wrists, feet, and ankles where the spatial-peak SAR shall not exceed 4 W/kg, as averaged over any 10 grams of tissue. The safety guidelines being proposed for the European Union are more lax and peak SARs of 2.0 W/kg for any 10 grams of tissue are considered acceptable for exposures of the general public (European Committee for Electrotechnical Standardization [CENELEC], 1995) for tissues other than hands, wrists, feet, and ankles, where the safety guidelines are similar to those of ANSI/IEEE (ANSI/IEEE, 1992).

In this paper we present a review of the numerical as well as experimental methods that may be used not only for compliance testing but also for design of cellular telephones and other PCS devices that minimize energy absorbed in the body

56

and maximize radiated energy. It is clear that increasingly accurate models, both numerical and experimental, and calculation and measurement procedures will be needed as the wireless revolution progresses to the use of higher and higher frequencies for a myriad of present and future applications. We will also outline some of the challenges in this area, particularly for applications at the higher microwave frequencies.

Numerical Methods

Analytical and numerical methods have been developed over the last 40 years to understand coupling of electromagnetic fields to biological bodies (Lin & Gandhi, 1995). While the earliest of the models involved homogeneous and layered planar, spherical, cylindrical, prolate spheroidal, and ellipsoidal models, the focus in the last 20 years has been on development of increasingly sophisticated, anatomically-based models that are capable of providing information on induced current and SAR distributions from a variety of far-field and near-field sources from extremely low frequencies (ELF) to microwave frequencies (Gandhi, 1990, 1995). These models have been shown to be capable of predicting the frequencies and polarization conditions of highest absorption by the human body (the so-called resonant conditions) and the likely high SARs in the human legs for vertically polarized incident fields in the VHF range—results that have led to frequency-dependent safety standards and the more recent inclusion of the induced current limits in the various safety guidelines (ANSI/IEEE, 1992; CENELEC, 1995).

Several numerical methods such as the method of moments (MOM), multiple multipole method, volume-surface integral equation method, finite integration technique (FIT), finite-element time-domain method, and finite-difference time-domain method (FD-TD), etc., have been developed for calculation of SAR distributions (Gandhi, 1990; Lin & Gandhi, 1995; Simunic, 1995). As evidenced from the published literature (Dimbylow & Mann, 1994; Gandhi & Chen, 1995; Gandhi, Chen, & Wu, 1994; Jensen & Rahmat-Samii, 1995) and the proceedings of a recent COST 244 meeting (Simunic, 1995), a method of choice for calculations of SAR distributions for coupled near-field devices such as cellular telephones is the FD-TD method. This method is perhaps the most popular of the numerical electromagnetic methods at the present time and has been used for a myriad of other electromagnetic problems as well, such as RF microwave antennas and circuit design, radar scattering from objects of various types, and issues of electromagnetic compatibility and interference (Kunz & Luebbers, 1993; Taflove, 1995).

A major advantage of this method is that the computer memory requirement and the computation time increase linearly as the number of voxels (volume pixels) into which an interaction space of interest, including the cellular telephone and the coupled parts of the body, (e.g., the models of the head and the hand) can be divided. This is a considerable improvement over N^2 and N^3 for some of the methods, such as MOM. Highly discretized volumes with N on the order of 10^6-10^7, and with cell sizes on the order of 1-3 mm, can, therefore, be used to obtain SAR distributions for anatomically realistic models. The perceived advantages of the FD-TD method over other numerical techniques for mobile telephone dosimetry are given in the following.

1. It is considerably more efficient than traditional numerical electromagnetic methods such as the MOM, allowing use of realistic, anatomically-based models with resolutions on the order of 1-3 mm, using readily available computing workstations.

2. Since electrical properties such as the dielectric constants and conductivities of various tissues are not known with a high degree of precision, and accurate knowledge of these properties is evolving at the present time, it is relatively simple to incorporate these for dosimetric calculations using the numerical procedures.

3. It is also simple to alter the voxel sizes to calculate SAR distributions for heads of various sizes representative, for example, of women and children, and to use various postures of the telephones vis-à-vis the body.

4. Even though simple parallelepiped metal boxes covered with plastic have, to date, been used to model the handsets, the FD-TD procedure is perfectly capable of reading data files of software such as AutoCAD and Pro Engineer defining the exact geometry of the handset and its contents, albeit with a resolution of 1-3 mm, that is possible with the memories of today's readily available computing workstations. It has been alleged that this resolution may be inadequate to properly model the RF currents that may flow on internal substructures of the new transceivers, resulting in inaccurate SAR distributions. Our experience, however, has been that the microwave parts of the circuit are enclosed in a shielding metal box which in recent devices may only be a fraction of the handset. This can certainly be modeled in the FD-TD method.

5. Lastly, numerical procedures such as the FD-TD method permit calculations of the radiation patterns for a conceived wireless device coupled to the human body permitting, therefore, design of these devices that give desirable radiation patterns and lowest SARs that are within the safety guidelines.

Measurement Methods

Simple and more complex experimental models (phantoms) have and are being developed to obtain SAR distributions for actual operating wireless devices (Balzano, Garay, & Steel , 1978; Balzano, Garay, & Manning, 1995; Chatterjee, Gu, & Gandhi, 1985; Chou, personal communication, 1994; Cleveland & Athey, 1989; Gabriel, personal communication, 1994; Gandhi & Chen, 1995; Gandhi et al., 1994; Guy & Chou, 1986; Kuster & Balzano, 1992; Schmid, Egger, & Kuster, 1996; Stuchly, Spiegel, Stuchly, & Kraszewski, 1986). For the simplest of these models, homogeneous tissue-simulating gels or fluids are used in some sort of an insulating container which gives the phantom the shape of the body that is to be modeled (Balzano et al., 1978, 1995; Chatterjee et al., 1985; Guy & Chou, 1986; Schmid et al., 1996). For the more complex experimental models, several different tissue-simulant compositions representing the important regions such as the skin, skull, eyes, brain, etc. are used (C.K. Chou, personal communication, 1994; Cleveland & Athey, 1989; C. Gabriel, personal communication, 1994; Gandhi & Chen, 1995; Stuchly et al., 1986). In liquid or semi-solid forms, it is quite cumbersome to keep these materials of different compositions from mixing with each other to create more homogeneous properties. Procedures such as surrounding these materials with thin plastic wraps or other separators are therefore used. Since the human anatomy is quite complex, such phantoms consisting generally of two to four or five tissue types do not necessarily match the anatomical details of the head or any other region that is to be modeled. Some authors have, therefore, focused on using homogeneous tissue-simulating fluids and on realistic exposure conditions (actual handsets, spectacle frames, etc.). Fluids rather than gels are preferred to facilitate rapid movement of the internal E-field sensor which is driven by a stepper motor or a robot for determination of the 3-D SAR distribution from which 1- or 10-gram peak SARs can be obtained for compliance with the safety guidelines.

The resolution of the measurements is on the order of several millimeters because of the E-field sensor dimensions that are typically on the order of 4-5 mm (Balzano et al., 1995; Bassen & Babij, 1990; Bassen & Smith, 1983; Schmid et al., 1996). Since the amount of tissue-simulant material that is displaced by these sensors is quite significant (on the order of $\lambda_e/4$ in wet tissues at the PCS frequencies on the order of 1.8-2.2 GHz), this is likely to influence the field distribution that one is trying to measure, particularly at the higher frequencies. Smaller E-field sensors would therefore be needed for dosimetry at higher wireless communication frequencies.

The FD-TD Method

The FD-TD method has been described in several publications (Dimbylow & Mann, 1994; Gandhi, 1990, 1995; Gandhi & Chen, 1995; Gandhi et al., 1994; Jensen & Rahmat-Samii, 1995; Lin & Gandhi, 1995; Simunic, 1995) and a couple of recent textbooks (Kunz & Luebbers, 1993; Taflove, 1995). In addition to many applications in the various areas of microwave design and calculations (Kunz & Luebbers, 1993; Taflove, 1995), this method has also been used successfully to obtain SARs for anatomically based models of the human body for whole-body or partial-body exposures to spatially uniform or nonuniform (far-field or near-field) electromagnetic fields from ELF to microwave frequencies (Gandhi, 1990, 1995; Lin & Gandhi, 1995). In this method, the coupled Maxwell's equations in differential form are solved for all points of the absorber (model of the human head and neck and the approximate model of the hand), as well as the space including the plastic-covered handset, the antenna embedded in a dielectric sheathing and the region to the absorbing boundaries which are generally taken to be at least 10 cells away from the telephone-head/neck coupled region (Dimbylow & Mann, 1994; Gandhi & Chen, 1995; Gandhi et al., 1994; Jensen & Rahmat-Samii, 1995). Various absorbing boundary conditions such as Mur's second-order boundary condition (Mur, 1981), retarding-time boundary condition (Berntsen & Hornsleth, 1994), and, more recently, Berenger's perfectly matched layer boundary condition (Berenger, 1994) have been used by the various authors. Negligible differences in the calculated SAR distributions or the radiation patterns are obtained regardless of the boundary conditions that are used (Cui, Chen, & Gandhi, 1995).

Even though the FD-TD method has been thoroughly tested against analytical solutions, measured data, and other numerical techniques for far-field exposures, it has not, until recently, been subjected to such rigorous validation for near-field exposures. We have recently started to focus on this issue. In the following section we give some near-field test cases where excellent agreement is found between the results obtained using the FD-TD method and other analytical and/or other procedures (Furse & Gandhi, 1995).

Validation Test Runs

Dipole Antenna Near a Two-Layered Half-Space

The first validation was for a dipole antenna very near a layered half-space. The geometry is shown in Figure 1. An exact, analytical solution, based on expansion of the fields from the dipole and enforcement of the boundary conditions at the planar surfaces, is given in King (1993). For the specific case given, the frequency is 900 MHz, the dipole is of length $l = 12$ cm, and is located at a distance $d_o = 2$ cm away from the first layer. The first layer is 1-cm-thick skull-equivalent material, with $\varepsilon_r = 5.977$ and $\sigma = 0.09913$ S/m. The second layer is infinitely thick brain-equivalent material with $\varepsilon_r = 50.2852$ and $\sigma = 1.3423$ S/m.

For the FD-TD method, a cell size of 5 mm is used in the horizontal (x, y) directions, and 9.23 mm in the vertical (z) direction. This gives an antenna 13 cells long, with the feedpoint in the center cell, and a distance of 4 cells between the antenna and the first layer, which is 2 cells thick. The second layer is supposed to be infinitely thick, which is modeled by a thickness of 24.5 cm (49 cells), which is sufficiently thick to attenuate all of the fields to well below 1 percent of their peak values before the end of the material is reached. The infinite nature of the two-layered half-space in the x- and z-directions was modeled by considering a sufficiently large box so that the fields were very small at the edges. This box is taken to be 12 cm (24 cells) in the x-direction and 33.3 cm (36 cells) in the z-direction. The simulation was run for 10 cycles, but convergence was observed at about eight cycles.

Figure 2 shows the magnitude of the electric field along the y-axis, comparing the analytical solution (see Table 1 of King, 1993) with the values calculated by the FD-TD method. Values are normalized to a feedpoint current of 100 mA rms.

A similar test geometry is given in Figure 10 of Kuster and Balzano (1992). This simulation is made at 840 MHz, with a half-wave dipole antenna located 1.5 cm from the first layer, which is 1-cm-thick bone-equivalent material, having properties $\varepsilon_r = 5$, $\sigma = 0.15$ S/m. The second layer is brain with properties $\varepsilon_r = 42$, $\sigma = 0.75$ S/m. The

60

FD-TD simulation is run with a horizontal cell size of 5 mm and vertical cell size of 5.9655 mm. The infinite absorbing material is modeled as before, using a large box of dimensions x = 12 cm, y = 30 cm (including both layers), and z = 39.4 cm. The simulation is run for 10 cycles.

Figure 3 shows the SAR values along the y-axis comparing the MMP method of Kuster and Balzano (1992) and the FD-TD results. Values are normalized to a feedpoint current of 100 mA rms. The close agreement of FD-TD solutions to the analytical and MMP solutions for a dipole antenna in front of an infinite layered space give good confidence in FD-TD's ability to correctly model antennas in close proximity to an absorbing material. The following simulation analyzes the effect of a finite-sized model on the FD-TD solution.

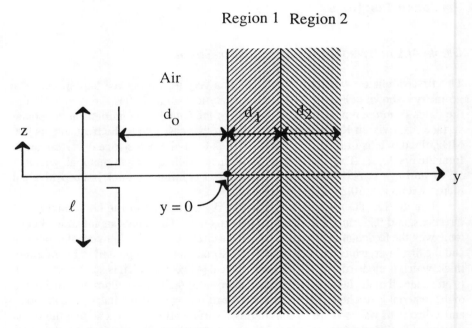

Figure 1. A dipole antenna in front of a layered half-space. For the test case in King (1993), the frequency is 900 MHz, $\ell = 12$ cm, $d_0 = 2$ cm, $d_1 = 1$ cm, $d_2 = \infty$ (24.5 cm), $\varepsilon_{r1} = 5.977$, $\sigma = 0.09913$, $\varepsilon_{r2} = 50.2852$, $\sigma_2 = 1.3423$. The FD-TD simulation uses $\Delta x = \Delta y = 5$ mm, $\Delta z = 9.23$ mm.

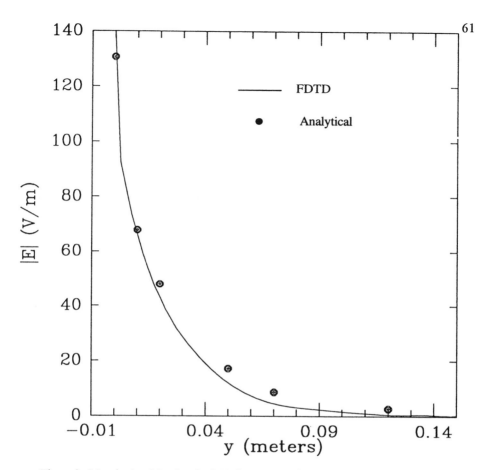

<u>Figure 2.</u> Magnitude of the electric field along the y axis for the model shown in
Figure 1. Values are compareed for the FD-TD simulation and analytical data from
King (1993).

A Dipole Antenna Near an Absorbing Box of Finite Dimensions

The second validation was for a dipole antenna near an absorbing box of finite
dimensions. This was similar to the first validation, except that the finite nature of the
box was accurately modeled, and measured data was available (see Figure 3 of Kuster
& Balzano, 1992) for comparison. The frequency was 840 MHz, and the dipole was
17.3 cm long. It was located a distance d_o from the box, with the feedpoint centered
in front of the box, which was $15 \times 30 \times 50$ cm^3 in the x, y, z directions, respectively.

The box was made of 5-mm-thick acrylic glass (assumed to be polystyrene with
$\varepsilon_r = 2.55$). Since the cell sizes used in this simulation were slightly larger than the
thickness of the acrylic, an effective dielectric constant for the glass was calculated
from the formula (Gandhi et al., 1994):

62

$$\varepsilon_{\textit{eff}}^{1} = \frac{\varepsilon_r \Delta}{\varepsilon_r (\Delta - W) + W}$$

where Δ is the size of the FD-TD cell, W is the thickness of the acrylic, and ε_r is the dielectric constant of this material. This formula is derived by finding the average fields at the air-dielectric interface and setting them equal to the fields in a larger-sized cell, giving the smaller effective dielectric constant given above. The box is filled with brain-simulating material with $\varepsilon_r = 53$ and $\sigma = 1.4$ S/m (Kuster & Balzano, 1992).

Figure 4 shows the SAR distributions along the y-axis comparing the FD-TD simulations and measurements made by Kuster and Balzano (1992) for various

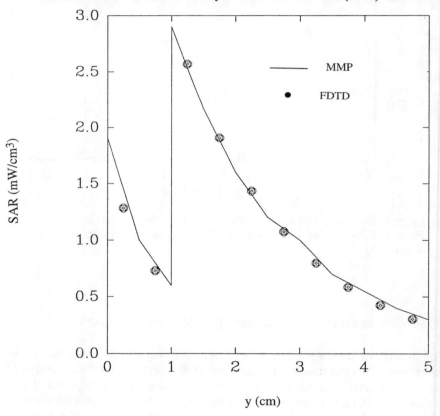

Figure 3. Magnitude of the electric field along the y-axis for the model shown in Figure 1 with a frequency of 900 MHz, $d_0 = 1.5$ cm, $d_1 = 1$ cm, $d_2 = \infty$ (39.4 cm), $\ell = 17.3$ cm, $\varepsilon_{r1} = 5.0$, $\sigma_1 = 0.15$, $\varepsilon_{r2} = 42$, $\sigma_2 = 0.75$. The FD-TD simulation uses $\Delta x = \Delta y = 5$mm, $\Delta z = 5.9655$ mm. Values are compared with the MMP results of Kuster and Balzano (1992).

distances, d_o, between the dipole and the box. The FD-TD simulations use a cell size of $\Delta z = 5.9655$ mm, and $\Delta x = \Delta y = 5.133$, 5.1, 6.35, and 7.6 mm for the separation distances between the antenna and the box of $d_o = 15.4$, 20.4, 25.4, and 30.4 mm, respectively. The vertical cell size, Δz, was chosen to precisely model the height of the antenna, and the horizontal cell size, Δx, Δy, was chosen to precisely model the separation distance, d_o. Values which are used for ε_{eff} are 2.388, 2.426, 1.918, and 1.666 for the four different cells' sizes, respectively. Simulations are run for 2500 time steps, and convergence is observed at about 1500 time steps. Values are normalized to a feedpoint current of 100 mA rms.

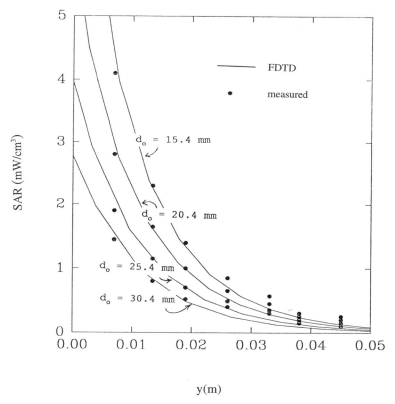

Figure 4. SAR distribution along the y-axis for the dipole antenna in front of the phantom box. Frequency = 840 MHz. Values are given for different separation distances, d_o, between the dipole and box, as compared with measured data from Kuster and Balzano (1992).

An Infinitesimal Dipole Near a Sphere

The test case simulations for cases 1 and 2 give good confidence in the FD-TD method's ability to correctly predict the field or SAR distribution within a planar phantom as a function of distance between the antenna and phantom. These simulations do not require modeling of curved surfaces that are associated with the high-resolution head models in cellular phone studies. The test cases 3 and 4 demonstrate FD-TD's ability to correctly analyze fields within spherical objects that do require modeling of curved surfaces. For this FD-TD analysis, the curved object was modeled using "stair stepping," or cubical cells filling the curved object. Thus, the smaller the sphere relative to the cell size, the coarser the modeling approximation.

For this test case, an infinitesimal dipole is located 1.5 cm away from a 20-cm-diameter brain-equivalent sphere (Dhondt & Martens, 1994). The frequency is 900 MHz, and the properties taken for the sphere are $\varepsilon_r = 43$ and $\sigma = 0.83$ S/m. The infinitesimal dipole is modeled as a single feedpoint location, without the surrounding antenna from the previous test cases. The FD-TD cell size is $\Delta x = \Delta y = \Delta z = 5$ mm, which makes the sphere 40 cells in diameter.

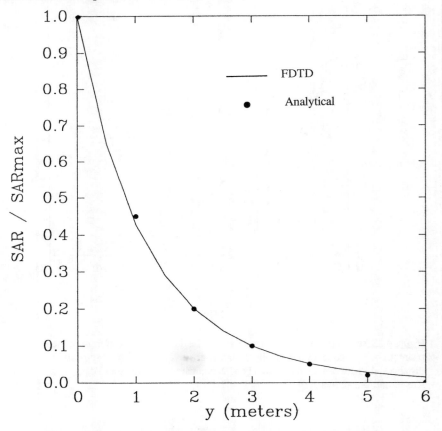

Figure 5. Relative SAR distribution along the y-axis of the homogeneous brain-equivalent sphere excited by an infinitesimal dipole. Analytical data is taken from Dhondt and Martens (1994).

Figure 5 shows the relative SAR along the y-axis from the front edge of the sphere calculated using the FD-TD method and compared to an analytical solution based on the Bessel function expansion (Dhondt & Martens, 1994). The excellent agreement here again adds confidence that the FD-TD method can accurately model curved absorbing models. The following simulation adds to that confidence by examining a full-sized antenna near a sphere, comparing not only the trend of the field distribution, but its absolute magnitude as well.

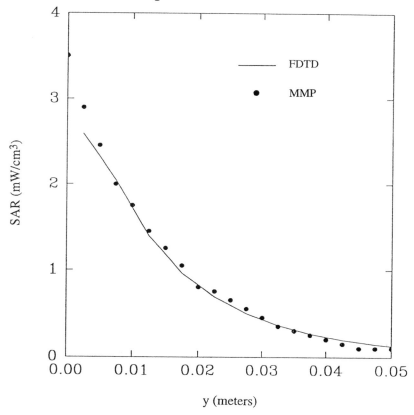

Figure 6. SAR distribution along the y-axis of the homogeneous brain-equivalent sphere excited by a 17.3 long dipole antenna. Values are compared with the MMP solution of Kuster and Balzano (1992). Diameter = 10 cm; frequency = 840 MHz.

A Dipole Antenna Near a Lossy Sphere

The next test case was for a dipole antenna near a homogeneous brain-equivalent sphere. The frequency is 840 MHz, and the approximately half-wave-long dipole antenna (l = 17.3 cm) is located 2.5 cm from the sphere. The sphere has a radius of 10 cm. This is modeled with an FD-TD cell size of $\Delta x = \Delta y = 5$ mm, and $\Delta z = 5.9655$ mm, and the simulation was run for 1500 time steps. The dielectric properties used for the sphere are $\varepsilon_r = 55$, $\sigma = 1.4$ S/m. Figure 6 shows the SAR distribution along the y-axis from the front edge of the sphere, for the two different sizes of the sphere. The FD-TD simulations are compared to MMP simulation data from Kuster and Balzano (1992). Once again, the excellent comparisons give confidence that FD-TD can accurately model antennas in the very near field of curved absorbing objects.

Anatomic Models of the Human Body

As aforementioned, heterogeneous anatomically-based models, particularly of the human head, are needed to obtain the SAR distributions due to mobile telephones. Based on magnetic resonance imaging (MRI) and/or computed tomography (CT) scans, millimeter-resolution anatomic models of the human body are becoming increasingly available and are being used for dosimetry of cellular telephones (Dimbylow & Mann, 1994; Gandhi, 1990, 1995; Gandhi & Chen, 1995; Gandhi et al., 1994; Jensen & Rahmat-Samii, 1995; Lin & Gandhi, 1995). Whereas a somewhat cruder model of the human head with a resolution of 6.56 mm was used in Jensen and Rahmat-Samii (1995), a higher-resolution MRI-based model with a 2-mm cell size has been used by Dimbylow and Mann (1994).

We have developed a millimeter-resolution model of the human body (Gandhi, 1995; Gandhi & Chen, 1995; Gandhi et al., 1994) from the MRI scans of a male volunteer of height 176.4 cm and weight 64 kg. The MRI scans were taken with a resolution of 3 mm along the height of the body and 1.875 mm for the orthogonal axes in the cross-sectional planes. Even though the height of the volunteer was quite appropriate for an average male, the weight was somewhat lower than an average of 71 kg, which is generally assumed for an average male. This problem can, to some extent, be ameliorated by assuming that the pixel dimensions for the cross sections are larger than 1.875 mm by the ratio of $(71/64)^{1/2} = 1.053$, (i.e., 1.974 mm instead of 1.875 mm). Using a software package from the Mayo Clinic called ANALYZE, the MRI scans of the human body were converted into images involving 30 tissue types whose electrical properties (ε_r, σ) can then be prescribed at the mobile telephone midband frequencies of 835 MHz or 1900 MHz. The 30 tissues taken for the whole-body model are: muscle, fat, regular bone, compact bone, cartilage, skin, nerve, intestine, spleen, pancreas, heart, blood, parotid gland, liver, kidney, lung, bladder, cerebrospinal fluid, eye humour, eye sclera, eye lens, stomach, erectile tissue, prostate gland, spermatic cord, testicle, ligament, brain, pineal gland, and pituitary gland. Since only the model of the head and neck is used for the present calculations, only 15 of these tissues are involved in this model. The theoretical weights of each of the major tissues were calculated based on specific gravities defined by the International Council on Radiation Protection and Measurements (International Council on Radiation Protection and Measurements [ICRP], 1992) and the number of voxels of each tissue in the model. These weights are given in Table 1 and are compared to the weights of the tissues of the average "reference" man (ICRP, 1992). Most of the comparisons are excellent. The reasons for some of the discrepancies between the reference man and model weights are given in the footnotes of Table 1.

Tissue Type	Mass Density g/cm³	No. of Voxels	Weight in grams Model	reference man (ICRP, 1992)
muscle	1.047	2,604,370	31,871	28,000
fat	0.916	1,388,947	14,873	13,500
bone[1]	1.465	564,906	9,675	10,000
cartilage	1.097	13,839	177[2]	2,500
skin[3]	0.983	289,720	3,329	2,600
nerve	1.038	5,410	65.6[4]	30[5]
intestine	1.042	104,204	1,270[9]	1,010[10]
pancreas	1.045	9,394	114.8	100
heart	1.030	59,236	713.1[9]	450[10]
blood	1.058	58,074	718[6]	5,500
liver	1.030[8]	146,074	1,759	1,800
kidney[7]	1.050	24,780	304	310
lung[7]	0.347	242,731	983.8	1,000
bladder	1.030	18,053	217.4[9]	150-250
stomach	1.05	47,914	588[9]	150[10]
prostate gland	1.045	2,830	34.5	16
testicle[7]	1.044	7,223	88.1	60
ligament	1.220	29,472	420	1,500
pineal gland	1.048	18	0.2	0.18
pituritary gland	1.066	22	0.3	0.6
brain	1.035	138,188	1,673	1,400

[1] Compact and regular bone combined. [2] Major cartilage regions (ear, nose) only. No bone-end cartilage. [3] 1-voxel thick layer around entire body except eyes and ear canal. [4] Spinal cord, optic nerve, other large nerves included. [5] Spinal cord only. [6] Major arteries and vessels only. [7] Pair. [8] No value given. Estimate based on tissue content. [9] Full (contents are not differentiated from organ). [10] Empty (organ only).

Table 1. Comparison of weights of tissues/organs in the MRI-based model with "reference man" (ICRP, 1992)

68

The new dielectric properties assumed for the various tissues at 835 and 1900 MHz are given in Table 2. These are taken from the unpublished data of C. Gabriel (personal communication, 1994). Also included at the bottom of Table 2 are the lower dielectric properties for fat, bone, and cartilage previously reported in the literature (Durney, Massoudi, & Iskander, 1986; Stuchly & Stuchly, 1980). We have considered two orientations of the handset, one that is held vertically relative to the head (tilt angle of 0°) and another that is held at a tilt angle of 30° relative to the head (see Figure 7). To simulate a handset that is typically tilted forward by 30° for a vertically erect head, we have modified the MRI-based model so that it is tilted forward by 30°. As described in Lazzi and Gandhi (1997), the forward tilt is accomplished by a "best fitting" technique wherein each of the cells of the present model is assigned to a new corresponding cell only if no other cells have a better fitting to the new one. An error matrix proportional to the distance of the rotated cells from the cell centroid of the new cell is used and minimized to obtain the original cells that may occupy the new cell location. The 30° forward-tilted head thus obtained is shown in Figure 7 together with the original untilted head model. For the tilted model, a vertical orientation of the handset and the antenna allows more accurate modeling of their shapes and dimensions. Models for each of the antennas and the handsets were assumed to be covered with insulating materials of ε_r =4.0. Because of the different cell sizes used, particularly for the smaller models representative of 10- and 5-year-old children, different values of ε_{eff} obtained from Equation 1 have been used for the various simulations for these cases.

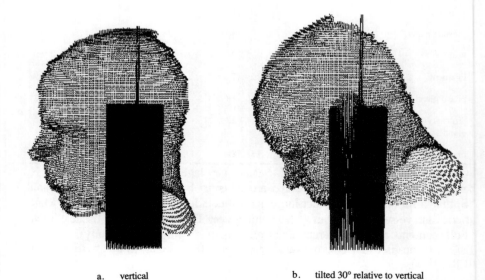

a.   vertical   b.   tilted 30° relative to vertical

Figure 7. The two head models with the telephone used for the calculations.

Tissue	Spec. Gravity 10^3kg/m^3	835 MHz		1900 MHz	
		ε_r	σ S/m	ε_r	σ S/m
muscle	1.04	51.76	1.11	49.41	1.64
fat	0.92	9.99	0.17	9.38	0.26
bone (skull)	1.81	17.40	0.25	16.40	0.45
cartilage	1.10	40.69	0.82	38.10	1.28
skin	1.01	35.40	0.63	37.21	1.25
nerve	1.04	33.40	0.60	32.05	0.90
blood	1.06	55.50	1.86	54.20	2.27
parotid gland	1.05	45.25	0.92	43.22	1.29
CSF	1.01	78.10	1.97	77.30	2.55
eye humour	1.01	67.90	1.68	67.15	2.14
sclera	1.17	54.90	1.17	52.56	1.73
lens	1.10	36.59	0.51	42.02	1.15
pineal gland	1.05	45.26	0.92	43.22	1.29
pituitary gland	1.07	45.26	0.92	43.22	1.29
brain	1.04	45.26	0.92	43.22	1.29
		Old properties (Durney et al., 1986; Stuchly & Stuchly, 1980)		Old properties (Durney et al., 1986; Stuchly & Stuchly, 1980)	
fat	0.92	7.20	0.16	9.70	0.27
bone (skull)	1.81	7.20	0.16	8.40	0.15
cartilage	1.10	7.20	0.16	9.70	0.27

Table 2. Dielectric properties and specific gravities of the various tissues assumed at the midband mobile telephone frequencies of 835 and 1900 MHz (Gabriel, 1996). Also included are the lower dielectric properties for fat, bone, and cartilage previously reported in the literature (Durney, Massoudi, & Iskander, 1986; Stuchly & Stuchly, 1980).

Because of the proximity of the hand to the telephone, it is essential to also model the hand for numerical calculations. For calculations to date we have modeled the hand by a region of 2/3 muscle-equivalent material of thickness 1.974 cm (10 δ_y) wrapped around the handset on three sides, with the exception of the side facing the head, with height two-thirds that of the handset.

By scaling the cell sizes of the MRI-based model, we have developed smaller models of the head, neck, and hand to correspond to dimensions characteristic of 10- and 5-year-old children, respectively. In the Dosimetry Handbook (Durney et al., 1986), the heights and weights for average 10- and 5-year-old children are given as 1.38 and 1.12 m and 32.5 and 19.5 kg, respectively. These heights and weights are also in agreement with the averages for the boys given in Lentner (1984). To obtain models of these needed heights, we have scaled the cell size $\delta_z = 3$ mm of the MRI-based model of the adult male of height 176.4 cm to new dimensions $\delta_z = 2.3469$ and 1.9048 mm, respectively. Also, maintaining the square shapes of the pixels in the cross-sectional planes as for the MRI-based model, we have altered the dimensions $\delta_x = \delta_y$ from 1.875 mm of the adult male model of weight 64.0 kg to new cell sizes $\delta_x = \delta_y = 1.51$ and 1.2989 mm to obtain models of 10- and 5-year-old children of weights 32.5 and 19.5 kg, respectively. The approximate hand dimensions have been similarly scaled through these cell sizes so that the hands cover less than two-thirds of the heights of the assumed handsets for models of 10- and 5-year-old children.

It is well-known that considerably lower values of ε_r and σ have previously been reported for fat, bone, and cartilage in the published literature (Durney et al., 1986; Stuchly & Stuchly, 1980) as compared to the higher values that have recently been determined by C. Gabriel (1996). These lower values of ε and σ reported for fat, bone, and cartilage, given at the bottom of Table 1, have been taken instead of the newer values for some of the runs (see Table 6) to determine the effect of tissue properties on SAR distributions.

We are aware of a preprint of a paper that has recently been submitted for publication (Hombach, Meier, Burkhardt, Tay, & Kuster, 1996). As referred to in the companion article by Kuster (1998), three different anatomically based models, two of these with a resolution as low as 1 mm, have been used for dosimetric calculations (Hombach et al., 1996) using the FIT implemented in the commercially available package MAFIA (CST, 1994). As given by the authors, "the lower part of the head was assigned to only one tissue type." The more serious problems for this paper pertain to the elimination of the ear in these models "to avoid increased effects caused by different ear modeling" and use of dipole antennas rather than the handset. It is well known that the highest SARs are obtained for the ear and the volumetric region of the tissues behind it. For all of the calculations given in this paper (see Tables 3 and 4, and also Dimbylow & Mann, 1994; Gandhi & Chen, 1995; Jensen & Rahmat-Samii, 1995), we have not only included the ear but assumed it to be squished against the head. Furthermore, the SAR distribution is sensitive to the exact modeling of the antenna, the handset, and the posture of the handset vis-à-vis the human head.

Even though models with resolution on the order of 1 mm are now becoming available, models with 2-3 mm resolution are quite adequate for frequencies of 1-2 GHz since it has previously been shown that FD-TD cell sizes as large as $\lambda_e/5$ are perfectly capable of giving accurate SAR distributions (Gandhi, Gu, Chen, & Bassen,

1992). For a frequency of 2 GHz, the wavelength λ_e in high-water tissues such as muscle, skin, and brain is about 23 mm and cell sizes on the order of 2-3 mm certainly observe the aforementioned requirement. It is recognized that finer-resolution models would indeed be needed for still higher-frequency wireless devices. Toward this end, we are presently developing the next-generation model of the human body with a resolution of 0.9375 mm along each of the three orthogonal axes.

	New properties	Old properties	Homogeneous model
Peak 1-voxel SAR (W/kg)	10.86	8.52	15.98
Peak 1-g SAR (W/kg)	2.93 (1.00g)	2.05 (1.00g)	4.17 (1.03 g)
Peak 1-g SAR for brain (W/kg)	1.13 (1.09 g)	0.86 (1.02 g)	---
Power absorbed by head and neck	45.0%	44.0%	41.5%
Power absorbed by "hand"	9.2%	11.9%	8.4%
Peak 1-voxel SAR for brain (W/kg)	1.62	2.11	---
CSF average (mW/kg)	72.7	62.6	---
Brain average (mW/kg)	72.3	62.9	---
Humour average (mW/kg)	31.8	32.9	---
Lens average (mW/kg)	11.3	12.8	---
Sclera average (mW/kg)	17.8	19.4	---

Table 3. SAR distributions for different properties of the various tissues. A $\lambda/4$ antenna above a handset is taken for the calculations at 835 MHz. Radiated power = 600 mW.

The Peak 1-Gram SAR

According to the ANSI/IEEE C95.1-1992 RF safety guideline for uncontrolled environments, the spatial-peak SAR should not exceed 1.6 W/kg for any 1 gram of tissue defined as a tissue volume in the shape of a cube (ANSI/IEEE, 1992). Because of the irregular shape of the body (e.g., the ears) and tissue heterogeneities, a tissue volume in the shape of a cube of, say, $1 \times 1 \times 1$ cm will have a weight that may be in excess of, equal to, or less than 1 gram. Larger or smaller volumes in the shape of a cube may, therefore, need to be considered to obtain a weight of about 1 gram. Furthermore, for an anatomic model such as ours using unequal cell sizes (1.974 ×

	$\lambda/4$ antenna	$3\lambda/8$ antenna
Peak 1-voxel SAR (W/kg)	3.90	2.66
Peak 1-g SAR (W/kg)[1]	0.52 (1.01 g; 98.7%)	0.32 (1.01 g; 98.7%)
Peak 1-g SAR (W/kg)[2]	1.11 (1.03 g; 81.0%)	0.69 (1.06 g; 86.0%)
Peak 1-g SAR (W/kg)[3]	1.03 (1.10 g; 82.4%)	0.69 (1.11 g; 86.1%)
Peak 1-g SAR for brain (W/kg)[2]	02.0 (1.00 g)	0.16 (1.00 g)
Peak 1-g SAR for brain (W/kg)[3]	0.19 (1.05 g)	0.16 (1.00 g)
Power absorbed by head and neck	35.6%	29.4%
Power absorbed by "hand"	13.8%	7.0%
Peak 1-voxel SAR for brain (W/kg)	0.29	0.26
CSF average (mW/kg)	8.0	8.3
Brain average (mW/kg)	7.6	7.6
Humour average (mW/kg)	3.2	2.6
Lens average (mW/kg)	1.5	1.3
Sclera average (mW/kg)	1.8	1.5

[1] 5 x 5 x 3 cells; 0.987 x 0.987 x 0.9 cm; 0.88 cm^3
[2] 5 x 5 x 4 cells; 0.987 x 0.987 x 1.2 cm; 1.17 cm^3
[3] 6 x 6 x 3 cells; 1.184 x 1.184 x 0.9 cm; 1.26 cm^3
It was not possible to obtain 1-g weight of the brain for subvolume 1; hence., the 1-g SAR for brain for this case is not given.

Table 4. SAR distributions for the squished-ear model of the adult male for $\lambda/4$ and $3\lambda/8$ antennas at 1900 MHz. Time-averaged radiated power = 125 mW.

1.974 × 3 mm), it is not very convenient to obtain exact cubical volumes even though nearly cubic shapes may be considered. We have, therefore, considered 5 × 5 × 3, 5 × 5 × 4, and 6 × 6 × 3 cells for the model of the adult male to obtain subvolumes on the order of 1 cm^3. For each of these subvolumes selected close to and around the regions of the high SARs, we have divided the absorbed powers by the weights calculated for the individual subvolumes to obtain 1-gram SARs. Furthermore, we have considered only those subvolumes where at least 80 percent of the cells are occupied by the tissues and no more than 20 percent of the cells are in air. As expected, there is a great deal of variability in the 1-gram SARs that are obtained. In keeping with the ANSI/IEEE safety guidelines, weights equal to or in excess of 1 gram are considered to obtain the spatial-peak SARs that are given in Table 4 for two assumed lengths of monopole antennas above a metal box of dimensions 14 δ_x × 28 δ_y × 51 δ_z (2.76 × 5.53 × 15.3 cm) and 1-cell thickness δ of plastic covering of effective dielectric constant ε_{eff} given by Equation 1, which is somewhat lower than the dielectric constant ε_r of the actual insulation layer of thickness w (generally 1 mm).

In Table 4, it is interesting to note that even though the peak 1-gram SARs for the superficial tissues are highly variable (by almost 2:1), the corresponding values for the internal tissues, such as the brain, are nearly identical regardless of the subvolumes that are considered. The reason for the highly variable peak 1-gram SARs for the superficial tissues is that various subvolumes of, say, 0.8-1.2 cm³ in the shape of a cube may each give a weight of about 1 gram, depending on the amount of air in such subvolumes. For our case, larger subvolumes such as 5 × 5 × 4 and 6 × 6 × 3 cells with volumes of 1.17 and 1.26 cm³, respectively, involve more of air and the ear tissues and still have weights of at least 1 gram, whereas the smaller subvolumes of 5 × 5 × 3 cells with a total volume of 0.88 cm³ must have more of the non-ear head tissues in order to get weights of 1 or more grams of weight. Since the subvolumes to consider for peak 1-gram SARs have not been clearly defined in the ANSI/IEEE safety guidelines (ANSI/IEEE, 1992), the variability in the peak 1-gram SARs given in Table 4 is hard to resolve and is clearly troublesome. All three peak 1-gram values have, therefore, been given in Table 4. For each of the cases, the weights and percentage of tissues by volume are given within parentheses of the peak 1-gram SARs.

This problem of lack of definition of the subvolume to consider was brought to the attention of the Dosimetry Working Group[2] of Wireless Technology Research (WTR), LLC. At its meeting in Duarte, California, on 30 October 1995, the working group decided to recommend to ANSI/IEEE that the tissue subvolume to consider should not extend beyond the most exterior surfaces of the body (e.g., the upper, lower, and side boundaries of the ear) but may include the air that is contained therein (e.g., the air in the crevices of the ear). Also, the weight of the subvolume may not be smaller than 1 gram, but preferably as close to it as possible. For the SAR data given in Table 4, this corresponds to case 2 with a peak 1-gram SAR of 1.11 W/kg for the λ/4 antenna and 0.69 W/kg for the 3 λ/8 monopole antenna above the handset.

Comparison with Calculations of Dimbylow and Mann

Even though all of our calculations have been done for plastic-covered handsets and antennas, we have made a limited number of runs using the same configurations as previously used by Dimbylow and Mann (1994). The objectives of these runs were to verify that the SAR distributions obtained at the European GSM frequencies of 900 MHz and 1800 MHz were fairly similar to those obtained by another research group which had used a very different model of the head and neck. For these test runs we used the tissue properties given in Table 5, which were taken from the paper as far as possible and likewise assumed the handset dimensions of 2.4 × 6 × 15 cm. Unlike the cubical cell sizes of 2 mm used by Dimbylow and Mann, we have taken a voxel size of 1.974 × 1.974 × 3 mm for our calculations. The summaries of the results obtained for the four test cases without the hand are given in Tables 6 and 7 for 900 and 1800

MHz, respectively. Also given as footnotes are the data calculated by Dimbylow and Mann for comparison. Since the exact weights of the $1 \times 1 \times 1$ cm subvolume were not prescribed, we have considered the various subvolumes 1, 2, and 3 that were previously considered for the data given in Table 4. Also, even though the exact placements of the assumed handset vis-à-vis the ear were not exactly prescribed, it is interesting to note that the peak 1-gram SARs calculated for our model are fairly similar both at 900 and 1800 MHz. For our calculations we have assumed the feed points to be in the cross-sectional plane 6 mm below the top of the ear.

Tissue	Spec. Gravity 10^3kg/m^3	835 MHz		1900 MHz	
		ε_r	σ S/m	ε_r	σ S/m
muscle	1.04	58.00	1.21	56.00	1.76
fat	*0.92	*9.99	*0.17	*9.38	*0.26
bone (skull)	1.85	8.00	0.11	8.00	0.15
cartilage	1.10	35.00	0.60	32.00	0.57
skin	1.10	35.00	0.60	32.00	0.57
nerve	*1.04	*33.4	*0.60	*32.05	*0.90
blood	1.06	64.00	1.24	64.00	1.80
parotid gland	*1.05	*45.25	*0.92	*43.22	*1.29
CSF	1.06	72.00	2.13	72.00	2.50
eye humour	1.01	73.00	1.97	74.00	2.27
sclera	1.01	66.00	1.93	62.00	2.28
lens	1.05	44.00	0.80	42.00	1.19
pineal gland	*1.05	*45.26	*0.92	*43.22	*1.29
pituitary gland	*1.07	*45.26	*0.92	*43.22	*1.29
brain	1.03	49.00	1.10	47.00	1.42

* These values were not prescribed in Dimbylow and Mann (1994).
Table 5. Dielectric properties and specific gravities assumed for test runs for comparison with the calculations of Dimbylow and Mann (1994).

	No hand λ/4 antenna above handset	No hand λ/2 dipole
Peak 1-voxel SAR (W/kg)	7.57	9.13
Peak 1-g SAR (W/kg)[1]	2.07* (1.00 g; 92.0%)	2.10[†] (1.00 g; 92.0%)
Peak 1-g SAR (W/kg)[2]	2.49* (1.07 g; 83.0%)	2.71[†] (1.07 g; 83.0%)
Peak 1-g SAR (W/kg)[3]	2.45* (1.18 g; 86.1%)	2.47[†] (1.13 g; 81.5%)
Peak 1-g SAR for brain (W/kg)[2]	1.36 (1.01 g)	1.54 (1.01 g)
Peak 1-g SAR for brain (W/kg)[3]	1.31 (1.10 g)	1.48 (1.10 g)
Power absorbed by head and neck	51.7%	52.0%
Peak 1-voxel SAR for brain (W/kg)	4.6	2.6
CSF average (mW/kg)	62.3	60.7
Brain average (mW/kg)	74.4	88.0
Humour average (mW/kg)	50.6	42.8
Lens average (mW/kg)	26.5	19.8
Sclera average (mW/kg)	43.4	33.1

Superscripts 1, 2, and 3 are for cell numbers and subvolumes given in the footnote of Table 4.
* SAR scaled from Table 2 of Dimblyow and Mann (1994) = 2.17 W/kg.
† SAR scaled from Table 2 of Dimbylow and Mann (1994) = 2.02 W/kg.
Table 6. SAR distributions for the Utah model of the adult male without squished ear for comparison with data obtained by Dimbylow and Mann (1994) using the NRPB model. Frequency = 900 MHz. Radiated power = 600 mW. Distance of the source point to the ear = 1.38 cm (7 δ) as against 1.4 cm in Dimbylow and Mann (1994).

Effect of Tissue Properties on SAR Distributions

As given in Table 2, with both the old and the new values of dielectric properties, considerably higher values of ε_r and σ have recently been reported for fat, bone, and cartilage by C. Gabriel (1996). The ear is composed mainly of cartilage that is covered by the skin. In Table 3 we compare the salient features of the SAR distributions at 835 MHz that are obtained using both the new and old dielectric properties for these tissues. For this table and for Tables 8-10, we give the SARs that are calculated using the procedure suggested by the Dosimetry Working Group of WTR (see above).

Since some measurement systems for SAR evaluations use a homogeneous phantom model, also shown for comparison in Table 3 are the SARs obtained for the homogeneous model with properties identical to that of the brain at 835 MHz (see Table 2). It is interesting to note that the homogeneous model overestimates the peak 1-gram SAR by 42% as compared to that obtained using the anatomically based model. Use of homogeneous models could, therefore, lead to rejection of devices which would be considered in compliance with safety guidelines, had more realistic, anatomically-based models been used.

	No hand $\lambda/4$ antenna above handset	No hand $\lambda/2$ dipole
Peak 1-voxel SAR (W/kg)	1.54	1.90
Peak 1-g SAR (W/kg)[1]	0.53* (1.00 g; 98.7%)	0.55[†] (1.00 g; 98.7%)
Peak 1-g SAR (W/kg)[2]	0.87* (1.03 g; 80.0%)	0.81[†] (1.04 g; 81.0%)
Peak 1-g SAR (W/kg)[3]	0.83* (1.13 g; 81.5%)	0.76[†] (1.16 g; 83.3%)
Peak 1-g SAR for brain (W/kg)[2]	0.27 (1.04 g)	0.41 (1.01 g)
Peak 1-g SAR for brain (W/kg)[3]	0.27 (1.02 g)	0.40 (1.07 g)
Power absorbed by head and neck	45.4%	46.4%
Peak 1-voxel SAR for brain (W/kg)	0.50	0.64
CSF average (mW/kg)	7.8	9.0
Brain average (mW/kg)	10.4	13.2
Humour average (mW/kg)	8.8	7.4
Lens average (mW/kg)	2.5	2.0
Sclera average (mW/kg)	5.7	4.5

Superscripts 1, 2, and 3 are for cell numbers and subvolumes given in the footnote of Table 4.
* SAR scaled from Table 3 of Dimblyow and Mann (1994) = 0.70.
[†] SAR scaled from Table 3 of Dimbylow and Mann (1994) = 0.78.
Table 7. SAR distributions for the Utah model of the adult male without squished ear for comparison with data obtained by Dimbylow and Mann (1994) using the NRPB model. Frequency = 1800 MHz. Radiated power = 125 mW. Distance of the source point to the ear = 1.38 cm (7 δ) as against 1.4 cm in Dimbylow and Mann (1994).

	Adult male	10-year-old child	5-year-old child
Peak 1-voxel SAR (W/kg)	10.86	16.82	31.73
Peak 1-g SAR* (W/kg)	2.93 (1.00g)	3.21 (1.02 g)	4.49 (1.00 g)
Peak 1-g SAR for brain* (W/kg)	1.13 (1.09 g)	1.42 (1.00 g)	1.56 (1.00 g)
Power absorbed by head and neck	45.0%	42.6%	39.5%
Power absorbed by "hand"	9.2%	10.7%	5.5%
Peak 1-voxel SAR for brain (W/kg)	1.62	3.02	4.62
CSF average (mW/kg)	72.7	187.2	283.2
Brain average (mW/kg)	72.3	160.3	239.8
Humour average (mW/kg)	31.8	78.2	117.3
Lens average (mW/kg)	11.3	33.6	52.5
Sclera average (mW/kg)	17.8	48.7	73.7

* 5 x 5 x 4 cells; 0.987 x 0.987 x 1.200 cm; 1.170 cm^3 for the adult male
  7 x 7 x 4 cells; 1.057 x 1.057 x 0.939 cm; 1.049 cm^3 for the 10-year-old child
  8 x 8 x 5 cells; 1.039 x 1.039 x 0.950 cm; 1.026 cm^3 for the 5-year-old child

Table 8. Comparison of SAR distributions for models of an adult male and 10-year- and 5-year-old children. Frequency = 835 MHz. Time-averaged radiated power = 600 mW. A $\lambda/4$ antenna above a handset is taken for the calculations.

For each of the calculations given in Table 3, we have considered a quarter-wave monopole antenna above a handset of dimensions $2.96 \times 5.73 \times 15.5$ cm ($14 \delta_x \times 28 \delta_y \times 51 \delta_z$ for the metal box covered with 1-mm-thick plastic on all sides) and the model of the adult male. The telephone is held against the left side of the head. The driving point of the monopole is located at the top of the handset, in the center of the 5.73 cm side furthest from the ear on the edge of the 2.96 cm side. The thin monopole antenna is assumed embedded in a covering sheath of dielectric material $\varepsilon_r = 4.0$ which, in the FD-TD formulation, is modeled by a 2×2 cell square stack of dielectric cells of cross-sectional dimensions 3.95×3.95 mm. New dielectric properties of the various tissues given in Table 2 are used for the results given in column 1 for these and all further cases considered in this paper.

Even though very similar fractional powers absorbed by the whole head are obtained for all three models, the peak 1-voxel SARs are considerably higher for the models using the newer higher conductivities for the cartilage (Table 2). Furthermore, the homogeneous model grossly overestimates the SAR and is also incapable of providing tissue-relevant SAR distributions.

	Adult male	10-year-old child	5-year-old child
Peak 1-voxel SAR (W/kg)	3.90	4.9	6.20
Peak 1-g SAR* (W/kg)	1.11 (1.03 g)	0.90 (1.02 g)	0.97 (1.07 g)
Peak 1-g SAR for brain* (W/kg)	0.20 (1.00 g)	0.25 (1.07 g)	0.31 (1.00 g)
Power absorbed by head and neck	35.6%	34.4%	32.2%
Power absorbed by "hand"	13.8%	9.4%	6.8%
Peak 1-voxel SAR for brain (W/kg)	0.29	0.42	0.61
CSF average (mW/kg)	8.0	20.6	33.4
Brain average (mW/kg)	7.6	19.6	32.9
Humour average (mW/kg)	3.2	17.4	39.2
Lens average (mW/kg)	1.5	7.6	17.8
Sclera average (mW/kg)	1.8	9.9	20.5

* 5 x 5 x 4 cells; 0.987 x 0.987 x 1.200 cm; 1.170 cm^3 for the adult male
7 x 7 x 4 cells; 1.057 x 1.057 x 0.939 cm; 1.049 cm^3 for the 10-year-old child
8 x 8 x 5 cells; 1.039 x 1.039 x 0.950 cm; 1.026 cm^3 for the 5-year-old child

Table 9. Comparison of SAR distributions for models of an adult male and 10-year- and 5-year-old children. Frequency = 1900 MHz. Time-averaged radiated power = 125 mW. A $\lambda/4$ antenna above a handset is taken for the calculations.

Effect of Head Size on SAR Distributions: Comparison for Adult and 10- and 5-year-old Children

As previously described in the section regarding anatomic models of the human body, we have developed smaller models of the head, neck, and "hand" by reducing the voxel size $1.974 \times 1.974 \times 3.0$ mm of the MRI-based model to new voxel sizes of $1.51 \times 1.51 \times 2.3469$ mm and $1.2989 \times 1.2989 \times 1.9048$ mm in order to obtain dimensions characteristic of 10- and 5-year-old children, respectively. In Tables 8 and 9, we give the salient features of the SAR distributions obtained for quarter-wave monopole antennas mounted as discussed earlier at irradiation frequencies of 835 and 1900 MHz, respectively. It is interesting to note that even though the peak 1-gram SARs are fairly similar for the three models at 1900 MHz, the 1-gram SARs are considerably higher for the smaller head sizes at 835 MHz (Table 8). Also, the peak 1-voxel SARs are higher and a larger in-depth penetration of absorbed energy or higher SARs are obtained for the smaller models both at 835 and 1900 MHz. The fact that there is a larger in-depth penetration of SARs for the models of 10- and 5-year-old children as compared to those for the model of the adult is illustrated in Figures 8 and 9 for 835 and 1900 MHz, respectively. Because of a larger depth of penetration of EM fields at 835 MHz into the heads of the smaller subjects, increasing SARs are obtained for smaller models at this frequency. A similar trend of increasing 1-gram SARs for the smaller models at 835 MHz has also been observed for a longer 3 λ/8 antenna for which the SAR distributions are given in Table 10. The higher 1-voxel SARs for the smaller models in Table 8-10 are likely due to the thinner ears, which results in the antennas being somewhat closer to the region of highest SARs that are observed generally at the points of contact of the squished ear to the scalp of the head.

	Adult male	10-year-old child	5-year-old child
Peak 1-voxel SAR (W/kg)	5.97	7.65	12.75
Peak 1-g SAR* (W/kg)	1.60 (1.00 g)	1.49 (1.00 g)	1.88 (1.00 g)
Peak 1-g SAR for brain* (W/kg)	0.65 (1.05 g)	0.78 (1.00 g)	0.85 (1.00 g)
Power absorbed by head and neck	33.7%	28.8%	25.5%
Power absorbed by "hand"	5.6%	4.3%	2.8%
Peak 1-voxel SAR for brain (W/kg)	0.93	1.40	2.01
CSF average (mW/kg)	79.8	170.6	244.5
Brain average (mW/kg)	63.9	125.5	183.0
Humour average (mW/kg)	21.4	46.5	69.8
Lens average (mW/kg)	7.9	20.6	31.2
Sclera average (mW/kg)	12.0	29.3	43.3

* 5 x 5 x 4 cells; 0.987 x 0.987 x 1.200 cm; 1.170 cm³ for the adult male
7 x 7 x 4 cells; 1.057 x 1.057 x 0.939 cm; 1.049 cm³ for the 10-year-old child
8 x 8 x 5 cells; 1.039 x 1.039 x 0.950 cm; 1.026 cm³ for the 5-year-old child
Table 10. Comparison of SAR distributions for models of an adult male and 10-year- and 5-year-old children. Frequency = 835 MHz. Time-averaged radiated power = 600 mW. A 3λ/8 antenna above a handset is taken for the calculations.

80

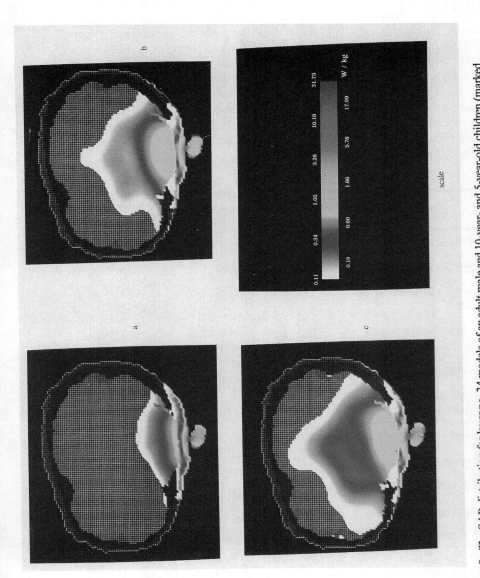

Figure 8. The SAR distribution for layer no. 34 models of an adult male and 10-year- and 5-year-old children (marked a, b, c). This layer contains the feed point and is two cells lower than the cross-sectional plane passing through the top of the ear for each of the models. Frequency = 835 MHz. Radiated power = 600 mW.

81

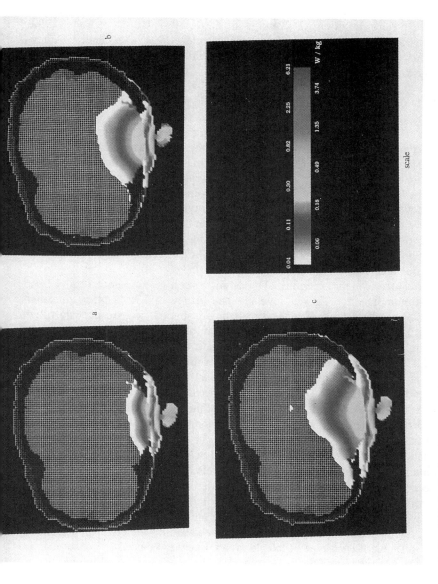

Figure 9. The SAR distribution for layer no. 34 for models of an adult male and 10-year- and 5-year-old children (marked a, b, c). This layer is two cells lower than the cross-sectional plane passing through the top of the ear for each of the models. Frequency = 1900 MHz. Radiated power = 125 mW.

Experimental Models

As previously mentioned in in the section on measurement methods, experimental methods have been used for over 25 years to obtain SAR distributions for far-field and near-field exposure conditions (Balzano et al., 1978, 1995; Bassen & Babij, 1990; Chatterjee et al., 1985; Chou, personal communication, 1994; Cleveland & Athey, 1989; Gabriel, personal communication, 1994; Gandhi & Chen, 1995; Gandhi et al., 1995; Guy & Chou, 1986; Johnson & Guy, 1972; Stuchly et al., 1986; Kuster & Balzano, 1992; Schmid et al., 1996; Stuchly & Stuchly, 1995). Tissue-simulant materials, both in the form of liquids and semi-solid gels (Chan, unpublished data; Cheung & Koopman, 1976; Chou, Chen, Guy, & Luk, 1984; Hartsgrove, Kraszewski, & Surowiec, 1987; Johnson & Guy, 1972) have been developed, the latter permitting tissue-dependent heterogeneous representation of the exposed models. For mobile telephone dosimetry, as shown in Table 3, use of homogeneous models can result in SARs that are considerably higher than those for heterogeneous, anatomically correct models. The lower peak 1-gram SARs for the anatomically based models are likely due to somewhat lower SARs for the cartilage-dominated region of the ear and the considerably smaller SARs for the relatively thick (approximately 1 cm), lower-conductivity region of the skull. For compliance testing, use of homogeneous models may result in rejection of devices which would be considered in compliance if heterogeneous thicker-skull models are used.

To provide realism for experimental modeling, several investigators, (e.g., Chou, personal communication, 1994; Cleveland and Athey, 1989; Gabriel, personal communication, 1994), have developed realistically shaped, heterogeneously-filled models that are filled with biological phantom materials simulant of tissues such as skull, brain, muscle, eyes, etc. All of these models use skull-shaped shells with substantial thicknesses that are representative of the human skull. Even though these models do not have the anatomical details such as are possible with computer-based numerical procedures, they are a considerable improvement over homogeneous models in not increasing the SARs artificially. Simplicity of the model and convenience in its use have often been cited as the reasons for using homogeneous models for compliance testing of mobile telephones. It is claimed that for certain types of antennas, the overestimation of the spatial-peak SAR averaged over 1 gram is within 33% of the values obtained using anatomically correct models (Hombach et al., 1996; Kuster 1998). But this last statement cannot be considered to be based on any rigorous scientific arguments. Indeed, the overestimation provided by the homogeneous model may vary with frequency and the nature of the antenna and the handset. Since compliance testing of mobile telephones being introduced into society is an important issue and millions of each type of telephone are likely to be used by consumers, it makes no sense to take shortcuts by using homogeneous experimental models when heterogeneous models are available and are being increasingly used for such testing.

Concluding Remarks

Since it is a near-field problem, both the calculations and the measurements of SAR distributions are sensitive to the placement of the source vis-à-vis the body and the models that are used. Small differences in the reported SAR distributions are, therefore, likely due to both of these issues. Compliance testing is much easier if a given device results in peak 1-gram or 10-gram SARs that are well within the safety guidelines (ANSI/IEEE, 1992; CENELEC, 1995). The problem is considerably harder for devices for which the SARs are close to the limits of the safety guidelines. In the absence of testing procedures defined by the consensus standard-setting groups such as ANSI/IEEE, expert groups such as the Dosimetry Working Group of WTR and others need to define procedures that may be used for compliance testing of wireless communication devices.

Acknowledgments

The author gratefully acknowledges the contributions of his colleagues, Gianluca Lazzi and Cynthia M. Furse, to this work. The validation test runs described were done by Cynthia Furse (Furse & Gandhi, 1995), while the data given in Tables 3-10 was obtained by Gianluca Lazzi. The graphics for Figures 7-9 were done by Vishram Pandit.

Notes

[1] The effective dielectric constant ε_{eff} is derived by noting that the dielectric fields close to the metallic surface such as that of a handset are primarily normal, and only a part of the FD-TD cell width is actually filled with the dielectric material. The required continuity of the normal component of $D = \varepsilon E$ with outer region can be used to obtain ε_{eff}.

[2] Dosimetry Working Group of WTR consists of the following individuals: A. W. Guy (Chairman), C. K. Chou, C. Gabriel, O. P. Gandhi, N. Kuster, R. Petersen, P. Polson, V. Santomaa, Q. Balzano, and A. Taflove.

References

American National Standards Institute/Institute of Electrical and Electronics Engineers (ANSI/IEEE). (1992). Standard for safety levels with respect to human exposure to radio frequency electromagnetic fields, 3 kHz to 300 GHz (Rep. C95.1-1992). New York: Institute of Electrical and Electronics Engineers, Inc.

Balzano, Q., Garay, O., & Steel, F. R. (1978). Energy deposition in simulated human operators of 800-MHz portable transmitters. IEEE Transactions on Vehicular Technology, 27(4), 174-181.

Balzano, Q., Garay, O., & Manning, T. (1995). Electromagnetic energy exposure of simulated users of portable cellular telephones. IEEE Transactions on Vehicular Technology, 44, 390-403.

Bassen, H. I., & Babij, T. M. (1990). Experimental techniques and instrumentation. In O. P. Gandhi (Ed.), Biological effects and medical applications of electromagnetic energy (pp. 141-173). Englewood Cliffs, NJ: Prentice Hall.

Bassen, H. I., & Smith, G. S. (1983). Electric field probes: A review. IEEE Transactions on Antennas and Propagation, 31(5), 710-718.

Berenger, J. P. (1994). A perfect matched layer for the absorption of electromagnetic waves. Journal of Computational Physics, 114, 185-200.

Berntsen, S., & Hornsleth, S. N. (1994). Retarded time absorbing boundary conditions. IEEE Transactions on Antennas and Propagation, 42, 1059-1064.

CENELEC European Prestandard ENV 50166-2, (1995). Human Exposure to Electromagnetic Fields: High Frequency (10 kHz to 300 GHz), CENELEC Central Secretariat: rue de Stassart 35, B-1050, Brussels, Belgium.

Chan, K.W. Microwave phantoms. Unpublished report.

Chatterjee, I., Gu, Y. G., & Gandhi, O. P. (1985). Quantification of electromagnetic absorption in humans from body-mounted communication transceivers. IEEE Transactions on Vehicular Technology, 34(1), 55-62.

Cheung, A. Y., & Koopman, D. W. (1976). Experimental development of simulated biomaterials for dosimetry studies of hazardous microwave radiation. IEEE Transactions on Microwave Theory and Technique, 24, 669.

Chou, C. K., Chen, G. W., Guy, A. W., & Luk, K. H. (1984). Formulas for preparing phantom muscle tissue at various radiofrequencies. Bioelectromagnetics, 5, 435-441.

Cleveland, R. F., & Athey, T. W. (1989). Specific sbsorption rate (SAR) in models of the human head exposed to handheld UHF portable radios. Bioelectromagnetics, 10(2), 173-186.

CST. (1994). The MAFIA Collaboration. User's Guide Mafia Version 3.x. Darmstadt, Germany: CST GmbH.

Cui, Y., Chen, J. Y., & Gandhi, O. P. (1995, June). Comparison of various boundary conditions for SARs and radiation patterns of cellular telephones [abstract]. In The seventeenth annual meeting of the Bioelectromagnetics Society, Boston, Massachusetts abstract book, 31.

Dhondt, G. & Martens, L. (1994, November). A canonical case with an analytical solution for the comparison of electromagnetic field solvers. In D. Simunic (Ed.), Proceedings of the COST 244 Meeting on Reference Models for Bioelectropmagnetic Test of Mobile Communication Systems, Rome, Italy, 98-104.

Dimbylow, P. J., & Mann, S. M. (1994). SAR calculations in an anatomically based realistic model of the head for mobile transceivers at 900 MHz and 1.8 GHz. Physics in Medicine and Biology, 39, 1537-1553.

Durney, C. H., Massoudi, H., & Iskander, M. F. (1986). Radiofrequency radiation dosimetry handbook (4th ed., Rep. No. USAF SAM-TR-85-73). Brooks Air Force Base, TX: USAF School of Aerospace Medicine, Aerospace Medical Division.

Federal Communications Commission. (1994, June). Amendment of the Commission's rules to establish new personal services (No. FCC, 94-144). Washington, DC: Federal Communications Commission.

Furse, C. M., & Gandhi, O. P. (1995, October). Validation of the FDTD method for canonical problems with near-field sources (Interim Report No. 1). Submitted to Wireless Technology Research, LLC, Washington, D.C.

Gabriel, C. (1996). Compilation of the Dielectric Properties of Body Tissues at RF and Microwave Frequencies (AL/OE-TR 1996-0037). Brooks Air Force Base, TX: Occupational and Environmental Health Directorate, Radiofrequency Radiation Division.

Gandhi, O. P. (1990). Numerical methods for specific absorption rate calculations. In O. P. Gandhi (Ed.), Biological effects and medical applications of electromagnetic energy (pp. 113-140). Englewood Cliffs, NJ: Prentice Hall.

Gandhi, O. P. (1995). Some numerical methods for dosimetry: Extremely low frequencies to microwave frequencies. Radio Science, 30, 161-177.

Gandhi, O. P., & Chen, J. Y. (1995). Electromagnetic absorption in the human head from experimental 6-GHz handheld transceivers. IEEE Transactions on Electromagnetic Compatibility, 37, 547-558.

Gandhi, O. P., Chen, J. Y., & Wu, D. (1994, September). Electromagnetic absorption in the human head for mobile telephones at 835 and 1900 MHz. In Proceedings of the International Symposium on Electromagnetic Compatibility EMC '94, Rome, Italy, 1-5.

Gandhi, O. P., Gu, Y. G., Chen, J. Y., & Bassen, H. I. (1992). SAR and induced current distributions in a high-resolution anatomically based model of a human for plane-wave exposures 100-915 MHz. Health Physics, 63, 281-290.

Gandhi, O. P., Sedigh, K., Beck, G. S., & Hunt, E. L. (1976). Distribution of electromagnetic energy deposition in models of man with frequencies near resonance. In Biological effects of electromagnetic waves (Publication No. 77-8011, pp. 44-67). Rockville, MD: Bureau of Radiological Health, Food and Drug Administration, U. S. Department of Health, Education and Welfare.

Guy, A. W., & Chou, C. K. (1986). Specific absorption rate of energy in man models exposed to cellular UHF mobile antenna fields. IEEE Transactions on Microwave Theory and Technique, 34(6), 671-680.

Hartsgrove, G., Kraszewski, A., & Surowiec, A. (1987). Simulated biological materials for electromagnetic radiation absorption studies. Bioelectromagnetics, 8, 29-36.

Hombach, V., Meier, K., Burkhardt, M., Tay, R., & Kuster, N. (1996). The dependence of EM energy absorption upon human head modeling at 1800 MHz. IEEE Transactions on Microwave Theory and Technique, 44, 1865-1873.

International Council on Radiation Protection (ICRP). (1992). Report of the task group on reference man (Rep. No. 23). New York: Pergamon Press.

Jensen, M. A., & Rahmat-Samii, Y. (1995). EM interaction of handset antennas and a human in personal communications. Proceedings of the IEEE, 83, 7-17.

Johnson, C. C., & Guy, A. W. (1972). Nonionizing electromagnetic wave effects in biological materials and systems. Proceedings of the IEEE, 60, 692-718.

King, R. W. P. (1993). The electromagnetic field of a horizontal electric dipole in the presence of a three-layered region: Supplement. Journal of Applied Physics, 74, 4845-4848.

Kunz, K. S., & Luebbers, R. J. (1993). The finite-difference time-domain method in electromagnetics. Boca Raton, FL: CRC Press.

Kuster, N. (1998). Compliance testing of handheld mobile communications equipment. In G. L. Carlo (Ed.), Wireless phones and health: Scientific progress (pp. 47-54). Norwell, MA: Kluwer Academic Press.

Kuster, N., & Balzano, Q. (1992). Energy absorption mechanism by biological bodies in the near field of dipole antennas above 300 MHz. IEEE Transactions on Vehicular Technology, 41(1), 17-23.

Lazzi, G., & Gandhi, O. P. (1997). Realistically tilted and truncated anatomically based models of the human head for dosimetry of mobile telephones. IEEE Transactions on Electromagnetic Compatibility, 39(1), 55-61.

Lentner, C. (Ed.). (1984). Geigy scientific tables. Basle, Switzerland: CIBA-GEIGY Limited.

Lin, J. C., & Gandhi, O. P. (1995). Computational methods for predicting field intensity. In C. Polk & E. Postow (Eds.), Handbook of biological effects of electromagnetic fields (pp. 337-402). Boca Raton, FL: CRC Press.

Mur, G. (1981). Absorbing boundary conditions for the finite-difference approximation of the time-domain electromagnetic-field equations. IEEE Transactions on Electromagnetic Compatibility, 23, 337-382.

Schmid, T., Egger, O., & Kuster, N. (1996), Automated E-field scanning systems for dosimetric assessments. IEEE Transactions on Microwave Theory and Technique, 44 (1), 105-113.

Simunic, D. (Ed.). (1994, November). Reference models for bioelectromagnetic test of mobile communication systems. Proceedings of the COST 244 Meeting, Rome, Italy.

Stuchly, M. A., Spiegel, R. J., Stuchly, S. S., & Kraszewski, A. (1986). Exposure of man in the near field of a resonant dipole: Comparison between theory and measurements. IEEE Transactions on Microwave Theory and Techniques, 34, 26-31.

Stuchly, M. A., & Stuchly, S. S. (1995). Experimental radio and microwave dosimetry. In C. Polk & E. Postow (Eds.), Handbook of biological effects of electromagnetic fields (2nd ed., pp. 295-336). Boca Raton, FL: CRC Press, Inc.

Stuchly, M. A., & Stuchly, S. S. (1980). Dielectric properties of biological substances -- Tabulated. Journal of Microwave Power, 15, 19-26.

Taflove, A. (1995). <u>Computational electrodynamics: The finite-difference time-domain method.</u> Dedham, MA: Artech House.

II

BIOLOGICAL RESPONSES INDICATIVE OF GENETIC EFFECTS

Editor's Note:

Traditional approaches to assessing carcinogenic effects rely in large part on the assessment of genetic impact. However, assessment of the genetic impact of low-power radio frequency radiation is tedious, with hundreds of possible approaches, some scientifically valid, and some not.

A series of papers by Drs. Henry Lai and N.P. Singh at the University of Washington have caused a stir in the popular media, in particular, regarding potential genetic effects from radio frequency radiation and their impact on the users of wireless phones. The debate regarding the significance of the original work by Drs. Lai and Singh lives on while investigators around the world attempt to confirm their findings. Results of much of this work are expected in early 1999.

Nonetheless, a large body of relevant scientific work exists regarding the genetic impact of low-power radio frequency radiation. The papers by Drs. Brusick, Verschaeve, Meltz, Roti Roti and colleagues, and Wolff present a useful summary of existing science and nuances necessary for appropriate interpretation of the information as regards public health protection. It is important to note that positive genetic effect studies are not sufficient to independently lead to public health intervention. Positive results must be interpreted in the context of other complementary studies in a weight-of-evidence context.

G. L. C.

6
GENOTOXICITY OF RADIOFREQUENCY RADIATION
David Brusick

Abstract

Concerns have been raised regarding potential adverse effects from exposures to radiofrequency radiation (RFR). The focus of the concern has been directed at DNA interactions, producing a large number of publications describing the effects of RFR on the integrity of nucleic acids. Data from over 100 studies conducted in the range of 800-3000 megahertz (MHz) were reviewed and subjected to a weight-of-evidence evaluation. The results suggest that, although some subtle effects on DNA replication and transcription may be induced, RFR is not directly genotoxic and adverse DNA effects from RFR at high power intensities are predominantly the result of hyperthermia. This work was sponsored by Wireless Technology Research, LLC.

Introduction

Use of wireless communication devices such as cellular telephones is increasing dramatically in the United States, as well as internationally. Most current wireless devices operate by sending and receiving radio signals in the range of 800-900 MHz. Frequencies on newer devices may extend to 2000 MHz. Most cellular telephones currently in use employ continuous analog transmission technology; however, it is anticipated that use of digital equipment, which employs pulsed transmission of radio frequencies, will increase significantly in the next few years.

Expansion of this technology will result in substantial human exposure to radiofrequency radiation (RFR) on a chronic basis. During the past several years, concerns have been raised regarding the potential of RFR to initiate and/or promote tumor development, suppress components of the immune system, or induce genetic alterations (Elmer-Dewit, 1993; WHO, 1993). Research focused on safety issues of chronic exposure to RFR, particularly in the frequency range associated with wireless communication devices, is limited and inconclusive as to the interrogation of this research. To a large extent, confusion is the result of a lack of uniform exposure standards and measurement techniques and the small number of safety studies conducted in compliance with GLP regulations.

One of the most active areas of RFR testing is the assessment of direct and indirect effects on DNA. A published database containing results from over 100 studies exists. The types of studies conducted range from investigations of RFR interactions with purified DNA in vitro to assessment of chromosome damage in primary cells recovered from laboratory animals and humans exposed to RFR (WHO, 1993).

Electromagnetic fields within a frequency range of 300 Hz to 300 GHz interact with biological systems (WHO, 1993). Within this broad range, radiofrequencies encompass the range of frequencies from 30 kHz to 30,000 MHz. The most frequently studied radiofrequency, however, is 2450 MHz, the frequency associated with microwave ovens. This summary will concentrate on an analysis of the genotoxicity of RFR studies, with particular emphasis on those studies in the 800-1200 MHz range.

Studies summarized in this report include those conducted in microorganisms, cultured mammalian cells (both primary cultures and continuous cell lines), and in vivo assays (Table 1). Most of the studies are classified as hazard identification evaluations and include assessments for mutation induction, a wide range of chromosome alterations, cell transformation, and evidence for the induction of DNA repair processes. A smaller subset of the database consists of studies designed to detect cellular and molecular changes occurring in DNA exposed to RFR in situ or in similar extracellular matrices. These studies measured DNA responses not associated directly with genetic diseases and were, therefore, not viewed as highly relevant to assessments of genetic hazard or risk, although they may provide extremely useful mechanistic information.

Characteristics of the Database

Although the majority of the papers were published within the past ten years and use state-of-the-art techniques for assessing genotoxicity, some of the studies included in the database were published almost two decades ago. Since these older studies did not follow currently acceptable protocols, they have limited relevance. The database can be characterized as:

1. Heterogeneous with respect to target organisms, exposure methods, and genetic endpoints employed;

2. Complex with respect to the variation of responses across similar types of endpoints and target organisms; and

3. Redundant with respect to the frequency of replication of certain test methods (e.g., mutation induction in *S. Typhimurium*, chromosome aberration analyses in cultured human lymphocytes, mouse dominant lethal test).

Mechanism	Endpoint	Studies	Reported	
			Negative	Positive
DNA Disruption				
	DNA Breakage	14	9	5*
	Micronucleus	5	0	5
	Aberrations	30	17	13
	Dominant Lethal	6	3	3
Nucleotide Subsitution and Recombination	Gene Mutation	26	25	1
	SCE	17	15	2
Unknown				
	Chromosome Loss	2	2	0
	Spermhead Abnormality	2	1	1
	Cell Transformation	3	1	2
		105	73	32

*All in vivo

Table 1. Distribution of genotoxic effects by mechanism

Interpretation of results is also complicated by the high incidence of variables associated with RFR exposure. The most common variables are: (a) wave frequency, (b) power, (c) duration of exposure, (d) modulation, and (e) exposure temperature. Each of these parameters is critical for the interpretation of changes in biological activity and is potentially capable of affecting the outcome of an assay. For example, specific absorption rates (SARs) above 1-2 watts per kilogram (W/kg) are capable of raising the body temperature of most laboratory animals 1° C or more, which can lead to a wide range of adverse effects (WHO, 1993). Therefore, it is theoretically possible to generate different responses in two trials of the same in vivo test method if the SAR varies enough to give a 1° C temperature differential.

Strategy for Data Evaluation

A weight-of-evidence strategy was used to evaluate the database because of its size, redundancy of tests, and heterogeneity of test methods. Small data sets that are not redundant are more amenable to a micro-assessment strategy, because each assay exists once in the data set and an overall interpretation can be determined from the number and/or type of positive responses. Study redundancy accompanied by conflicting responses is commonly found in large data sets and makes interpretation difficult, because plausible explanations for divergent response generated by independent assay trials may not be possible. This situation characteristically results in selection of the positive (most conservative) response for use in the assessment. A system which focuses on positive responses may be self-fulfilling in that there are few, if any, agents with completely negative genotoxicity profiles.

Mutation is a low frequency event and bioassays used to detect DNA alterations have intrinsic rates of sporadic positive responses; therefore, the process of selecting the positive (most conservative) response for decision making can exclude valid conflicting data and may lead to erroneous conclusions about the genotoxicity of agents. Reviews of assay performance covering several in vitro assays (Kirkland & Dean, 1994) and the in vivo mouse micronucleus assay (Shelby et al., 1993) document the occurrence of sporadic positive responses. Estimates of the incidences of sporadic (nonreproducing) positive responses provided in these reviews were approximately 8% for the Ames test, 20% for the Mouse Lymphoma assay, and about 15% for in vitro chromosome aberrations in CHO. The incidence of sporadic (nonreproducing) positive responses in the mouse micronucleus test was 10%. The causes of these sporadic responses are numerous, but they can often be attributed to marginally positive, nonreproducible responses associated with target organism toxicity or responses associated with atypical concurrent control values in one of the trials. Some endpoints, such as mammalian cell transformation, mouse sperm head abnormalities, and plant cell clastogenicity, have high rates of sporadic positives due presumably to the susceptibility of these techniques to the production of change by nongenotoxic events (e.g., high osmolality, low pH, hyperthermia), whereas other assays, such as mutation in Drosophila, dominant lethal mutations in mice, and some DNA repair assays, appear to be more consistent. A thorough discussion of the rationale for using a weight-of-evidence approach for large, heterogenous, complex genotoxicity data sets has been published in a special issue of *Mutation Research* (Vol. 266, No. 1, 1992). An example of the application of this weight-of-evidence approach to an evaluation of a large genetic toxicity database resistant to micro-assessment was published by Brusick (1994).

Exposure Considerations

The most frequently-encountered confounding variable in the database was that of exposure conditions. RFR emitting sources used to conduct the studies covered in this review ranged from relatively unsophisticated converted microwave ovens to highly reliable and calibrated exposure systems.

RFR doses are expressed as specific absorption rates (SARs). SARs quantify the energy absorbed by the target organism and are expressed in W/kg. SARs define both peak and average values for exposure. Because of the associated adverse physiological changes produced in the target organism by RFR exposures, reliable comparisons and interpretations were difficult for studies not reporting SARs.

In addition to frequency, RFR exposure parameters that may influence the outcome of a study include modulation, polarization, and intermittent versus continuous emission. Invariably, one or more of these parameters differed among independent studies with a given assay. Consequently, dose comparisons were not possible.

Kerbacher et al. (1990) reviewed the relationship between SAR and thermal effects for in vitro exposures at 2450 MHz and a SAR of 33.8 W/kg. The conclusions of the authors were that many of the positive clastogenicity findings could be due to secondary thermal effects, and, if thermal effects are eliminated, RFR alone is not capable of inducing chromosome damage. Berman et al. (1980) attempted to provide similar information for germ cell damage in vivo following exposures to 2450 MHz RFR. The authors concluded that male rats exposed to RFR (5 mW/cm^2) from day 6 of gestation to 90 days of age were not at risk for DNA damage to their sperm.

Macro Assessment of the Database

Table 2 summarizes the qualitative responses in the database including the number of expected sporadic positive responses for specific assay types. With the exception of two test types—dominant lethality in mice and in vivo chromosome breakage—the actual incidence of positive responses in the RFR database is close to the number expected from sporadic responses. This suggests that the basis of concern for RFR DNA damage can be explained as normal variability found in a large sample of study responses. This explanation is not intended to trivialize the relevance of the published investigations, but it highlights some of the insights that may be derived from a macro-assessment strategy. (The increased incidences of chromosome breakage in somatic and germ cells have been attributed to hyperthermia-induced DNA strand breakage associated with microwave exposures [Leonard et al., 1983; Saunders et al., 1988].)

Risk Analysis Needs

The existing database is probably too heterogenous to provide reliable risk estimates for RFR. It also lacks a meaningful number of studies using RFR in the range of most wireless devices (Table 3). It will be necessary to differentiate between primary and secondary DNA damage if one is to develop a rational assessment of risk from exposure to RFR. Thus, a combination of in vitro and in vivo tests must be conducted under carefully controlled and monitored exposure conditions.

Summary

The data included in this review are derived from studies which evaluate the toxicological effects of RFR, as well as studies addressing basic biological responses to RFR at the cellular and molecular level. Some studies directed towards assessing the toxicological potential of RFR have reported alterations in primary DNA integrity and chromosome replication.

Adverse DNA effects following exposure of organisms to high frequencies and high power intensities of RFR appear to be predominantly the result of hyperthermia; however, there may be some subtle effects on the replication and/or transcription of genes under relatively restricted exposure conditions. While few studies indicate that

Bioassay Type	Intrinsic Sporadic Positives	Number of Times Used	Expected Positives	Observed Positives
Microbial	5%	24	1.2	1
In vitro cytogenetic	30%	32	9.6	12
Cell Transformation	50%	3	1.5	1
Mouse Lymphoma	20%	1	0	0
Drosophila	5%	12	<1	0
UDS in vitro	5%	4	<1	0
Plant cytogenetic	75%	1	1	1
Dominant Lethal	5%	6	0	3*
In vivo cytogenetic	10%	18	1.8	8*
Spermhead Abnormalities	50%	2	1	1

*Probably thermal effects: high temperature known to produce developmental effects and chromosome instability in vivo.

Table 2. Expectations for positive responses in the database due to sporadic positives.

RFR alters cell proliferation or differentiation, at least one set of studies suggests interaction with promoting agents such as TPA. The importance of these findings is not clear, since they occur under very restrictive exposure scenarios. Although adequate epidemiology studies directed toward cancer have not been completed, animal cancer studies conducted at 2450 MHz do not support concerns that RFR is an initiator, co-carcinogen, or promoter (Salford, 1993; Wu et al., 1989). In general, the data from a wide range of standard genetic test methods involving both mammalian and nonmammalian assays do not support the concern that RFR poses nonthermal genotoxic risk to somatic or germ cells of humans under normal exposure scenarios. It is clear that additional confirmatory and new studies assessing the direct effects of RFR on DNA are needed. These studies must be conducted with more robust study designs and with exposure systems capable of accurately defining dose and reducing and/or eliminating secondary thermal effects.

Endpoint	System	Frequency	Result	SAR	Reference
Aberration	CHO	1200 MHz	negative	24.33 w/kg	Meltz et al., 1990
	CHO	850 MHz	negative	14.4 w/kg	Meltz et al., 1990
	Human lymphocytes	954 MHz	positive	1.5 w/kg	Maes et al., 1995
SCE	CHO	1200 MHz	negative	24.33 w/kg	Meltz et al., 1990
	CHO	850 MHz	negative	14.4 w/kg	Meltz et al., 1990
	Mouse	800 MHz	negative	4 w/kg	Brown & Marshall, 1982
DNA Repair	MRC-5	1200 MHz	negative	4.5 w/kg	Meltz et al., 1987
	MRC-5	850 MHz	negative	4.5 w/kg	Meltz et al., 1987

Table 3. Summary of effects from exposure to RFR frequencies ranging from 800-1200 MHz

98

References

Berman, E., Carter, H. B., & House, D. (1980). Tests for mutagenesis and reproduction in male rats exposed to 2,450-MHz (CW) microwaves. Bioelectromagnetics, 1, 65-76.

Brown, R. F., & Marshall, S. V. (1982). Sister chromatid exchange in marrow cells of mice exposed to RFR (400, 800, and 1200 MHz CW) [abstract]. BEMS, 4th Bioelectromagnetics Society Annual Meeting - Abstracts, 51.

Brusick, D. J. (1994). An assessment of the genetic toxicity of atrazine: Relevance to human health and environmental effects. Mutation Research, 317, 133-144.

Elmer-Dewit, P. (1993, February). Dialing "P" for Panic. Time Magazine, 8, 42.

Kirkland, D. J., & Dean, S. W. (1994). On the need for confirmation of negative genotoxicity results in vitro and on the usefulness of mammalian cell mutation tests in a core battery: Experiences of a contract research laboratory. Mutagenesis, 9, 491-501.

Leonard, A., Berteaud, A. J., & Bruyere, A. (1983). An evaluation of the mutagenic, carcinogenic and teratogenic potential of microwaves. Mutation Research, 123, 31-46.

Maes, A., Collier, M., Slaets, D., & Verschaeve, L. (1995). Cytogenetic effects of microwaves from mobile communication frequencies (954 MHz). Electro Magnetobiology, 14, 91-98.

Meltz, M. L., Walker, K. A., & Erwin, D. N. (1987). Radiofrequency (microwave) radiation exposure of mammalian cells during UV-induced DNA repair synthesis. Radiation Research, 110, 255-266.

Meltz, M. L., Eagan, P., & Erwin, D. N. (1989). Absence of mutagenic interaction between microwaves and mitomycin C in mammalian cells. Environmental and Molecular Mutagenesis, 13, 294-303.

Salford, L. G., Brun, A., Persson, B. R. R., & Eberhardt, J. (1993). Experimental studies of brain tumour development during exposure to continuous and pulsed 915 MHz radio frequency radiation. Bioelectrochemistry and Bioenergetics, 30, 313-318.

Saunders, R. D., Kowalczuk, C. I., Beechey, C. V., & Dunford, R. (1988). Studies of the induction of dominant lethals and translocations in male mice after chronic exposure to microwave radiation. International Journal of Radiation Biology, 53, 983-992.

World Health Organization. (1993). Environmental health criteria 137: Electromagnetic fields (300 Hz to 300 GHz) (pp.80-180). Geneva, Switzerland: World Health Organization.

Wu, R. Y., Ghiang, H., & Shao, B. J. (1989). The effects of 2.54 GHz radiation on DMH-induced colon cancer in mice [abstract]. Bioelectromagnetics Society 11th Annual Meeting - Abstracts, (No. P-2-34).

7

SOME CONSIDERATIONS ON THE GENOTOXICITY OF RADIOFREQUENCY RADIATION

Luc Verschaeve

Abstract

According to most scientific data, it may be anticipated that radiofrequency radiation is in itself not capable of breaking DNA or being genotoxic, especially when exposure is under so-called athermal conditions. Yet, occasionally, significant genetic changes (e.g., increased chromosome aberration frequencies) are found which may be ascribed to small differences in biological samples and/or in the exposure conditions. Experiments using well defined exposure conditions and materials should therefore be encouraged. Furthermore, up to now, little attention was paid to potential synergistic effects with chemical mutagens/carcinogens. Also, the choice of the investigated genetic endpoint is important. This is often not sufficiently taken into consideration when results are evaluated. Finally, experiments on biomonitoring should also consider the presence of possible hypersensitive subjects in the test population.

Adverse health effects of nonionizing radiations have been investigated for several decades. However, it is still not possible to clearly estimate some of these effects. This is especially so for genetic effects and cancer. One of the reasons for the presence of inconsistent results is that, in addition to frequency, other exposure parameters are usually different from one investigation to the other. This is, for example, the case for the power, time of exposure, mode of exposure (pulsed or continuous emission), temperature, etc. At present, more attention is now being paid to these parameters; however, further attention and standardization must be encouraged.

Despite these shortcomings or difficulties, a review of the data obtained so far on genetic effects of radiofrequency (RF) radiation suggests that RFs are not directly genotoxic except maybe in extreme conditions where thermal effects are anticipated. This general conclusion is expected, since it is well known that the energy of RF radiation and other nonionizing radiations is too low to directly induce DNA breakage or damage (e.g., Léonard, Berteaud, & Bruyere, 1983). Yet, some considerations must be made with respect to possible indirect effects leading to a genotoxic event.

Synergism

It may be anticipated that RF radiation is in itself not capable of breaking DNA or being genotoxic in any way, especially when exposure is under so-called athermal conditions. However, it is clear that nonionizing radiations in general (e.g., extremely low frequencies [ELF], with even lower energies) can have biological effects. Some applications in the treatment of pathologies (e.g., Hinsenkamp, 1994) may be cited as an example. In addition, laboratory investigations in vivo and in vitro have shown that RF radiation may influence particular cellular processes and, for example, act on cell membranes (e.g., Saunders, Kowalczuk, & Sienkiewics, 1991; Tarricone, Cito, & D'Inzeo, 1993). These effects are usually classified as reversible, but they may have irreversible results when the cell is not only exposed to the RF field but also to another factor, e.g., a chemical mutagen or carcinogen. For example, we have repeatedly found a clear synergistic effect of mobile telephone frequencies with mitomycin C. Indeed, when human blood cells were exposed for two hours to 954 MHz waves (approximate SAR 1.5 W/kg) and then cultivated in the presence of mitomycin C, a marked increase in sister chromatid exchange frequency was found compared to cells that were cultivated in the same conditions but not RF-exposed (Maes, Collier, Slaets, & Verschaeve, 1996; Verschaeve, Slaets, Van Gorp, Maes, & Vankerkom, 1994). Similar results were found by Damiani et al. (1995), although negative results were reported when other test procedures were used (e.g., Ciaravino, Meltz, & Erwin, 1987). Although no mechanistic investigations have been performed which might explain the above synergistic action, these results are sufficiently clear to show that possible synergisms should be taken into account. RF radiation may theoretically sensitize cells to the action of chemical mutagens or carcinogens, increasing their harmful effect.

Hypersensitivity

In the last few years, serious consideration has been given to the possibility that populations exist that are hypersensitive to particular electromagnetic fields (Simunic, 1995). Hypersensitivity has not yet been extensively studied with regard to genotoxic effects and cancer susceptibility and deserves more attention, for example, in human biomonitoring studies.

Use of the Most Appropriate Cell Type

Although a number of cell types will always be used for genetic and other research because of their accessibility and ease of use (lymphocytes, fibroblasts, etc.), the use of particular cell types that may be considered target cells should be encouraged. With respect to mobile telephony, brain cells are a particularly relevant cell type, as the antenna from a cellular phone is held close to the head. In addition, the brain is particularly sensitive to the emitted electromagnetic fields. Although the absorbed energy is small even in worst case situations, local SAR values may exceed the accepted values (Anderson, Johansen, Pedersen, & Raskmark, 1995). In this respect, recently published investigations where effects of 2450 MHz microwaves were studied in rat brain cells with the "comet assay" are particularly interesting (Lai & Singh, 1995, 1996). Single-strand DNA breaks and alkali labile sites were found to be higher in brain cells from rats that were exposed to the microwaves for a short period of time compared to nonexposed animals. It was hypothesized that free radicals are involved in the RF radiation-induced DNA damage (Lai & Singh, 1997). These results may be considered of particular importance if confirmed, although the consequences of this finding remains unclear at present.

enetic Endpoints

stigated using a great number of in vitro or in vivo assays.
.g., easy to perform, inexpensive) and disadvantages (e.g.,
;," difficult to extrapolate the results to humans). Each test
o detect one of several genetic events (e.g., chromosome
tations or aneuploidy). Therefore, several test systems are
city test programs. Finally, some tests are more sensitive
of a genotoxic effect. This may be of particular importance
ctor is investigated that is by definition (theoretically) not
y a weak mutagen. In such cases, as is undoubtedly so for
cluding RF fields, the choice of the test system may be
well known that the evaluation of the frequency of sister
ore sensitive than that of chromosome aberrations when
it ionizing radiations, are considered (Evans, 1977). In this
that 2450 MHz microwaves (SAR 79 W/kg) behave like
nduce chromosome aberrations rather than sister chromatid
e, Arroyo, De Wagter, & Vercruyssen, 1993). Therefore,
(Cohen, Kunska, Astemborski, & McCulloch, 1985;
, RF fields (Maes et al., 1993) do not induce sister chromatid exchanges may not immediately be interpreted as a lack of genotoxicity of the particular radiation. Some of the genetic endpoints used so far may be not sensitive enough for this kind of investigation.

References

Andersen, J. B., Johansen, C., Pedersen, G. F., & Raskmark, P. (1995). On the possible health effects related to GSM and DECT transmissions: A tutorial study. Aalborg, Denmark: Aalborg University, Institute of Electronic Systems, Center for Perskommunikation.

Ciaravino, V., Meltz, M. L., & Erwin, D. N. (1987). Effects of radiofrequency radiation and simultaneous exposure with mitomycin C on the frequency of sister chromatic exchanges in chinese hamster ovary cells. Environmental Mutagenesis, 9, 393-399.

Cohen, M. M., Kunska, A., Astemborski, J. A., & McCulloch, D. (1985). The effect of low-level 60Hz electromagnetic fields on human lymphoblastoid cells. II. Sister chromatic exchanges in peripheral blood lymphocytes and lymphoblastoid cell lines. Mutation Research, 172, 177-184.

Damiani, G., Laurenti, P., Marchetti, M., Capelli, G., Ossola, P., & Tofani, S. (1995). Potential genotoxic effect of elf-modulated radiofrequency magnetic fields on peripheral lymphocytes. In D. Simunic (Ed.), Electromagnetic hypersensitivity (pp. 19-29). Proceedings of COST 244 meeting (EEC, DGXIII/72/95-EN). Brussels, Belgium: European Economic Community.

Evans, H. J. (1977). Molecular mechanisms in the induction of chromosome aberrations. In D. Scott, B.A. Bridges, & F.H. Sobels (Eds.), Progress in genetic toxicology (pp. 57-74). Amsterdam: Elsevier.

Hinsenkamp, M. (1994). Stimulation electromagnetique de l'osteogenese et de la consolidation des fractures (Duculot edition) [Electromagnetic stimulation of osteogenesis and fracture healing]. Gembloux, Belgium: Academie Royale de Belgique.

Lai, H., & Singh, N. P. (1995). Acute low-intensity microwave exposure increases DNA single-strand breaks in rat brain cells. Bioelectromagnetics, 16, 207-210.

Lai, H., & Singh, N. P. (1996). DNA single- and double-strand breaks in rat brain cells after acute exposure to low-level radiofrequency electromagnetic radiation. International Journal of Radiation Biology, 69, 513-521.

Lai, H., & Singh, N. P. (1997). Melatonin and a spin-trap compound block radiofrequency electromagnetic radiation-induced DNA strand breaks in rat brain cells. Bioelectromagnetics, 18, 446-454.

Léonard, A., Berteaud, A. J., & Bruyere, A. (1983). An evaluation of the mutagenic, carcinogenic and teratogenic potential of microwaves. Mutation Research, 123, 31-45.

Maes, A., Collier, M., Slaets, D., & Verschaeve, L. (1996). 954 MHz microwaves enhance the mutagenic properties of mitomycin C. Environmental and Molecular Mutagenesis, 28, 26-30.

Maes, A., Verschaeve, L., Arroyo, A., De Wagter, C., & Vercruyssen, L. (1993). In vitro cytogenetic effects of 2450 MHz waves on human peripheral blood lymphocytes. Bioelectromagnetics, 14, 195-501.

Rosenthal, M., & Obe, G. (1989). Effects of 50-Hz electromagnetic fields on proliferation and on chromosomal alterations in human peripheral lymphocytes untreated or pretreated with chemical mutagens. Mutation Research, 210, 329-335.

Saunders, R. D., Kowalczuk, C. I., & Sienkiewics, Z. J. (1991). Biological effects of exposure to nonionizing electromagnetic fields and radiation. III. Radiofrequency and microwave radiation (NRPB-R240). Chilton, Didcot, Oxfordshire, UK: National Radiological Protection Board.

Simunic, D. (Ed.). (1995). Electromagnetic hypersensitivity. Proceedings of COST 244 meeting, (EEC, DGXIII/72/95 -EN). Brussels, Belgium: European Economic Community.

Tarricone, L., Cito, C., & D'Inzeo, D. (1993). Ach receptor channel's interaction with MW fields. Bioelectrochemistry & Bioenergetics, 30, 275-285.

Verschaeve, L., Slaets, D., Van Gorp, U., Maes, A., & Vankerkom, J. (1994). In vitro and in vivo genetic effects of microwaves from mobile telephone frequencies in human and rat peripheral blood lymphocytes. In D. Simunic (Ed.), Mobile communications and extremely low frequency fields & instrumentation and measurements in bioelectromagnetic research: Proceedings of COST 244 meetings (pp. 74-83), (EEC,DGXIII/J31/94-FR). Brussels, Belgium: Euopean Economic Community.

8

STUDIES ON MICROWAVE INDUCTION OF GENOTOXICITY: A LABORATORY REPORT

Martin L. Meltz

Abstract

An extensive series of investigations has been undertaken to determine, using standard genetic toxicology assay protocols, whether or not microwave radiation can cause genetic damage at power density and specific absorption rate (SAR) levels at or above the guidelines existing at the time the studies were initiated. Using both pulsed wave and continuous wave exposures at 350, 850, and 1200 MHz, DNA repair could not be induced in normal human fibroblasts exposed in vitro. In addition, microwave exposure did not interfere with the DNA repair synthesis occurring after UV radiation. Where the medium temperature increased by 3 ° C, microwave radiation exposures at 2450 MHz, pulsed wave, at higher SAR levels did not induce mutation at the thymidine kinase locus in L5178Y mouse leukemic cells, or chromosome aberrations or sister chromatid exchanges in CHO cells. For all three endpoints, the cells were treated simultaneously with genotoxic chemicals and microwave radiation, the effect of the chemicals alone was the same as treatment with the chemicals alone. Several different chemicals were examined, each with a different known mechanism of action. Comments will be made as to the relationship of positive reports from laboratories and their obvious or likely association with heating of the exposed cells.

These studies, performed by members of the scientific staff of the University of Texas Health Science Center at San Antonio, were funded by the U.S. Air Force. The exposures and dosimetry were performed by Air Force technical personnel at the U.S. Air Force Research Laboratory (formerly Armstrong Laboratory), Brooks Air Force Base, Texas. Both institutions are Associate members of the Center for Environmental Radiation Toxicology (CERT), which is comprised of more than 55 scientists and staff members from the University of Texas Health Science Center at San Antonio, the U.S. Air Force Research Laboratory, Trinity University, the Southwest Research Institute, the Southwest Foundation for Biomedical Research, and the University of Texas at San Antonio. These scientists represent the highest concentration of experts in the field of nonionizing radiation in the world, with knowledge of the sources, dosimetry, bioeffects and health effects of microwave radiation, extremely low frequency fields, ultraviolet light, and laser emissions.

To address the immediate concern about potential health hazard, the investigation of genotoxicity was given a higher priority than investigations of other bioeffects. To investigate genotoxicity, several different endpoints were selected: DNA damage and inhibition of DNA repair; sister chromatid exchange (SCE) induction; chromosome aberration induction; and phenotypic mutation induction. This series of studies represents the most comprehensive investigation of the genotoxicity of microwave radiation ever performed by one laboratory.

We also pursued the investigation of potential microwave hazard by taking another very important experimental step. Assuming that no direct genotoxic effects of microwave radiation would occur, the last three assays were also used to determine whether microwave radiation altered the genotoxicity of three chemical mutagens, known to interact with DNA by different mechanisms, during or as a result of a simultaneous exposure with microwave radiation. The chemical mutagens used included Mitomycin C, Adriamycin, and Proflavin. Publications describing this extensive series of studies are listed at the end of this report.

One of the investigations (Meltz, Waslker, & Erwin, 1987) attempted to determine whether or not continuous or pulsed wave microwave radiation exposures, at 350 MHz, 850 MHz, or 1200 MHz, and at power densities including 10 mW/cm^2, can induce DNA repair. The studies were conducted with medium temperatures maintained at either 37° C or 39° C during the microwave exposure using water bath heating. If DNA repair were detected, it would indicate that the microwave exposure had damaged the DNA; however, it was not observed to occur. We then redirected our hypothesis based on what is know about the disease Xeroderma pigmentosum. Persons with this genetically inherited disorder have defects in DNA repair, and are at increased risk for sunlight-induced skin cancer. We therefore first damaged the DNA of normal, diploid human fibroblasts by exposure of the cells to ultraviolet light, and examined whether subsequent microwave radiation exposure inhibited the resulting DNA repair. No effect of the microwave radiation exposure on the DNA repair process, which involves a series of several different enzymatic actions, was observed.

Two papers by Meltz et al. (1989, 1990) describe our investigation of whether or not pulsed microwave radiation exposures at the frequency of 2450 MHz, delivered at higher power densities and SARs than used in the DNA repair studies, can cause phenotypic mutations. This was examined using the standardized thymidine kinase locus mutation assay in L5178Y mouse leukemia cells (mammalian cells). As an important extension to the microwave-only exposures, we expanded the studies to investigate whether a simultaneous exposure of the cells to microwave radiation during treatment with the genotoxic chemicals Adriamycin, Mitomycin C, or Proflavin could change the extent of the chemically-induced mutation frequency. The studies demonstrated that the microwave radiation exposures—at a power density and SAR high enough to cause an increase in the medium temperature—did not cause any mutations when the cells were exposed to the RFR alone, and most importantly, did not alter any of the mutation frequencies upon simultaneous exposure to chemical mutagens (i.e., compared to that resulting from the chemical treatment alone).

Two other papers from our laboratory (Ciaravino, Meltz, & Erwin, 1987, 1991) describe related studies using sister chromatid exchange induction upon exposure of Chinese hamster ovary cells as the endpoint. The potential interaction of the pulsed wave 2450 MHz RFR with the chemicals Mitomycin C and Adriamycin was examined. Again, no effect of the pulsed wave RFR exposure alone on SCE frequency was observed, and no interaction of the RFR exposure was observed with the chemical induction of the SCEs.

The final paper (Kerbacher, Meltz, & Erwin, 1990) describes studies using the same 2450 MHz pulsed wave RFR exposure of Chinese hamster ovary cells, but in this case using the more classical examination of chromosome aberration induction as the endpoint. The potential interaction of RFR with the chemicals Mitomycin C and Adriamycin was again examined. Induction of chromosome aberrations by the RFR exposure alone was not observed. An extremely small but statistically significant difference was observed in the number of aberrant cells during RFR exposure and Adriamycin treatment, but the temperature control (performed in the same experiment) revealed that the increase was the result of the elevated temperature, and not due to the RF radiation per se.

All of these studies were performed with the greatest attention to the exposure parameters, the power density and SAR, and the temperature during the microwave exposure. As appropriate, replicate independent treatment flasks for each exposure condition and/or replicate experiments were used or performed.

Specific Studies

DNA Repair

Figure 1 of Meltz et al. (1987) shows the DNA repair which occurs in MAC-5 normal human fibroblasts (in units of dpm/microgram of isolated DNA) over time after a UV exposure of 21 J/m^2. If the repair is allowed to occur at medium temperatures (water bath heating) of either 37° or 39° C, no difference is observed in the repair labeling.

The ability of RFR exposure to interfere with the DNA repair which occurs immediately after exposing cells to ultraviolet light was investigated by exposing the cells to RFR during the repair labeling period. As is observed in Figures 2, 3, and 4 of Meltz et al. (1987), for power densities of either 1 or 10 mW/cm^2 and exposure times of 1, 2, and 3 hours:

(i)   350 MHz, 850 MHz, or 1200 MHz continuous wave (CW) exposures at 37° C do not interfere with UV-induced DNA repair (by comparison of the RFR exposed vs. control values). Also,

(ii)   cells exposed to pulsed wave (PW) exposures at 37° C and at the same three frequencies also do not interfere with UV-induced DNA repair.

The 350 MHz exposures in the above experiments were performed in a TEM cell. The pulsed repetition rate was 5000 pps; the pulse width was 10 μs; the duty factor was 0.05. At 10 mW/cm^2, the peak power density was 200 mW/cm^2. The SAR was 0.39±0.15 W/kg. The 850 MHz and 1200 MHz experiments were performed in an anechoic chamber in the far field with downward exposure from an antenna horn. The repetition rate at 850 MHz was again 5000 pps; for a 10 mW/cm² average power density, the pulse width was 100 s and the duty factor was 0.5. This resulted in a peak power density of 20 mW/cm². The average SAR was 4.5±0.3 W/kg. For the 1200 MHz exposure, and a 10 mW/cm² average power density, the pulse repetition rate was 80,000 pps. With a 3 µs pulse width, this resulted in a duty factor of 0.24. The peak power density was 41.7 mW/cm². The average SAR was 2.7±1.6 W/kg.

Part of the study was repeated (Table I in Meltz et al., 1987) with an attempt made to "pre-stress" the cells by incubating them at 39° C after the UV light exposure, and during the simultaneous repair labeling period and microwave exposure period. Again, there was no effect of the PW RFR exposures on the DNA repair labeling.

In a second type of investigation, the ability of 350, 850 and 1250 MHz RFR exposures, CW or PW, to alone (without UV light damage) induce DNA repair was examined (Table II in Meltz et al., 1987). After 3 hour repair-labeling intervals, there was no evidence that RFR exposure at 10 mW/cm², at any of the three frequencies, induced DNA repair. This suggests (but does not prove) that repair-inducing DNA damage did not result from the RFR exposure.

Since neither induction of DNA repair, nor inhibition of repair in UV-damaged cell DNA had been observed upon exposure of the cells at these frequencies and the maximum 10 mW/cm² power density—which at the time was at approximately the level of the existing guidelines for RFR exposures—we switched frequencies to 2450 MHz, focused our studies on PW exposures (since there was at least a hypothesis that PW might be more likely to cause bioeffects than CW exposures), and considerably raised the power density and SAR. These changes resulted in a temperature increase in the cell culture medium in the exposure flasks. Typical exposure parameters in these studies include an average net forward power of approximately 600 W, power densities of approximately 50 mW/cm², SARs of approximately 34 W/kg, a pulse repetition rate of 25,000 pulses per second, a pulse width of 10 µs, and a duty factor of 0.25 (see individual experiments for exact values). The exposure time was 2-4 hours, depending on the type of experiment.

RFR Exposure and Sister Chromatid Exchange (SCE) Induction

Figure 1 in Ciaravino et al. (1987) shows the temperatures in the medium in an RFR exposed flask, a 37°C control flask, and a temperature control flask (i.e., use of water-bath heating to give a medium temperature similar to that in the RFR-exposed flasks).

Table III in Ciaravino et al. (1987) summarizes the results for six exposure conditions, with three replicate flasks per exposure condition, and for four completely independent experiments.

The data in this table indicates that:

(1)   MMC induces SCEs (comparing B to A);

(2)   neither RFR exposure or temperature control increases the frequency of the SCEs beyond that in the 37° C control (comparing E to C to A); and

(3)   even if RFR + MMC gives more SCEs than 37° C + MMC, the same result is seen with the temperature increase in the temperature control due to the water bath heating (comparing F to D to B).

In a completely different set of seven experiments, with Adriamycin at two different concentrations as the genotoxic chemical (Ciaravino et al., 1991), very similar results are seen, although the temperature increase has less of an effect.

RFR Exposure and Chromosome Aberration Induction

In these investigations, the RFR exposure parameters (Table I in Kerbacher et al., 1990) were virtually the same as listed above. The RFR exposure time was two hours.

The data summarized in Table II of Kerbacher et al. (1990), show that under these exposure conditions, pulsed wave microwave radiation does not cause chromosome aberrations of any type examined. Extending these studies to look for an interaction between simultaneous 2450 MHz PW RFR exposure and Mitomycin C (chemical clastogen) treatment (at two different chemical concentrations), Tables III and IV of Kerbacher et al. (1990) do not indicate any effect of the RFR exposure on the chemical induction of chromosome aberrations.

Subsequent experiments were performed with a chemical clastogen which interacts with DNA through a different mechanism, Adriamycin. Table IV of Kerbacher et al. (1990) summarizes the results of a simultaneous Adriamycin and RFR exposure and shows only one statistically significant difference between 37° C control + AdR and RFR + AdR. This difference was in "total aberration events per 100 cells." The same increase, however, was seen in the temperature control, and therefore was not due to the RFR as a form of radiation, but rather as a source of increased temperature.

RFR Exposure and Phenotypic Mutation

The L5178Y mutation assay was performed using exposure parameters which were only slightly different from those used in the SCE and chromosome aberration studies (see Meltz et al., 1989, 1990). The exposure time was increased to four hours.

Table I of Meltz et al. (1989) shows a comparison of the mutation frequency per 10^6 viable cells, in 5 different (independent) experiments, for RFR-exposed vs. temperature control vs. 37° C conditions. In this assay, it was understood that a doubling of the mutation frequency compared to the 37° C control is required to indicate that the treatment-agent was a weak mutagen. This is clearly not the case for RFR exposure. This same result was seen in three more experiments, performed in a separate investigation (Table 1, Meltz et al., 1990). In the latter study, the induced mutant frequency, which is obtained by subtracting the 37° C control mutant frequency from the experimental mutant frequency, also demonstrated this absence of RFR induction of mutation.

The possible effect of simultaneous RFR exposure on chemical induced mutation was examined for Mitomycin C (Meltz et al., 1989) and proflavin (Meltz et al., 1990). In both cases, there were no statistically significant differences between the RFR, the temperature control, and the 37° C exposure conditions during the simultaneous treatment.

The conclusions from this series of investigations are as follows:

1) Microwave radiation exposures without an elevation of temperature appear not to be genotoxic. Radio frequency radiation exposure therefore cannot act as an initiator for cancer induction (to the extent that the initiation, promotion, progression model is relevant).

2) Microwave radiation exposures, at least at the frequency of 2450 MHz, also are not able to alter the induction of SCEs, chromosome aberrations, or phenotypic mutations resulting from a simultaneous chemical mutagen treatment.

These observations imply that:

a) the uptake of genotoxic chemicals into the cells was not affected;

b) the ability of the different chemicals to reach the DNA was not affected;

c) the ability of the chemicals to damage the DNA was not affected; and

d) the ability of the cells to perform those biochemical steps which would result in the expression of SCEs, chromosome aberrations, or phenotypic mutations was not affected. (The steps involved include, for chromosome aberrations, breakage reunion during and/or subsequent to the exposure period; for mutation, the steps include error prone repair occurring during the exposure and subsequent expression period.)

Issues Relevant to Recent Positive Reports of Genotoxicity

Considering the abundance of evidence, including the studies described above, demonstrating that microwave radiation exposures at a variety of frequencies are not genotoxic without an elevation of temperature, several recent reports suggesting otherwise need to be examined for their technical merit. These include reports by Maes, Verschave, Arroyo, De Wagter, and Vercruyessen (1993), Garaj-Vrhovac, Horvat, and Koren (1990, 1991), and Garaj-Vrhovac, Fucic, and Horvat (1992).

In the Maes et al. (1993) study, which reported microwave induction of chromosome aberrations in human lymphocytes, a metal thermistor probe enclosed in a syringe needle was immersed in the sample during the exposure. Correct technique requires the use of non-microwave interactive probes (and no metal) in the sample being irradiated. The metal thermistor/shielding syringe needle was basically an antenna, and the heating pattern in its vicinity is unknown.

With respect to the series of reports by Garaj-Vrhovac et al. (1990, 1991, 1992), with exposures at 7.7 GHz, after which chromosome aberrations were reported, careful reading of one of the manuscripts reveals that the authors themselves state that the temperature of the cells during the exposure was not known. The experimental details are so poorly stated that it is unclear if the exposures were properly performed. The cells were said to be irradiated "in a semi-permeable membrane," but it is not stated if the membrane was in a tissue culture container and immersed under medium during the exposure (and, if so, how much medium was present), or if the membrane was simply placed under the antenna on the supporting table. One set of survival curves presented in one of the papers appears to be similar to standard thermal survival curve data, i.e., demonstrating increased killing at elevated temperatures with time. Unfortunately, no temperature measurements during the exposure are described.

References

SISTER CHROMATID EXCHANGE INDUCTION

Ciaravino, V., Meltz, M. L., & Erwin, D. N. (1987). Effects of radio frequency radiation and simultaneous exposure with Mitomycin C on the frequency of sister chromatid exchanges in Chinese hamster ovary cells. Environmental Mutagenesis, 9, 393-399.

Ciaravino, V., Meltz, M. L., & Erwin, D. N.. (1991). Absence of a synergistic effect between moderate-power radio-frequency electromagnetic radiation and Adriamycin on cell-cycle progression and sister-chromatid exchanges. Bioelectromagnetics, 12(5), 289-298.

Kerbacher, J.J., Meltz, M.L., & Erwin, D.N. (1990). Influence of Radio frequency radiation on chromosome aberrations in CHO cells and its interaction with DNA-damaging agents. Radiation Research, 12, 311-319.

DNA REPAIR INDUCTION (INDICATING DNA DAMAGE), AND DNA REPAIR INHIBITION

Meltz, M. L., Walker, K. A., & Erwin, D. N. (1987). Radio frequency (microwave) radiation exposure of mammalian cells during UV-induced DNA repair synthesis. Radiation Research, 110, 255-266.

MUTATION INDUCTION AT THE THYMIDINE KINASE LOCUS

Meltz, M. L., Eagan, P., & Erwin, D. N. (1989). Absence of mutagenic interaction between microwaves and Mitomycin C in mammalian cells. Environmental and Molecular Mutagenesis, 13, 294-303.

Meltz, M. L., Eagan, P., & Erwin, D. N. (1990). Proflavin and microwave radiation: Absence of a mutagenic interaction. Bioelectromagnetics, 11, 149-157.

REPORTS CONSIDERED FOR TECHNICAL MERIT

Garaj-Vrhovac, V., Fucic, A., & Horvat, D. (1992). The correlation between the frequency of micronuclei and specific chromosome aberrations in human lymphocytes exposed to microwave radiation in vitro. Mutation Research, 281, 181-186.

Garaj-Vrhovac, V., Horvat, D., & Koren, Z. (1990). The effect of microwave radiation on the cell genome. Mutation Research, 243, 87-93.

Garaj-Vrhovac, V., Horvat, D., & Koren, Z. (1991). The relationship between colony-forming ability, chromosome aberrations and incidence of micronuclei in V79 Chinese hamster cells exposed to microwave radiation. Mutation Research, 263, 143-149.

Maes, A., Verschave, L., Arroyo, A., De Wagter, C., & Vercruyessen, L. (1993). In vitro cytogenetic effects of 2450 MHz waves on human peripheral blood lymphocytes. Bioelectromagnetics, 14, 495-501.

9

CONSIDERATIONS REGARDING THE USE OF IN VITRO TRANSFORMATION AND ALKALINE COMET ASSAYS TO ASSESS THE CARCINOGENIC POTENTIAL OF RADIOFREQUENCY RADIATION

Joseph L. Roti Roti, Robert S. Malyapa, and Eric Ahern

Transformation Assays

We are using the murine embryonic cell line (C_3H 10T½) system to measure the ability of certain agents to induce or promote neoplastic transformation according to the method described by Reznikoff, Bertram, Brankow, and Heidelberger (1973). One advantage of this system is that an international protocol has been established (International Agency for Research on Cancer/National Cancer Institute/U.S. Environmental Protection Agency Working Group, 1985). Further, the type II and III transformants which are scored have been shown to produce tumors when implanted into nude mice (Hall & Miller, 1977). Because carcinogenic agents, i.e., ionizing radiation, are also lethal, the dynamic range of the assay can be limited (Hall & Hei, 1987). While this situation might appear to be a disadvantage, it in fact provides us with the means to determine how well the system is calibrated. With this method, care must be taken to ensure that variables are controlled or documented. Two obvious issues are the serum lot and minimizing the background. However, I would like to consider another source of variability as shown in the plot of transformation frequencies vs. γ-ray dose (Figure 1). It can be seen that the standard deviations on the irradiated samples are unacceptably large. While one could argue that the differences in the mean values are statistically different, the difference between the background value and that for 1.5 Gy is within the 95% confidence limit of the latter. The question then arises: "Is this error random or systematic?" Since transformation frequency is related to the number of viable cells plated in each flask (Figure 2), this uncertainty appears to be systematic. Further, the increase in transformation frequency with decreasing cell number is larger when cells have been irradiated. If limits (300-500) are set on the number of viable cells per flask, then the uncertainty associated with each of these transformation values is significantly reduced (Figure 3). Thus, the mean transformation frequency of the 1.5 Gy point is well beyond the 95% limits of the 0 and 4.5 Gy values. Clearly, the assay is sensitive enough to measure the initiation

114

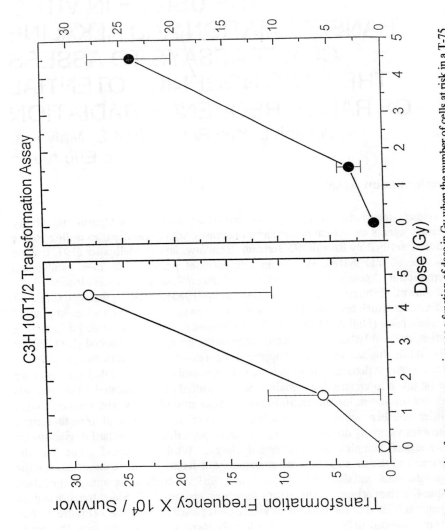

Figure 1. Transformation frequency per survivor as a function of dose in Gy when the number of cells at risk in a T-75 flask range from 250-700 cells (left panel) and 300-450 cells (right panel).

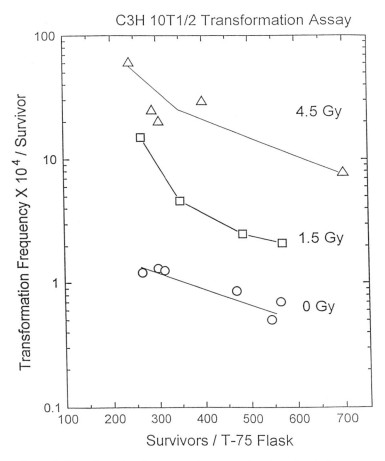

C3H 10T1/2 Transformation Assay

Transformation Frequency X 10^4 / Survivor

4.5 Gy

1.5 Gy

0 Gy

Survivors / T-75 Flask

Figure 2. Transformation frequency plotted as a function of radiation dose versus the number of survivors at risk.

of transformation by x-ray doses above 1 Gy. By adding a promoter (such as TPA), it is possible to push the sensitivity of this assay to approximately 0.3-0.5 Gy (Kennedy, Murphy, & Little, 1980). Thus, we believe that with proper controls, the observation of a reproducible dose-dependent response which is enhanced by promoters and reduced by suppressors would be unlikely to be sporadically positive.

DNA Damage Assays

In the neoplastic transformation assay, the frequency of tumorigenic cells arising from normal embryonic cells is a well characterized end point. In contrast, the alkaline comet assay appears to have a less well characterized end point. This assay was designed as a method to measure radiation-induced DNA damage on a cell-by-cell

116

basis (Olive, Wlodek, Durand, & Banath, 1992; Ostling & Johanson, 1984; Singh, Stephens, & Schneider, 1994; Tice, Andrews, & Singh, 1990). Further, it has been reported that brain cells removed from rats exposed to 1.2 W/kg of 2450 MHz electromagnetic radiation manifest DNA damage as measured by this assay (Lai & Singh, 1995). Therefore, additional efforts to characterize exactly what is being measured is of great interest. Clearly, the assay is very sensitive. Dose response curves of Chinese hamster fibroblasts clearly show that the assay can measure radiation-induced DNA damage following doses as low as 1.0 cGy (Figure 4). (In work with other cell lines, we were able to detect DNA damage following doses below 1 cGy; see below.) In this regard, it is also of interest to examine the size distributions of the comet lengths of the comets in these irradiated populations (Figure 5). As can been seen comparing the 0 cGy and 1 cGy distributions, the mean and the mode of the population clearly shifts up with radiation dose, and each of these distributions basically has one population of comets, although at the higher dose levels the tails present quite a long distribution. We also did a preliminary study with isolated brain cells, and the dose response curve (Figure 6) demonstrates that this assay is sensitive enough to measure a radiation dose response in excised in vivo tissue. However, it should be noted that the comet length of the untreated sample was a bit higher than that seen in the tissue culture cells. We pursued this issue further in the following pilot experiment. Two rats at a time were placed in the chamber and were euthanized by CO_2 asphyxiation. After the rats were dead, one rat was dissected first and the next rat was dissected second. The time difference was between 1 and 1-1/2 min. As one can see, the mean comet length obtained in these rat brain cells from both hippocampus and the cortex was very sensitive to the difference in dissection time (Figure 7). If we look at the distribution of these comet lengths (Figure 8), one can clearly see that there are two separate populations of cells, one with a size around 120 µm and the other with mean around 20 µm (see the lower panel). The population with the mean around 20 µm consists of comets without tails, i.e., undamaged ones. The viabilities by dye exclusion assays are shown in each of the panels. These populations have a very high level of viability and yet apparently DNA damage is being induced during the time interval between death and dissection. It is known that brain cells will respond to oxygen deprivation by inducing apoptosis. The apoptotic process includes controlled cutting of the DNA. These types of damage distributions may be indicative of apoptosis secondary to the method of euthanasia. It should be noted that this is not exactly the method that Lai and Singh used, but our intention was to confirm their results with an assay which theoretically should be equivalent.

Another study we have undertaken is to utilize Hoechst staining, which is known as a vital dye. In other words, there is "no" toxicity associated with this dye. It is used to fluorescently label cells for cell sorting. The sorted cells show only a small loss in clonogenicity. This method has been used in numerous studies. Surprisingly, we found that this method causes damage detectable by the alkaline comet assay. In Figure 9, various conditions are compared, i.e., cells which were: 1) unstained; 2) stained with Hoescht (2.5 µM), but not sorted; 3) sorted, but not stained; and 4) stained and sorted. Clearly, the cells that were stained and sorted manifested a great deal of damage by the alkaline comet assay. This damage appears not to be lethal. Further, given the possible mechanism of induction, it is unlikely that the damage is single-

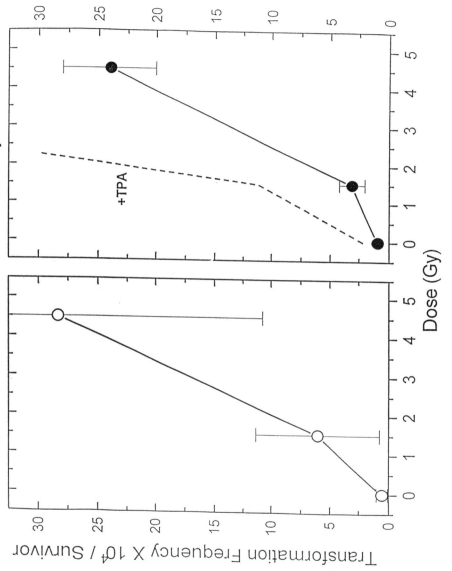

<u>Figure 3.</u> The effects of tumor promoter TPA (0.1 µg/ml) on radiation-induced neoplastic transformation.

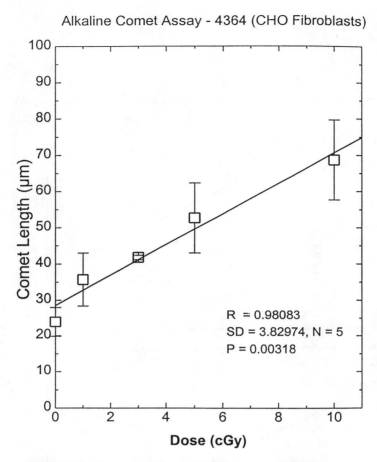

Figure 4. Alkaline comet assay—relationship between tail-length and radiation dose on CHO fibroblsats. Note that the sensitivity is 1 cGy.

strand DNA breaks. Another possibility is that basic sites have been induced which are alkaline labile bonds. The point of these studies is to illustrate the need for any positive result obtained with the alkaline comet assay to be verified by other methods. In our work, we include at least two other assays to attempt to characterize any damage to which this assay responds. As above, we believe that a well characterized response detected by these assays is unlikely to be a "sporadic positive."

Program Overview

The goal of our project is to assess the carcinogenic potential and related biological

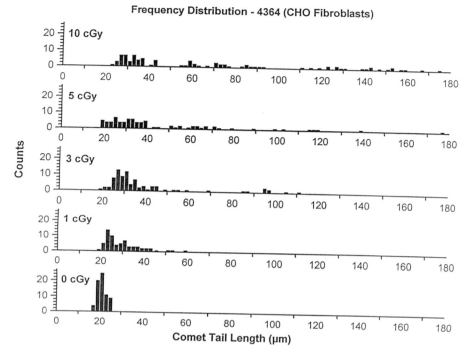

Figure 5. Frequency distribution of comet tail lengths irradiated from 0 to 10 cGy.

effects of 850 and 2450 MHz electromagnetic radiation. In our group, since we deal with ionizing radiation, we chose to use the acronym NIEMR for nonionizing electromagnetic radiation. We plan to accomplish this goal through of a series of interrelated research and testing projects which are intended to cover a wide variety of possible biological effects. Basically, the project is divided into teams. The various teams are responsible for the completion of two to four projects. Also, there are two support cores: an Engineering team and an FCM team. Our group spends a lot of time studying cell proliferation and a good FCM team is critical to this endeavor.

The biological portion of the project is divided into four teams. First, there is an in vivo team, and it has the goal of assessing the possible promotion effect and tumor-bed effect of NIEMR. This team has two projects: a tumor-bed effect project using the 9L rat glioma system and a promotion study with ENU as the inducer. We have a Genotoxicity team responsible for three projects. One is a project to confirm the work of Lai and Singh (1995). Another project is to directly measure any possible in vitro promotion and induction of neoplastic transformation. The third project is to determine if there are any changes induced in nuclear matrix proteins. We have a Gene Expression team. Their projects include studies to measure oncogene expression, studies to measure the binding of transcription factors, testing for effects on differentiation signaling, and testing to determine if there is any altered mRNA expression. We have a Signal Transduction and Cell Physiology team. They have

120

three projects, including a study of intracellular communication and signaling, a study of the effects of RFR on oxidative stress and the cells' response to oxidative stress, and a project to look at any effects on cellular or cell membrane physiology.

Our research plan is to conduct a series of standardized and established tests concurrently with parallel research projects designed to understand the mechanisms of any positive response that a given test might detect. In this context, we are going to assume positive responses are telling us something that needs to be understood rather than being statistical outliers. Our overall philosophy is that an integrated research and testing program, in the long run, will be the most cost-effective manner to produce definitive answers regarding the health effect of NIEMR.

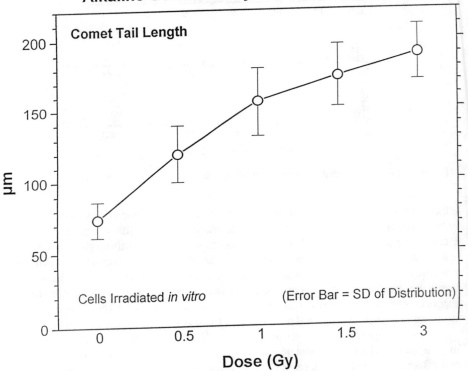

Figure 6. Radiation dose response of rat hippocampus cells irradiated in vitro.

Updated Results with the Alkaline Comet Assay

The alkaline comet assay, according to the method of Olive et al. (1992), was used to measure DNA damage in rat lymphocytes isolated from whole blood following low doses of γ-radiation, 0.5 cGy. The comet parameters, normalized comet moment, and

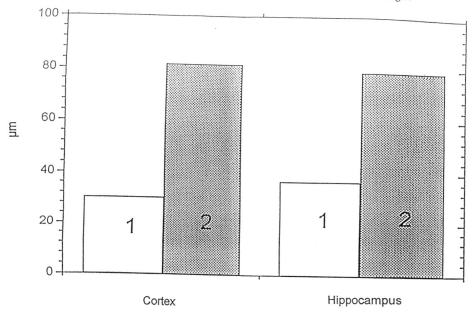

Figure 7. Effect of time of brain dissection on comet tail length of cells isolated from either the cortex or the hippocampus of sham treated Sprague-Dawley rats. "1" refers to the group of rats dissected first after euthanasia, and "2" refers to the group dissected second.

comet length described by Kent, Eady, Ross, and Steel (1995) were obtained by image analysis and used as measures of DNA damage. These results from rat lymphocytes and those from C3H 10T1/2 cells and U87MG cells (see below) are comparable with data obtained using the alkaline comet assay according to the method of Singh et al. (1994). It was observed that the alkaline comet assay can detect DNA damage at doses as low as 0.6 cGy. Therefore, we conclude that the Olive version of the alkaline comet assay is as sensitive as the Lai and Singh modification of the comet assay and should be equally able to detect DNA strand breaks. (A manuscript describing this work has been submitted for publication.)

Our first NIEMR studies were to determine if exposure of cultured mammalian cells in vitro to 2450 MHz radiation causes DNA damage. The alkaline comet assay was used to measure DNA damage after in vitro 2450 MHz irradiation of exponentially growing U87MG and C3H 10T1/2 cells. Exposures were done in specially-designed radial transmission lines (RTLs) that provided relatively uniform microwave exposure. Specific absorption rates (SARs) were 0.7 and 1.9 W/kg. Temperatures were monitored continuously in real time and remained at $37 \pm 0.3°$ C. Every experiment included sham exposure(s) in an RTL. Positive controls were irradiated with 0.3 - 3 cGy of γ-rays. Cells were irradiated for 2 hours, 2 hours, followed by a 4 hour

Frequency Distribution - Effect Of Time Of Dissection On Comet Tail Length
(Note: "1" refers to rat dissected first and "2" to rat dissected second)

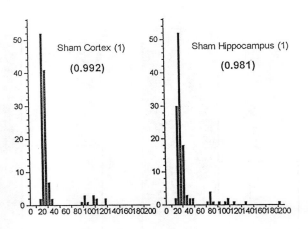

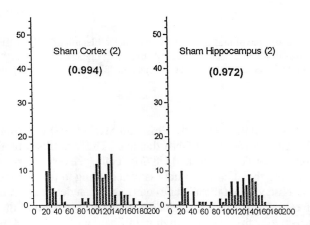

Comet Tail Length (μm)

Figure 8. Shows the frequency distribution of comet tail lengths from the brain of rats dissected first and those dissected second.

incubation at 37° C in an incubator, 4 hours and 24 hours. After these treatments, samples were analyzed by the alkaline comet assay as described by Olive et al. (1992). Images of comets were digitized and analyzed using a PC-based image analysis system. The normalized comet moment and comet length were determined. No significant differences were observed between the exposed group and the controls after exposure to 2450 MHz continuous wave (CW) irradiation. Thus, 2450 MHz irradiation does not appear to cause DNA damage in cultured mammalian cells as measured by the alkaline comet assay. (A manuscript describing this work has been accepted by *Radiation Research*.)

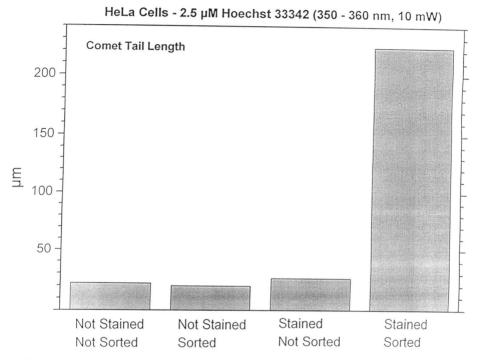

Figure 9. Shows the effect of UV and Hoechst 33342 on the comet tail length.

Mouse C3H 10T1/2 fibroblasts and human glioblastoma U87MG cells were exposed to cellular phone communication frequency radiations in order to determine if such exposure produces DNA damage in in vitro cultures. Two frequency modulations were studied: frequency modulated continuous wave (FMCW), with a carrier frequency of 835.62 MHz, and code division multiple access (CDMA), centered on 847.74 MHz. Exponentially growing (U87MG and C3H 10T1/2 cells) and plateau phase cultures (C3H 10T1/2 cells) were exposed to either FMCW or CDMA for periods of time up to 24 hours in specially-designed RTLs at an SAR of 0.6 W/kg. Temperatures in the RTLs were monitored continuously and maintained at $37 \pm 0.3\,^\circ C$. Sham exposure of cultures in an RTL (negative control) were included with every experiment, while ^{137}Cs irradiated cell samples were used as positive controls. The alkaline comet assay as described by Olive et al. (1992) was used to measure DNA damage. No significant differences in comet length or normalized comet moment were observed between cells exposed to either FMCW or CDMA or sham treated cells. Our results indicate that exposure of cultured mammalian cells to cellular phone communication frequencies with these modulations at an SAR of 0.6 W/kg does not cause DNA damage measurable by the alkaline comet assay. (A manuscript describing this work has been accepted by *Radiation Research*).

To confirm the reported observation that low intensity, acute exposure to 2450 MHz radiation causes DNA single-strand breaks (Lai & Singh, 1995), male Sprague-Dawley rats weighing approximately 250 g were irradiated with 2450 MHz, CW microwaves for 2 hours at an SAR of 1.2 W/kg in a cylindrical wave guide system (Guy, Wallace, & McDougall, 1979), with no associated temperature rise in the core body temperature of the rats. After irradiation or sham treatment, rats were euthanized by either CO_2 asphyxia or by guillotine (8 pairs of animals per euthanasia group). The brains were then removed and immediately immersed in cold Ames saline; the cells from the cerebral cortex and the hippocampus were dissociated separately and subjected to the alkaline comet assay. Irrespective of the euthanasia method, no significant differences were found between the sham treated and brain cells from either the cerebral cortex or the hippocampus of the exposed rats in terms of the comet length or the normalized comet moment. However, the data from the CO_2 asphyxiated rats showed more intrinsic DNA damage and more experiment-to-experiment variation than did the data from rats euthanized by guillotine. Therefore, the guillotine method of euthanasia is the most appropriate for studies of DNA damage. We were unable to confirm the observation that DNA damage is produced in cells of the rat cerebral cortex or the hippocampus after a 2 hours exposure to 2459 MHz, CW microwaves or at 4 hours after the exposure. (A manuscript describing this work has been submitted.)

References

Guy, A. W., Wallace, J., & McDougall, J. A. (1979). Circular polarized 2450 MHz waveguide system for chronic exposure of small animals to microwaves. Radio Science, 14, 63-74.

Hall, E. J., & Miller R. C. (1977). The how and why of in vitro oncogenic transformation. Radiation Research, 87, 452.

Hall E. J., & Hie, T. K. (1990). Modulation factors in the expression of radiation-induced oncogenic transformation. Environmental Health Perspectives, 88, 149.

International Agency for Research on Cancer/National Cancer Institute/U.S. Environmental Protection Agency Working Group. (1985). Cellular and molecular mechanisms of cell transformation and standardization of transformation assays of established cell lines for the prediction of carcinogenic chemicals: Overview and recommended protocols. Cancer Research, 45, 2395-2399.

Kennedy, A. R., Murphy, G., & Little, J. B. (1980). Effect of time and duration of exposure to 12-0-Tetradecanoylphorbol-3-acetate on x-ray transformation of C3H 10T1/2 cells. Cancer Research, 40, 1915-1920.

Kent, C. R. H., Eady, J. J., Ross, G. M., & Steel, G. C. (1995). The comet moment as a measure of DNA damage in the comet assay. International Journal of Radiation Biology, 67, 655-660.

Lai, H., & Singh, N. P. (1995). Acute low-intensity microwave exposure increases DNA single-strand breaks in rat brain cells. Bioelectromagnetics, 16, 207-210.

Olive, P. L., Wlodek, D., Durand, R. E., & Banath, J. P. (1992). Factors influencing DNA migration from individual cells subjected to gel electrophoresis. Experimental Cell Research, 198, 259-267.

Ostling, O., & Johanson, K. J. (1984). Microelectrophoresis study of radiation-induced DNA damage in individual mammalian cells. Biochemical and Biophysical Research Communications, 123, 291-298.

Reznikoff, C. A., Bertram, J. S., Brankow, D. S., & Heidelberger, C. (1973). Quantitative and qualitative studies on chemical transformation of cloned C3H mouse embryo cells sensitive to post-confluence inhibition of cell division. Cancer Research, 33, 3239-3249.

Singh, N. P., Stephens, R. E., & Schneider, E. L. (1994). Modifications of alkaline microgel electrophoresis for sensitive detection of DNA damage. International Journal of Radiation Biology, 66, 23-28.

Tice, R. R., Andrews, P., & Singh, N. P. (1990). The single cell gel assay: A sensitive technique for evaluating intercellular differences in DNA damage and repair. Basic Life Science, 53, 291-301.

10

COMMENTS ON "GENOTOXICITY OF RADIOFREQUENCY RADIATION"
Sheldon Wolff

Concerns have been raised about the possible genotoxic (and therefore carcinogenic) effects of radiofrequency radiations (RFRs). These concerns have prompted the initiation of a research program to ascertain whether or not RFRs are indeed mutagenic. To understand the nature of the genotoxic effects, it is first necessary to illustrate the various types of genetic damage manifested as mutations.

Induced mutations can be broadly classified into two groups: those that are true point mutations or intragenic mutations and those that are gross chromosomal changes or intergenic mutations. The latter class, when induced by physical agents, comprises by far the largest group of mutations obtained. The reason for this lies in the difference in size between a single locus, which is used in the usual mutation study, and a whole genome. To fix our ideas on this, we can compare a very large gene, which could contain 30 kB of DNA (30,000 bases), to the entire genome, which contains three billion bases. Thus, gross chromosomal changes observable in cells are 100,000 to 1 million times larger than a single locus.

True point mutations, in the purest sense, would consist of a single base change in the gene. Each amino acid in a protein is specified in the DNA as a three-letter code consisting of a permutation of three of the four bases adenine (A), thymine (T), guanine (G), and cytosine (C). An analogy attributed to L. Lerman, based on the three-letter DNA code, represents the code for a protein by the sentence THE CAT SAT AND ATE THE RAT ... If there is a single base change, it could result in a missense mutation in which a different amino acid would be substituted in the protein. Such a missense mutation could be seen if the C in the second word is substituted with a B so that the sentence would now read THE BAT SAT AND ATE THE RAT ... Other mutations could be the result of the deletion or addition of a single base. For instance, deletion of the E in the first word would result in a frameshift or nonsense mutation, in which every subsequent amino acid and thus the whole protein is changed, i.e., THC ATS ATA NDA TET HER AT...

Small deletions of this type or small insertions cannot be visualized in cytological preparations of cells in which the chromosomes can actually be seen with the aid of a compound microscope. Thus, these changes are still considered point mutations. As deletions or insertions become larger, however, this class of mutation grades into those that would be visible, and, therefore, would be classified as gross chromosomal changes. Also included in this latter class are exchanges between different parts of chromosomes, which include not only the insertions, but also the formation of dicentric chromosomes, ring chromosomes, and translocations, which come from the breakage of the chromosome and the subsequent rejoining of the broken pieces in abnormal ways.

The most commonly studied physical agent for the induction of mutations has been ionizing radiations, which include X-rays. Biophysical studies had earlier shown that irradiation of antibodies with electrons of different energies only inhibited binding to antigens at energy levels over the ionization potential of 1.5 electron volts (ev).

With ultraviolet light, on the other hand, one can get thymine dimers and other photoproducts in the DNA that will cause errors in replication when the cells enter the S phase. Therefore, with UV light, if one looks for the types of cytogenetically observable mutations or aberrations, one finds that they are chromatid types of aberrations rather than full chromosome aberrations.

With the use of ionizing radiations, which have enough energy to break chemical bonds, it has been found that chromosomes are usually broken by clusters of ionizations. It should be noted that a single ionization has an energy level of approximately 32 ev, whereas a carbon-carbon bond in an organic molecule has an energy level of only about 4-5 ev.

Over the years, it had been inferred that most mutations were indeed chromosomal in origin, i.e., were deletions or other chromosomal changes. The reasons for this were that most induced mutations were homozygous lethals, and that densely ionizing radiations such as neutrons or alpha rays, which are more efficient at producing chromosomal effects, have a high relative biological effectiveness in the induction of mutations. With recent molecular techniques whereby one can actually study the changes observed at the DNA level, this inference has been borne out in that most induced mutations, indeed, are chromosomal in origin.

The types of aberrations induced by ionizing radiations vary depending on the part of the cell cycle irradiated. If cells in G_1 (the part of the cell cycle before DNA is synthesized) are irradiated, the chromosomes react to radiation as though they are a single strand, even though they are composed of a DNA double helix and associated proteins. Thus, one gets simple breaks in chromosomes. If these are allowed to enter the S phase (where DNA is synthesized) before any repair has gone on, then the broken chromosome is replicated so that at metaphase the full chromosome (i.e., both chromatids) are broken. Such chromosome aberrations increase linearly with the dose of radiation, indicating that they are one-hit phenomena. Such aberrations are produced at the time of the single "hit" and thus are independent of the time over which the radiation is given; that is, they are independent of the intensity of the radiation or whether or not the radiation is fractionated into several small doses.

Other aberrations, however, such as translocations, dicentrics, and ring chromosomes, come about from the production of two separate breaks in the chromosomes, followed by the illegitimate rejoining, or misrepair, that leads to the broken ends rejoining not with themselves, but with other broken ends. Since such aberrations require the production of two breaks, they have been found to increase as the square of the dose—as expected, since the probability (p) of getting a single break is directly proportional to dose (D), and the chance, therefore, of getting two breaks would be p x p and would be proportional to p^2 or D^2.

Furthermore, because a large proportion of the single breaks become repaired or restitute, such two-hit aberrations, when induced with sparsely ionizing radiations, are subject to an intensity or dose fractionation effect, whereby fewer aberrations are produced as the intensity of the radiation is lowered or if there is time for repair between individual fractions of the dose. That is, because of repair, breaks produced at the first part of the dose will not be present in the cell at the time additional breaks are produced by the latter parts of the dose. Because the breaks are not in the cell concurrently, they cannot interact with one another to form gross chromosomal changes. Therefore, the yield of this type of mutation is dependent both upon the total dose and the time the dose is delivered.

Up until now, the aberrations commonly used for dosimetric purposes have been the dicentrics produced in human lymphocytes in the peripheral blood. The use of this cell has many advantages. In the first place, dicentrics are produced when two broken chromosomes exchange parts and leave behind an acentric fragment that will not be included in the daughter cells when the lymphocytes divide. Thus, the daughter cells will be genetically imbalanced and will die. This means that there is a very low background of dicentrics in peripheral blood lymphocytes. The peripheral blood lymphocyte is also a long-lived cell in which all the chromosomes are in G_o (i.e., cells that are not cycling) and thus are not subject to cell stage sensitivity differences. Further, the cells can be obtained by simple venipuncture, which is essentially a noninvasive technique.

The corollary type of aberration is the translocation, in which the acentric pieces of each broken chromosome rejoin with the centric pieces from the other chromosome so that genes from one chromosome are translocated to another. No material is lost and the cells usually are viable. This process then forms one type of actual mutation. When genes become translocated, they could become activated if they are moved next to a promoter, they could become inactivated, or they could even lead to the formation of a new type of protein. Until recently, quantitative studies of the induction of chromosomal changes, especially to determine doses, has relied upon the production of dicentrics, mainly because they could be determined unequivocally with the staining methods available. Translocations, on the other hand, could only be observed if the fragments exchanged were grossly unequal. The advent of new fluorescent in situ hybridization methods show great promise for changing this so that translocations and insertions will be able to be seen with great precision irrespective of their size.

Another cytogenetic assay that has been used to estimate genetic change is the induction of micronuclei. As noted above, many of the chromosomal changes that are induced result in the deletion of large pieces of chromosomes. These pieces, not having a centromere, will not segregate to the poles of the dividing cell and will not be included in the daughter nucleus, but will form a separate micronucleus. Occasionally, nondisjunction of a whole chromosome will occur because of chromosomes lagging on the spindle, but this is a minor contribution to the numbers of micronuclei that are found. Although micronuclei are derived from chromosomal aberrations, their use as a measure of mutation suffers from many drawbacks that are not found when aberrations are observed. For instance, the background numbers of micronuclei found in peripheral blood lymphocytes is rather high and quite variable from person to person. It thus becomes impossible to tell what was induced in a given individual unless that individual had been sampled prior to the exposure. Furthermore, the shape of the dose curve is always linear with dose, even though a large proportion of the fragments come from the formation of dicentrics and other two-hit aberrations that should contribute a large two-hit or dose-squared component to the curves.

The fact that chromosome aberrations are the result of double-strand DNA breaks and not single-strand breaks raises serious conceptual concerns about the use of the single-cell-gel, or comet, assay that often is carried out under highly basic conditions that lead to the production of the single-strand breaks in DNA. Thus, the endpoint observed, although indicating that DNA damage can occur, might not be related to mutation.

As noted above, in order to produce a biological effect, energy has to be absorbed. In a simple sense, the dose then ordinarily would be considered to be the rate at which the energy is absorbed multiplied by the time over which it is absorbed. This then will give the total energy absorbed. With chemicals, a similar concept is used in that dose is considered to be the concentration of the chemical times the time that it is administered.

With RFRs, it has been observed that there is not enough energy to produce chromosome breaks or genetic changes directly. It has also been noted that to see any biological effects at all, high specific absorption rates (SARs) are needed. The SAR, however, does not really tell how much energy is being absorbed; it is only a rate. Exposure to a high SAR for one second will not be the same as exposure to that same high SAR for an hour. In the latter case, 3600 times as much energy will be absorbed.

With RFRs at higher frequencies, there is the possibility that there could be thermal effects, but even in this case, to get a biological effect, one needs to have the intensity times the time; that is, one needs to have a high enough SAR for a long enough period before there is enough energy in the cell to produce a thermal effect. This is largely because humans are homeothermic organisms, which have efficient mechanisms of reducing internal heat. Furthermore, extensive amounts of energy are needed to break chemical bonds directly, as most people who have toiled in organic chemistry laboratories and have watched vessels boil for long periods of time to drive many of the reactions can attest. It is true, however, that in biological systems this may be less important because many of the reactions are driven catalytically by enzymes. Therefore, enough heat to cause enzyme denaturation or inactivation could lead to a biological effect. Even under such circumstances, however, there is a need to maintain fairly high temperatures for a long time before effects can be seen on such processes as DNA synthesis or protein degradation. For instance, in studies of the effects of hyperthermia, cells often have to be kept at 44-45° C for 15 minutes before effects can be found. A simple 1° or 2° change from 37° C to 38° or 39° has not been effective.

Therefore, in conclusion, I would say that Dr. Brusick's analysis, which has shown that most studies do not show any genetic effects of RFRs, fits with expectations based on biophysical reasoning. Further, I would emphasize that SARs by themselves are inadequate measures of the "dose," which ultimately has to be related to the total energy absorbed.

III

BIOLOGICAL RESPONSES INDICATIVE OF CARCINOGENIC AND OTHER NON-GENETIC EFFECTS

Editor's Note:

Traditionally, animal bioassays with exposure durations ranging from 90 days to two years have been a reliable predictor of human health risk. Like genetic studies, however, animal bioassays must be interpreted in view of other relevant scientific information as part of the weight of evidence. Further, in the post-market surveillance context necessarily applied to wireless communication instruments, animal studies are rarely sufficient in themselves to show a path toward public health intervention.

The papers by Dr. Chiabrera and colleagues, and Drs. Sheppard, Veyret, Tenforde, and Sivak provide a comprehensive background for interpretation of animal bioassays and a summary of conclusions that can be drawn to date from completed studies. It is important to note that exposure systems capable of providing a range of doses for low-power radio frequency radiation have only recently become available. (See the paper by Dr. Chou in Section I). Pivotal bioassay results employing these new exposure systems will be forthcoming in the next three to five years.

Most recently, a special supplement to the *International Journal of Toxicology*, presented a series of papers addressing the relevance of radio frequency to tumor promotion in humans. (See Embrey, M. [Ed.]. [1998]. Relevance of radiofrequency to tumor promotion in humans. International Journal of Toxicology, 17,[Suppl. 3], 1-142.)

G. L. C.

11

RECENT ADVANCES IN THE BIOPHYSICAL MODELING OF RADIOFREQUENCY ELECTROMAGENTIC FIELD INTERACTIONS WITH LIVING SYSTEMS

Alessandro E. Chiabrera, Bruno Bianco, Elsa Moggia, Tullio Tommasi, and Jonathan J. Kaufman

Introduction

The waveforms of the electromagnetic (EM) fields generated by hand-held mobile telecommunication systems near and inside the user's head are rather complex, as they result from: (i) the modulation that transfers the vocal information to the carrier; (ii) the burst mechanism of the time division multiple access, which corresponds to an additional amplitude modulation superimposed on the voice-modulated carrier; (iii) the current drawn from the power supply during the on-time of each burst, which generates a stray magnetic field pulsating at the same repetition rate; and (iv) the burst duty factor.

Therefore, for a normal mode of operation, the corresponding spectrum in the frequency domain includes: (i) the ultrahigh frequency (UHF) carrier frequency surrounded by two side bands, whose width is in the bottom low frequency (LF) range and whose closest internal frequency spacing is related to the extremely low frequency (ELF) current burst and to its duty factor; and (ii) frequency components from ELF to LF related to the current burst and to its duty factor (Anderson, Johansen, Pedersen, & Raskmark, 1995).

As far as the field intensity is concerned, it is classified as low because, in most practical situations, it is well below the safety standard based on time and space averages of EM power deposition in biological tissues. However, the assessment of a biophysical basis for possible bioeffects cannot rely on a traditional interaction mechanism such as tissue heating. In fact, the actual field amplitudes in the time domain and at the tissue points where they reach the maximum values fall in intensity ranges for which some experimental claims exist in the literature about biological effects in electromagnetic exposure at the aforesaid frequencies generated by mobile telecommunication systems (Adey, 1980; Bawin & Adey, 1976; Blackman, Benane, Robinovitz, House, & Joines, 1985; Blackman, Blanchard, Benane, & House, 1995; Carpenter & Ayrapetyan, 1994; Lay, Horita, & Guy, 1994; Miklavcic, Karba,

Vodovnik, & Chiabrera, 1994; Simunic, 1993, 1995).

At present, there is no clear evidence supporting adverse health events. On the other hand, it would be irresponsible to deny a priori such a possibility, in view of the anticipated rapid increase of EM exposure due to the development of personal multimedia communication systems. A preliminary step toward the solution of the problem is to investigate if there exists any biophysical basis for interaction mechanisms between the kind of EM fields so far considered and some specific biological process.

Models of the Interaction Mechanisms

The biophysical models described focus on the understanding of the *first interaction step*, at the molecular level. Any attempt to model subsequent cellular processes seems premature (Chiabrera & Rodan, 1984). Few examples exist in the literature that circumvent the problem of the first interaction step by assuming a priori that it exists and by describing its effects on a phenomenological basis (Pilla, Nasser, & Kaufman, 1994; Tarricone, Cito, & D'Inzeo, 1993; Tsong & Gross, 1994).

The current state of the science suggests that the following elementary processes should be considered as the most likely candidates for the first interaction step:

i.   binding of a ligand ion to a receptor protein;
ii.   transport of a messenger ion through a protein.

The case of Ca^{++} messenger ions is a paradigmatic one. The binding of Ca^{++} ions to calmodulin is a classical example of an interaction step of type i), while its transport through a cell membrane channel is a classical example of type ii). Gated-channel operation and free-radical production are other examples. For instance, the formation of hydroxyl radical OH^- or its encountering a DNA site are elementary processes of type i) which can be related to the cancer issue, for example, if the RF exposure is able to affect the OH^- lifetime or its adsorption to DNA. Alterations of Na^+ and K^+ transport across excitable membranes can be important for brain functions. In general, a variety of proteins serve as active participants in oxidation-reduction processes, where the electron plays the role of a control ligand. The electron binding conditions are not well understood, but it should be kept in mind that even a ligand as small as an electron could be regarded as a potential actor in bioelectromagnetics. Another interesting example is offered by the channel, which runs down the center of the ring-shaped molecules formed where the complementary bases on DNA's two strands meet. At the 1995 meeting of the American Association for the Advancement of Science, experimental evidence was reported that electrons may be shooting down the central channel. Although the biological implications are not clear, the electron-DNA system could be a biological sensor of EM exposure.

In both processes i) and ii), the *system* under investigation is the ion-protein system. The two kinds of processes can be unified, to some extent, by the same modelling approach. The unified model includes an endogenous force $F_{end} = QE_{end}$ which attracts the ion of charge Q to the binding site or sweeps the ion along the channel. The distinction between the two processes stems from the specific spatial conformation of the electric field $\mathbf{E}_{end}(\mathbf{r})$. The spatial coordinate vector $\mathbf{r}$ is representative of the ion position with respect to a reference point in the protein, assumed as the coordinate origin. The evaluation of the value of $\mathbf{E}_{end}(\mathbf{r})$ in the absence of the ion and at thermodynamic equilibrium, denoted in the following by $\mathbf{E}_{th}$, can be obtained from any protein data bank.

Another basic force $\mathbf{F}_{bm} = Q\mathbf{E}_{bm}$, which affects the ion dynamics in the protein proximity, is due to the cell basal metabolism, which biases the system out of thermodynamic equilibrium. We assume that the electric field $\mathbf{E}_{bm}$ is, on average, a steady field so that it may depend on $\mathbf{r}$ only. In order to stress its importance, we quote the prophetic words of Linus Pauling: "We are so far from equilibrium that even *highly improbable reactions* can occur, without violation of the laws of thermodynamics. Many of these highly improbable reactions depend upon having a seed, a *template*, that directs the reaction." The force that could provide the high sensitivity to low-intensity EM fields of the *reaction* between ion and protein is $\mathbf{F}_{bm}$, while the previous force $\mathbf{F}_{end}$ plays the role of the Pauling *template*, which can be highly nonlinear.

The choice of the *state variables* of the system depends on the approach used, a classical or quantum one. We have developed an approximate criterion to establish which approach should be chosen. Let us consider the values taken by the previous field $\mathbf{E}_{end}$ at thermodynamic equilibrium, say $\mathbf{E}_{th}$. The corresponding endogenous potential energy $U_{th}(\mathbf{r})$ goes to zero at infinity and has one or more minima in the protein domain, whose order of magnitude is $(-U_0)$. The order of magnitude of the size of the potential wells is R_c. Then, if $4\pi^2 M R_c^2 U_0 / h^2 > 1$ (M is the ion mass and h is the Planck constant), the classical approach is applicable so that the quantum approach becomes optional. If $4\pi^2 M R_c^2 U_0 / h^2 < 1$, then the quantum approach is the only one to be used. In the case of coulombic potential energy, due to a point charge $(-Q)$, which is divergent for $\mathbf{r} = 0$, the effective value to be used for U_0 is $\{Q^2 / [2(2)^{1/2}\pi\varepsilon_B R_c]\}$, where ε_B is the equivalent dielectric permittivity of the protein, which is taken equal to the permittivity of its embedding medium.

In the classical case, the three components of the ion displacement vector $\mathbf{r}(t)$ and the three components of the ion velocity $d\mathbf{r}/dt$ are the six state variables necessary to describe the temporal evolution of the system. In the quantum case, the matrix components $\rho_{mn}(t)$ of the density operator ρ, represented in a suitable orthonormal base, are the state variables to be used. The reader must be aware that there is no physical analogy between the above classical state variables and the quantum ones. The average temporal evolution $O(t)$ of any observable operator O is given by the trace $O(t) = Tr(O\rho)$.

It is apparent that no explicit state variables are provided for the protein itself. The effects of the actual displacement of the protein charges and of any allosteric conformational change in the protein are incorporated into its dielectric properties and simulated by a correction of the thermodynamic equilibrium value of $\mathbf{E}_{end}$, as discussed in the section "The Endogenous Field."

The *input* signal is the exogenous EM field. If $\mathbf{A}(x, y, z, t)$ is the exogenous vector potential and $\phi(x, y, z, t)$ is the exogenous scalar potential, the input e.m field is given by:

138

$$E = -\nabla\phi - \partial A/\partial t \qquad (1a)$$

$$B = \nabla x A \qquad (1b)$$

where ∇ is the nabla operator, E is the exogenous electric field vector, and B is the exogenous magnetic induction vector. We assume that the values of A and ϕ in situ are derived from the exposure characteristics and that A satisfies the Coulomb gauge $\nabla \cdot A = 0$.

Another *input* to the system is thermal *white* noise, which arises from the random collisions of the system molecules with the thermal bath. In addition, a *coloured* noise due to the cell basal metabolism, which biases the system out of thermodynamic equilibrium, is superimposed on the aforesaid background white noise (Chiabrera, Bianco, Kaufman, & Pilla, 1992; Kaufman, Chiabrera, Hatem, Bianco, & Pilla, 1990; Weaver & Astumian, 1994).

The state variables, e.g., x(t), y(t), z(t) in the classical case or $\rho_{mn}(t)$ in the quantum case, may be chosen as the *output* of the system, in response to its inputs. More representative output variables are the ion binding probability (in process i) or the ion transit time (in process ii). When the messenger ion is close to or inside an allosteric protein, a conformational change may occur that is the signaling event of biological significance. Small conformational changes may imply far-reaching biological consequences. In this case, one should look for an alternative output variable which could reflect the allosteric change.

Once the output has been chosen, it must be evaluated in the absence and in the presence of the exogenous EM exposure. In both conditions, noise is present. *A comparison of the outputs in the two conditions gives an estimate of the exposure effectiveness on the first interaction step.*

The Classical Langevin-Lorentz State Equations

The classical approach to evaluating the first interaction step at the microscopic level is to study how the displacement $r(t)$ of a messenger ion is affected by EM exposure. The related state equations for the ion-protein system are:

$$dr/dt = v \qquad (2a)$$

$$dv/dt = -\beta v + \gamma (E_{end} + E_{bm}) + \gamma (E + v \times B) + n \qquad (2b)$$

For the sake of simplicity, the ion is modeled as a point charge Q with zero intrinsic electric and magnetic moments, $\gamma = Q / M$, and it is assumed that the protein does not generate any endogenous magnetic moment. In this paper, we consider Ca^{++} as a paradigmatic example. In this case, $Q = 3.2 \ 10^{-19}$ C, $M = 6.66 \ 10^{-26}$ kg, and $\gamma = 0.48 \ 10^{7}$ C/kg.

The viscous collision frequency tensor β is a nonlinear function of the components of the endogenous force ($Q\mathbf{E}_{end}$) and accounts for the energy loss of the ion colliding with the surrounding molecules while it is moving at velocity $\mathbf{v}$ (Chiabrera, Bianco, Kaufman et al., 1992). We assume that β is an isotropic diagonal tensor so that it reduces to a single scalar collision frequency. Furthermore, the collisions exert a random force ($M\mathbf{n}$) on the ion, whose ensemble average value is zero. Then β and $\mathbf{n}$ emulate, according to Langevin (Wax, 1954), the effects of the thermal bath on the ion-protein system. Accordingly, the statistical properties of $\mathbf{n}$ are related to β, as will be discussed in the section "NOISE." The noise $\mathbf{n}$ is thus a random input to the system. The exogenous electric field $\mathbf{E}$ and the magnetic induction $\mathbf{B}$ enter the Lorentz force [$Q(\mathbf{E} + \mathbf{v} \times \mathbf{B})$]. They are the known exogenous input signals to the system, as discussed in the section "Exogenous EM Input."

The above equations (2) can model the ion dynamics in various situations, depending on the choice of $\mathbf{E}_{end}(\mathbf{r})$. The important properties of $\mathbf{E}_{end}$ obtained, at thermodynamic equilibrium, from the Protein Data Bank are its very high intensity (on the order of 10 V/Å) and its strong dependence on the displacement components. The first property implies that it cannot be neglected in equation (2b). This argument could lead to the erroneous conclusion that any low-intensity EM exposure has negligible effects on the ion dynamics because the exogenous Lorentz force is small with respect to the endogenous force. Such a conclusion is incorrect because the components of the gradient tensor $\nabla \mathbf{E}_{end}$ are very large (e.g., 10^{11} V/Å^2 as an order of magnitude), and the effects of the exogenous exposure are related also to this tensor. We stress that the endogenous force is the main source of nonlinearity in equations (2), and this is the first paramount property necessary for explaining potential effects of low-intensity exposure in general and at radiofrequencies (RF) in particular. If $\mathbf{E}_{end}$ mimics the field inside the helicoidal path of a membrane channel, the ion cyclotron resonance model (Liboff, 1985; McLeod & Liboff, 1986) can be obtained. However, in the analyses performed by Liboff and McLeod, the authors considered a direct current (DC) magnetic induction $\mathbf{B}_0$ only, without an overall framework for taking into account the effects of the temporal variations in $\mathbf{B}$. They were therefore unable to indicate how the response might vary for different alternating current (AC) magnetic induction intensities and to correlate it with the helix pitch. Some of their results have been re-evaluated (Chiabrera, 1987).

If $\mathbf{E}_{end}$ emulates the field of a potential well, the Larmor precession model (Edmonds, 1993) is obtained. The classical Larmor equation is obtained from equations (2) by using cylindrical coordinates, under the simplifying hypotheses $\beta = 0$ and $\mathbf{B} = [B_0 + B_1(t)]\mathbf{i}_z$. The resulting noise immunity claimed afterwards in Edmonds is a tautology because a noise-immune process was already assumed ($\beta = 0$) as a working hypothesis. Moreover, the ion should probe only a specific portion of the wall of the potential well, in order to be biologically active. Thus, the potential well to start with should be anisotropic, while in Edmonds an isotropic well was considered.

If $\mathbf{E}_{end}$ simulates the restoring force of a binding site, the model described by some others is obtained (Bianco & Chiabrera, 1992; Bianco, Chiabrera, Morro, & Parodi, 1988; Chiabrera & Bianco, 1987; Chiabrera et al., 1985; D'Inzeo, Galli, & Palombo, 1993; Durney, Rushforth, & Anderson, 1988; Galt, Sandblom, & Hamnerius, 1993). These authors have offered the most detailed analysis of equations (2) so far available. In the case of B_0 parallel to $B_1(t) = B_{1M} \sin\omega t$, the relationship between ω and the AC and DC Larmor frequencies $\gamma B_{1M} / 4\pi$ and $\gamma B_0 / 4\pi$, has been found (Bianco & Chiabrera, 1992; Bianco et al., 1988; Chiabrera & Bianco, 1987; Chiabrera et al., 1985) for the maximal or minimal effectiveness (resonances and antiresonances) of the ELF exposure due to a pair of Helmholtz coils. More precisely (see, for example, Figure 3 in Bianco et al., 1988), the maximal effectiveness has been predicted for about integer odd values of the ratio between the AC cyclotron frequency and ω, i.e., $\gamma B_{1M} / \omega = (2n + 1)$, and for about integer values of the ratio between the DC cyclotron frequency and ω, i.e., $\gamma B_0 / \omega = n$, where $n \geq 0$ is any integer number. No effect is predicted for about integer even values $\gamma B_{1M} / \omega = 2n$ and if $\gamma B_0 / \omega$ is not zero nor an integer.

The weakness of the above closed form results, which could be relevant to the ELF exposure component from mobile telephones, is that they have been obtained by letting $\mathbf{E}_{end} = 0$. The same model has been studied in Bianco and Chiabrera (1992); Durney et al. (1988), and Galt et al. (1993), including an endogenous restoring force proportional to ion displacement. The aforesaid resonances and antiresonances were confirmed but the restoring proportionality constant must be smaller than the value expected from the Protein Data Bank. Another important criticism is that these results have not been evaluated taking into account thermal noise effects (Chiabrera, Bianco, Kaufman et al., 1992).

We point out that the values $\mathbf{E}_{th}$ taken by $\mathbf{E}_{end}$, as obtained from the Protein Data Bank, do not consider the so-called "reaction" field $\mathbf{E}_r$ due to both induced polarization and charge displacement, if any, induced by the messenger ion on the protein molecules. This additional contribution to $\mathbf{E}_{end} = \mathbf{E}_{th} + \mathbf{E}_r$ depends on the ion and plays a critical role, as shown in the section "The Endogenous Field."

The output of the ion-protein system can be evaluated from the ensemble average $< \mathbf{r \cdot r} >$ versus time. In the process i) (ligand binding), one assumes that the origin $\mathbf{r} = 0$ corresponds to the ion steady state position in the absence of any exposure. The ion is released at $t = 0$ in a *gedanken* experiment from the position $\mathbf{r} = 0$ at an average velocity $(Q\mathbf{E}_{bm} / M\beta)$. We assume that, if $(< \mathbf{r \cdot r} >) < R_c^2$, the ion is bound to the protein, R_c being the critical binding distance. The order of magnitude of R_c can be 1 nm. The time t^- when $< \mathbf{r \cdot r} > = R_c^2$ gives an estimate of the ion dissociation constant k^- because

$$t^- \cong 1/k^- \tag{3}$$

In the process ii) (messenger transport), the time course of $< \mathbf{r \cdot r} >$ can be used to evaluate the ion transit time t^t through a membrane channel.

The effectiveness of the EM exposure on the process considered is related to the relative difference in the values of the dissociation (transit) time t^- (t^t) in the presence and in the absence of the exogenous field, where noise is always present.

The Quantum Zeeman-Stark State Equation

The quantum mechanical approach to evaluating the first interaction step at the microscopic level is to study how the reduced density operator $\rho(x, y, z, t)$ of a messenger ion is affected by EM exposure. Once a suitable complete set of orthonormal base functions $\psi_n(x, y, z)$ has been chosen, any quantum-mechanical operator O can be described in terms of its matrix components $O_{mn} = \int \psi_m{}^* O \psi_n dx dy dz$, where * means complex conjugate and the integration is performed over the whole space.

Accordingly, the reduced density matrix $\rho(t)$, with elements $\rho_{mn}(t)$, evolves according to the state equation

$$d\rho/dt = -2\pi j[H_{end} + H_{bm} + H_1, \rho]/h - [T,[T,\rho - \rho_0]] \qquad (4)$$

where H_{end} is the endogenous Hamiltonian matrix related to the endogenous force (QE_{end}), H_{bm} is the Hamiltonian matrix related to the basal metabolic force (QE_{bm}), H_1 is the exogenous Hamiltonian matrix related to the scalar potential ϕ and to the vector potential $\mathbf{A}$, and ρ_0 is the steady state value of ρ when $H_1 = 0$. The commutator $[P,Q]$ of the operators P and Q is, by definition, PQ - QP. The lifetime operator T models the interaction with the thermal bath and its expression is given in (Chiabrera, Bianco, & Moggia, 1993). The elements of the double commutator $[T,[T,\rho - \rho_0]]$ contain suitable lifetimes θ_{mn}, τ_{mn}, which are the quantum-mechanical counterparts of the classical collision frequency β and allow the system relaxation to steady state when the exogenous field is removed. For example, the off-diagonal elements (m, n) of the double commutator are $(\rho_{mn} - \rho_{0,mn}) / \tau_{mn}$ (m $\neq$ n), and the resulting diagonal terms (m, m) are $\sum_n [(\rho_{mm} - \rho_{0,mm})/\theta_{h,mm} - (\rho_{nn} - \rho_{0,nn})/\theta_{h,nn}] / \theta_{mn}$. The lifetimes obey the conditions $\theta_{mn} = \theta_{nm} > \tau_{mn} = \tau_{nm} > 0$, for every m $\neq$ n. Finally, ρ_0 is the reduced density matrix in the steady state ($H_1 = 0$) sustained by the basal metabolism of the cell. Its value at thermodynamic equilibrium is ρ_{th}. The integration of equation (4) leads to the evaluation of the matrix $\rho(t)$ so that the observable value of any quantum operator can be computed.

Equation (4) can model the ion dynamics in various situations, depending on the choice of H_{end}. Letting $H_{bm} = 0$ and evaluating the contribution of the Zeeman component in H_1 due to the vector potential only, the ion parametric resonance model proposed in Lednev (1991), based on an earlier atomic spectroscopy theory, could be obtained. This model has been re-evaluated in Blanchard and Blackman (1994) and Lednev (1995). In both cases, the approach is rather heuristic because it is not related to the integration of equation (4). Instead, it is based on the direct computation of the probability transition of the ion between two putative energy levels (states) split by DC and AC Zeeman effects. Thus, the departure and arrival states of the ion (before and after transition) are assumed to be perfectly known (pure states). Such a hypothesis is per se inconsistent because the ion-protein system is open and exchanges energy with a thermal bath. The ion dynamics are instead characterized by a statistical mixture of states, and must therefore be described by the density operator. Furthermore, the ion parametric resonance model does not provide any relaxation mechanism from the excited state to the ground state.

A more satisfactory approach has been adopted in Bianco and Chiabrera (1992), Bianco, Chiabrera, D'Inzeo, Galli, and Palombo (1993), Chiabrera, Bianco, Kaufman, and Pilla (1991), and Chiabrera, Bianco, Tommasi, and Moggia (1992), where $H_{bm} = 0$ and $E_r = 0$, so that $H_{end} = H_{th}$ has been modelled by means of an endogenous attracting potential, of the Coulombic type, which emulates a binding site. The exogenous Hamiltonian has been evaluated in two situations: a Helmholtz exposure system at ELF (weak Zeeman effect) and a transverse electromagnetic (TEM) exposure at RF (combined weak Zeeman and Stark effects). In each situation, the binding probability of the ligand ion has been evaluated, in the presence and absence of exogenous exposure. By doing so, we have been able to prove that resonance effects are possible, but the change in binding probability due to the low-intensity exogenous exposure is negligible. On the other hand, the situation so far considered corresponds to thermal equilibrium ($H_{bm} = 0$). The conditions $H_{bm} = 0$ and $H_{end} = H_{th}$ implies that $\rho_0 = \rho_{th}$, where ρ_{th} is the thermodynamic equilibrium value of ρ. After introducing such a constraint in equation (4), the effect of any low-intensity exposure becomes negligible as compared with thermal noise. As already discussed, such a simplification is not acceptable for living systems, which are out of equilibrium. In our opinion, this is the key point to be addressed, letting $H_{bm} \neq 0$, otherwise, the most important aspect of any interaction mechanism is missed. The Hamiltonian H_{end} is the sum of a thermodynamic-equilibrium Hamiltonian H_{th} and a "reaction" Hamiltonian H_r which simulates the effects (on the ion) of the charge displacement induced by the ion itself on the protein. As previously pointed out, such a charge displacement could lead to an allosteric change of the protein conformation so that H_r also deserves special attention.

In process i), the output of the ion-protein system is $\rho_{mn}(t)$ or the binding probability $\wp(t) = Tr(P\rho)$. The entries of the matrix P are $P_{mn} = \int \psi_m^* \psi_n dxdydz$, where the integration domain is a binding sphere of radius R_c.

In practice, the integration of equation (4) with the boundary condition $\rho(0) = \rho_0$ gives the system transient behaviour $\rho(t)$, corresponding to the onset of the EM exogenous exposure H_1 at $t = 0$. Then, the time evolution of $\rho_{mn}(t)$ can be obtained. Sometimes it is more interesting to compute the limit $\wp_{av} = \lim t \to \infty (1 / t) \int \wp(t)dt$, where the integration domain is [0,t], and to compare it with the value $\wp_0 = Tr(P\rho_0)$ in the absence of any exposure.

In process ii), the transit time t^t across the channel can be computed from the ion displacement $r(t) = Tr(R_\alpha \rho)$, where $\alpha = x, y, z$. The entries of the displacement matrices R_α are $R_{\alpha,mn} = \int \psi_m^* \alpha \psi_n dxdydz$.

The Endogenous Field

In order to clarify the various and important aspects of the endogenous field, let us first consider the case of thermodynamic equilibrium. The importance of classical electrostatics as an approach to the study of charged and polar molecules has been widely recognized (Honig & Nicholls, 1995). On this basis, a reasonable and simple approximation of the endogenous force for a protein receptor is an isotropic restoring force for small values of r, namely:

$$F_{end} \cong QE_{th} \cong -M\omega_{end}^2 r \qquad (r<R_B) \qquad (5)$$

and a Coulombic force for large values of r, namely:

$$F_{end} \cong QE_{th} \cong -\xi r/r^3 \qquad (r>R_B) \qquad (6)$$

where R_B is the pertinent physical dimension of the protein site ($R_B \geq R_C$; Figure 1).

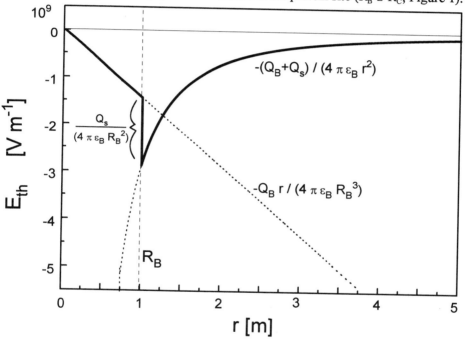

Figure 1. Plot of E_{th} (i.e., E_{end} at thermodynamic equilibrium) versus r, as given by equations (5, 7) and by equations (6, 8). The heavier lines indicate the ranges of validity of the equations. Equations (5, 7) give the electric field of a charge (-Q_B) corresponding to an uniform charge density [-$3Q_B$ / ($4\pi R_B^3$)] inside a sphere of radius R_B and of a charge (-Q_S) corresponding to a uniform surface charge density [-Q_S / ($4\pi R_B^2$)] on the surface of the sphere. Equations (6, 8) give the Coulomb electric field of a point charge - ($Q_S + Q_B$) at r = 0. The parameters chosen in the Figure are R_B = 1 nm, $Q_B = Q_S = Q/2 = 1.6 \times 10^{-19}$ C.

The order of magnitude of ω_{end} is 10^{12}-10^{14} r/s and that of ξ is 10^{-27} Jm for Ca^{++}. The intrinsic protein charge can be subdivided into an inner charge (-Q_B), uniformly distributed in a sphere of radius R_B, and a surface charge $(-Q_S)$, uniformly spread on the protein surface. The overall net protein charge is $[-(Q_B+Q_S)]$. Then, one can derive ω_{end} and ξ from Gauss' law, as follows:

$$\omega_{end} \cong [QQ_B/(4\pi\varepsilon_B MR_B^3)]^{1/2} \qquad (7)$$

$$\xi \cong Q(Q_B+Q_S)/(4\pi\varepsilon_B) \qquad (8)$$

where ε_B is the equivalent dielectric permittivity of the binding site, i.e., we assume that both the protein core and the protein embedding medium have about the same dielectric permittivity ε_B.

In the quantum case, the corresponding potential energies that enter the Hamiltonian are, respectively:

$$U_{end} \cong U_{th} \cong M\omega_{end}^2 r^2/2 \qquad (r<R_B) \qquad (9)$$

$$U_{end} \cong U_{th} \cong -\xi/r \qquad (r>R_B) \qquad (10)$$

as shown by the heavier lines in Figure 2, being $Q\mathbf{E}_{th} = -\nabla U_{th}$.

The choice of equations (5, 9) or (6, 10) and their ranges of application are dictated only by very practical reasons not related to physical reality, i.e., the closed form integrability of some solutions, requiring as a further inconsistency that their ranges of validity in space are extended to any value of r (Figures 1, 2). For example, equation (5) allows in some cases the closed form integration of equations (2) (Bianco et al., 1988; Chiabrera & Bianco, 1987; Chiabrera et al., 1985), while equation (10) allows choosing the well-known hydrogenoid eigenfunctions as orthonormal base for the solution of equation (4) (Bianco & Chiabrera, 1992; Bianco, Chiabrera, D'Inzeo et al., 1993; Chiabrera, Bianco, Kaufman et al., 1991; Chiabrera, Bianco, Tommasi et al., 1992; Chiabrera et al., 1993). In any case, the previous estimates of the values of ω_{end} and ξ are so large that any effect of low-intensity EM exposure seems negligible. However, the above relationships neglect the fact that the atomic charges of the protein are not immobile, put to the approaching ion by displacing their positions with respect to the ones at thermodynamic equilibrium. The evaluation of such an effect is rather cumbersome, and it is not considered in the Protein Data Bank, as it implies a dynamical model of the protein itself. If one considers the protein as a globe of radius R_B, surrounded by a thin dielectric shell of thickness D and dielectric permittivity ε_S, the parameter

$$\delta = (D/R_B)(\varepsilon_s/\varepsilon_B)/2 \tag{11}$$

plays the role of the effective dielectric thickness of the shell itself relative to R_B. Then we obtain:

$$F_{end} \cong -[QQ_B/(4\pi\varepsilon_B R_B{}^3)][1-4(Q/Q_B)\delta/(3+10\delta+6\delta^2)]r \tag{12}$$

In other words, from equations (5, 7), the endogenous field at thermodynamic equilibrium is derived as $\mathbf{E}_{th} = -[Q_B / (4\pi\varepsilon_B R_B{}^3)]\mathbf{r}$ and the "reaction" field is $\mathbf{E}_r = -2\mathbf{E}_{th}(Q/Q_B)\delta / (3 + 10\delta + 6\delta^2)$ so that the actual intensity of the endogenous field $\mathbf{E}_{end} = \mathbf{E}_{th} + \mathbf{E}_r$ can be reduced in comparison with $\mathbf{E}_{th}$. The ratio

$$E_{end}/E_{th} = 1 - 4(Q/Q_B)\delta/(3+10\delta+6\delta^2) \tag{13}$$

plays the role of a ratio $(\omega'_{end} / \omega_{end})^2$, where ω'_{end} is the actual value of ω_{end}. The plot of equation (13) is shown in Figure 3. Thus we have shown how the values obtained from the Protein Data Bank may give an estimate of $\mathbf{E}_{th}$ rather than of the actual $\mathbf{E}_{end}$. In fact, the true endogenous force seen by the ion can be much smaller, and this implies much smaller values of ω'_{end} as compared with ω_{end}. For our protein model, there exist ranges of Q / Q_B and of δ where the site repels the ion, instead of attracting it (Figure 3). The same argument holds true for the quantum model of the ligation process. An analogous approach can also be developed for the endogenous field in a channel. The corresponding spatial conformation is much more complex so that this case is not discussed in detail, but the results are similar.

The general conclusion is that, in proximity to the origin $\mathbf{r} = 0$, the endogenous force of the site can be dramatically reduced by the "reaction" field induced by the ion itself. As a consequence, low-intensity EM exposure can be of significance since low values of ω'_{end} are plausible. Also, some conclusions of Bianco and Chiabrera (1992), D'Inzeo et al. (1993), Durney et al. (1988), and Galt et al. (1993) must be re-evaluated because low values of ω'_{end} can cause an instability in the solution of equations (2) (under ELF sinusoidal magnetic induction), thereby leading to an extremely high sensitivity to the EM exogenous input signal.

So far, the protein polarizability has been described by constant parameters such as its inner dielectric permittivity ε_B and by the shell parameter δ. The protein may also undergo an allosteric conformational change induced by the approaching ion so that both ε_B and δ can be a function of $\mathbf{E}_{end}$ itself. This opens a completely new area of research, further enhancing the theoretical possibility of bioelectromagnetic effects at low intensities.

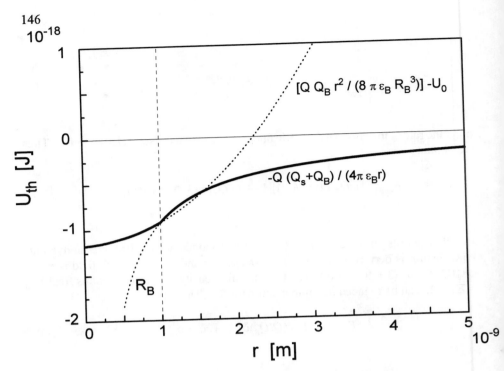

Figure 2. Plot of U_{th} (i.e., U_{end} at thermodynamic equilibrium) versus r, as given by equations (7, 9) and by equations (8, 10). The heavier lines indicate the ranges of validity of the equations. Same charges and parameters as in Figure 1.

Collision Frequency and Lifetimes

The collision frequency β of equation (2) and the lifetimes τ and θ which enter the matrix representation of the double commutator $[T,[T,(\rho - \rho_0)]]$ in equation (4) are related to the loss of energy of the ion-protein system (when it is out of thermodynamic equilibrium) because of its interactions with the thermal bath. Their orders of magnitude are linked by the relationship (Bianco, 1994):

$$\theta > \tau \cong 1/\beta$$

The value of β in bulk water can be evaluated to be as large as $0.5 \; 10^{14}$ Hz (Chiabrera, Bianco, Moggia, & Tommasi, 1994a). Such a value would clearly overwhelm any effect of low-intensity EM exposure (Hall, 1988). Such an argument is not applicable to the processes relevant to bioelectromagnetics because, as already pointed out, the ion moves inside a region surrounded by highly complex molecular structures. In the case of solvent polar molecules (e.g., water), the number of colliding solvent dipoles can be extremely small (Chiabrera, Morro, & Parodi, 1989) due to the large gradient of the endogenous electric field, which exerts a dielectrophoretic force on the dipoles and keeps them away from the region of large field intensities (Figure 4; Chiabrera, Bianco, Liebman, Kaufman, & Pilla, 1990; Chiabrera, Bianco, Parodi, Morro, & Liebman, 1991).

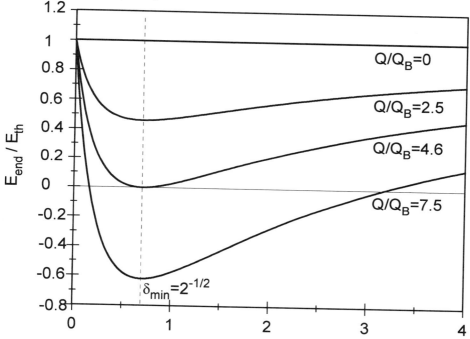

Figure 3. Plot of $E_{end} / E_{th} = (\omega'_{end} / \omega_{end})^2$ versus δ, as given by equation (13). Same charges and parameters as in Figure 1.

On the other hand, the surrounding molecular structures which generate $\mathbf{E}_{end}$ are, by definition, a spatial domain finite in size, say, a sphere of radius $R_B \geq R_C$, where the few colliding molecules move in the Knudsen ballistic regime. As a consequence, the mean free path cannot exceed the domain dimension R_B, irrespective of the low concentration of the colliding molecules. The resulting ion collision frequency (i.e., the effective viscosity) can be several orders of magnitude lower than in bulk water (Chiabrera et al., 1994a) as shown in Figure 5. This effect is separate and apart from those discussed in the section "The Endogenous Field." The collision frequency, as resulting from the Knudsen regime, implies that the surface of the crevice is closed, so that each time the ion reaches the surface, a collision occurs. This is not the case of the ion-protein systems considered in this paper, because the surface is permeable to the ion. A more realistic approach should define a ratio $p < 1$ between the actual surface portion that is impermeable to the ion, i.e., is responsible for the collisions, and the geometrical surface, i.e., $4\pi R_B^2$. Consequently, the low horizontal asymptotic

148

values given in Figure 5 should be multiplied by p, giving much lower values of β.

The key role of $\mathbf{E}_{end}$ becomes now fully apparent because small values of β (or $1/\tau$, $1/\theta$) can consistently occur if and only if $\mathbf{E}_{end}$ is very large and spatially not uniform in the region $r \cong R_B$. Then β or (τ, θ) can be approximated by small (large) constant values.

In conclusion, the collision frequency objection is refuted, and in this way also low intensity bioelectromagnetics may have the potential to affect ion-protein interactions.

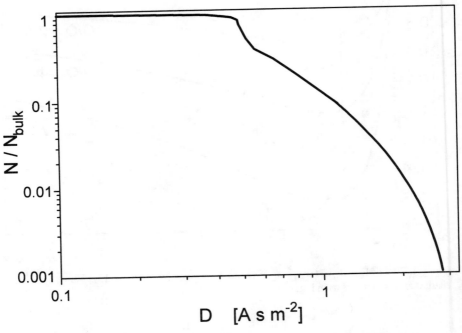

Figure 4. Plot of the ratio of the actual water concentration N in a molecular crevice to the bulk water concentration $N_{bulk} = 3.33 \ 10^{28}/m^3$ versus the electrical induction $D_{end} = \varepsilon_B E_{end}$ intensity (Chiabrera et al., 1989), with ε_B being the effective dielectric constant of the protein. The plot is right-bounded by a vertical asymptote.

Basal Metabolism Field

A problem to be solved in bioelectromagnetics is to devise a strategy for establishing how the out-of-thermodynamic equilibrium state of any living cell affects the ion-protein system. We strongly advocated the need for including the effects of the cell basal metabolism in the interaction models (Bianco, Chiabrera, & Kaufman, 1995; Chiabrera, Bianco, & Kaufman, 1995; Chiabrera, Bianco, Moggia, & Tommasi, 1994b). If they are neglected, any model for possible bioeffects of low intensity EM fields is fundamentally flawed. Basal metabolic processes fuelling the cell are the only source of steady power that can sustain signal "amplification" through the nonlinearities of the state equations for the ion-protein system.

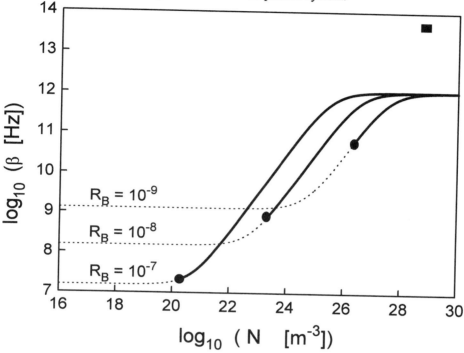

Figure 5. Plot of the collision frequency β versus the actual water concentration N in a molecular crevice of size R_B. The square corresponds to bulk water. The horizontal asymptote at $\beta \cong 10^{12}$ Hz corresponds to water vapour and the asymptotes at low N correspond to the Knudsen regime, when β becomes insensitive to large values of E_{end} (Chiabrera et al., 1994a). The actual values of β can be lower, as discussed in the text, because the protein surface is permeable to the ion. As a consequence, the effective surface that contributes to the Knudsen collisions is smaller. The heavier lines indicate the ranges of N where there exists more than one water molecule in the spherical crevice of radius R_B (binding site). The dots on each line correspond to one water molecule at the binding site.

Our approach considers protein embedded in a lipidic medium, e.g., a cell membrane. The cell basal metabolism sustains any biochemical process that requires an exogenous energy source, like ion pumps. A paradigmatic measure of such an out-of-thermodynamic equilibrium steady state of a living cell is the net voltage drop across the membrane, which reduces to zero at thermodynamic equilibrium (dead cell). Such a voltage drop is the integral of an electric field. In other words, one proof of the cell basal metabolic activity in the microenvironment surrounding a protein is the existence of an additional electric field component, $\mathbf{E}_{bm}$, which affects the ion-protein system. For simplicity's sake, we assume that $\mathbf{E}_{bm}$ is constant in time and space. As already discussed in the section "The Classical Langevin-Lorentz State Equations," E_{bm} enters directly equations (2) as an additive force $F_{bm} = QE_{bm}$, which drifts the ion. Moreover, it enters the solution $r(t)$ of equations (2) via the boundary conditions on the state variables. The dissociation (transit) time output is computed by releasing the ion at $r = 0$ at $t = 0$, with an initial velocity $v(0) = F_{bm} / M\beta$.

In the quantum case, F_{bm} enters the Hamiltonian H_{bm} and the steady state operator ρ_0. Without loss of generality, assuming that F_{bm} is directed along the z axis, we obtain for the operators:

$$H_{bm} \cong -QE_{bm}r\cos\theta \qquad (15)$$

$$\rho_0 = \{\rho_F + Q2E^2_{bm,z}(\rho_F - \rho_P)/(\beta^2 kTM) + \tfrac{1}{2}[(\rho_F - \rho_P)P_F + P_F(\rho_F - \rho_P)]\}/Z_0 \qquad (16)$$

where $P_F = [\dfrac{jhQE_{bmz}}{2\pi\beta kTM}]\dfrac{\partial}{\partial z}$; $\rho_F = \exp[-H_{th}/(kT) - P_F]$; $\rho_F = \exp\{\dfrac{h^2\nabla^2}{(8\pi 2kTM)} - P_F\}$; k is the Boltzmann constant and T is the absolute temperature. The value of the operator ρ_0 at thermodynamic equilibrium, i.e., ρ_{th}, becomes

$$\rho_{th} = \exp[-H_{th}/(kT)]/Z_{th} \qquad (17)$$

The denominators Z_0 and Z_{th} are the traces of the corresponding operators of the numerators $\{...\}$ in equations (16, 17) so that the traces of ρ_{th} and ρ_0 are equal to 1, as they must be. The operator $\rho_{bm} = \rho_0 - \rho_{th}$ indicates how far from thermodynamic equilibrium the ion-protein system is maintained by the basal metabolism.

When $F_{bm} = 0$, equation (16) reduces to its value ρ_{th} at thermodynamic equilibrium, as expected, and ρ_{bm} goes to zero. We recall that ρ_0 contributes both to equation (4) and to the boundary condition $\rho(0) = \rho_0$.

The endogenous field or Hamiltonian provides the nonlinearity which converts the power supplied by the metabolic sources via F_{bm} into the time-varying power necessary to affect the temporal evolution of the state variables by the low-intensity EM input signal.

The use of the five-state Zeeman-Stark model as an example (Bianco, Chiabrera, D'Inzeo et al., 1993; Chiabrera, Bianco, Kaufman et al., 1991; Chiabrera, Bianco, Tommasi et al., 1992; Lednev, 1995) and of the Coulombic potential energy (10) in H_{th} allows the contribution of H_{bm} to become important (as compared with H_{th}), if

$$E_{bm} > 10^{-2}(2\pi)^4 M^2\xi^3/(Qh^4) \qquad (18)$$

On the other hand, ρ_0 differs from ρ_{th} if

$$E_{bm} > 3(2\pi)M\xi B/(Qh) \qquad (19)$$

Both conditions are compatible with an acceptable order of magnitude of $\mathbf{E}_{bm}$, if the low values of ξ and β postulated in the sections "The Endogenous Field" and "Collision Frequency and Lifetimes" are allowed. Adopting the electronic jargon, we conclude that reasonable values of $\mathbf{E}_{bm}$ can *bias* the ion-protein system far enough from thermodynamic equilibrium, at an *operating point* of the non linear $\mathbf{E}_{end}(\mathbf{r})$ *characteristic* where the system may be potentially able to detect small EM input signals taking advantage of the *power supplied* by the basal metabolism of the cell itself via $\mathbf{E}_{bm}$, much like a transistor uses its power to amplify the time-varying signal applied to its input gate. The operating bandwidth is determined by the interplay of the time derivative at the left side of equations (2) or (4) with their right sides, respectively.

Noise

The interactions of the ion-protein system with the thermal bath are also reflected in random fluctuations of the state variables. These interactions are emulated, in equations (2), by the random force $(M\mathbf{n})$. The Boltzmann statistics and the fluctuation-dissipation theorem provide a classical guideline for the evaluation of the statistical properties of $\mathbf{n}$:

$$<\mathbf{n}> = 0 \qquad (20a)$$

$$<n_x(t)n_x(t')> = <n_y(t)n_y(t')> = <n_z(t)n_z(t')> = <\mathbf{n}(t)\cdot\mathbf{n}(t')>/3 = \frac{2\beta kT}{M}\delta(t-t') \qquad (20b)$$

The above equations describe the white-noise component of $\mathbf{n}$ (background noise), whose spectral density is uniform in the frequency domain. An additional coloured noise component is provided by the fluctuations of the out-of-equilibrium metabolic processes; this component is not addressed in this paper (Chiabrera, Bianco, Kaufman et al., 1992; Kaufman et al., 1990; Weaver & Astumian, 1994).

In quantum terms, the density operator is the correct tool for handling the interactions with the thermal bath. The Boltzmann statistics provide the value ρ_{th} of ρ_0 at thermal equilibrium ($H_{bm} = H_1 = 0$, and $E_r = 0$, so that $H_{end} = H_{th}$). Letting ε_i denote the energy eigenvalues of H_{th}, and choosing as an orthonormal base the eigenfunction of H_{th}, one obtains the matrix entries of ρ_{th} from equation (17). The so-called *populations* are:

$$\rho_{th,ij} = \exp(-\varepsilon_i/kT)/\Sigma_m \exp(-\varepsilon_m/kT) \tag{21}$$

and the so-called *coherences* are:

$$\rho_{th,ij} = 0 \qquad\qquad (i \neq j) \tag{22}$$

Recalling that $\rho_0 = \rho_{th} + \rho_{bm}$, it becomes apparent how white thermal noise is included in equation (4) and the boundary conditions via ρ_0.

We pointed out previously (Chiabrera, Bianco, Kaufman et al., 1992; Kaufman et al., 1990) that any bioelectromagnetic model must include thermal noise as input. The first task to be accomplished is the evaluation of the output when the exogenous EM exposure is absent in equations (2), i.e., $\mathbf{E} = \mathbf{B} = 0$, or in equation (4), i.e., $H_1 = 0$, so that noise is the only input acting on the system. The second task is the evaluation of the output when the exogenous EM exposure is active, and noise is always present. The third task is to compare, in relative terms, the outputs obtained in the two situations. Any conclusion about the effectiveness of the EM exposure on the ion-protein system must be drawn only as a consequence of such a comparison.

In the literature, many theoretical papers do not consider noise at all, and their authors perform the second task only in the absence of noise. These studies provide some information about the output dependence on the EM parameters (e.g., frequency, amplitude, etc.), but nothing can be inferred concerning the effectiveness of the EM exposure.

A further aspect is the possibility of stochastic resonance, which was reviewed in Chiabrera, Bianco, and Kaufman (1995). The ion-protein system retains all the necessary features for stochastic resonance (Poponin, 1995) so that one could expect that an optimal range of characteristic parameter values exist where the signal-to-noise ratio of the output is enhanced. The evaluation of the system state equations (2) or (4) naturally includes stochastic resonance, the study of which does not require any inherently different models.

Exogenous EM Input

We assume that $\mathbf{A}$ and ϕ are classically known. The exogenous EM input to the ion-protein system can be described by $\mathbf{A}(x, y, z, t)$ and $\phi(x, y, z, t)$, as pointed out in the section "Models of the Interaction Mechanisms." As a result, the classical and quantum cases can be discussed together. In order to specifically address the issue of mobile telecommunications, it is adequate to describe the EM field in terms of $\mathbf{A}$ only, letting $\phi = 0$. A reasonable approximation of the complex waveform discussed in the Introduction is to decompose $\mathbf{A}$ into an RF component $\mathbf{A}_{rf}$ related to the modulated carrier, into an ELF component $\mathbf{A}_b$ related to the burst repetition rate, and into a DC component A_0 related to the earth's magnetic field. We refer to a simple amplitude RF waveform of the type

$$[1+m\cos\omega_m t]\sin(\omega_c t) \tag{23}$$

where $f_c = \omega_c / (2\pi)$ is the RF carrier frequency, $f_m = \omega_m / (2\pi) << f_c$ is the modulation frequency, and m is the modulation depth. A linearly polarized TEM wave (Bianco, Chiabrera, Moggia, & Tommasi, 1993) propagating in a biological medium, whose average conductivity is σ, whose electric permittivity is $\varepsilon_0\varepsilon_r$, and whose magnetic permittivity is μ_0, is described by

$$A_{rf} \cong \sqrt{\frac{2\rho S}{\sigma(1+m^2/2)}} \{\frac{\exp(-\alpha_c y)}{\omega_c}\cos[\omega_c(t-y/v_c)] + \frac{m\exp(-\alpha_+ y)}{2\omega_+}\cos[\omega_+(t-y/v_+)] + \frac{m\exp(-\alpha_- y)}{2\omega_-}\cos[\omega_-(t-y/v_-)]\}i_x \tag{24a}$$

where S [W/kg] is the local specific absorption rate (SAR), ρ[kg/m³] is the local tissue density, $\omega_+ = \omega_c + \omega_m$ is the upper side band, and $\omega_- = \omega_c - \omega_m$ is the lower side band. The attenuation coefficient is

$$\alpha_i = \frac{\sigma}{\sqrt{2}} \frac{\varepsilon_0}{\mu_0} \{[\frac{\sigma}{\omega_i\varepsilon_0} + (\varepsilon_r^2 + \frac{\sigma^2}{\omega_i^2\varepsilon_0^2})^{\frac{1}{2}}]^{-\frac{1}{2}}\} \qquad (i = c, +, -) \tag{24b}$$

and the phase velocity is

$$v_i = \{\varepsilon_0\mu_0[\frac{\sigma}{\omega_i\varepsilon_0} + (\varepsilon_r^2 + \frac{\sigma^2}{\omega_i^2\varepsilon_0^2})^{\frac{1}{2}}]^{-\frac{1}{2}}\} \qquad (i = c, +, -) \tag{24c}$$

under the hypothesis $\varepsilon_r > \sigma / (\omega_0\varepsilon_0)$. As to the ELF magnetic induction field induced by the current burst (see section entitled, "Introduction"), it can be approximated by a sinusoidal field [$B_b\sin(\omega_b t)i_b$], so that:

$$A_b = [B_b\sin(\omega_{bt})i_b]\times(d+r)/2 \tag{25}$$

where d is a constant length vector which depends on the local tissue and i_b is the unit vector in the direction of B_b. A reasonable order of magnitude for d is a few millimeters or less. On a similar basis, the AC magnetic induction due to power line exposure and the earth's DC magnetic induction can be computed, respectively, from the vector potentials:

$$A_p = B_p i_p \times (d+r)/2 \qquad (26a)$$

$$A_0 = B_0 i_0 \times (d+r)/2 \qquad (26b)$$

where i_p and i_0 are the unit vectors in the direction of $\mathbf{B}_p$ and $\mathbf{B}_0$ respectively. To sum up, the exogenous EM input is given by $\mathbf{A} = \mathbf{A}_{rf} + \mathbf{A}_b + \mathbf{A}_p + \mathbf{A}_0$.

The corresponding electric and magnetic fields which enter equations (2) are obtained from equations (1). The Hamiltonian operator H_1 in equation (4) is given by (Bianco, Chiabrera, Moggia et al., 1993):

$$H_1 = j\gamma(h/2\pi)A\cdot\nabla \qquad (27)$$

RF Signal Demodulation

The nonlinearities of the ion-protein system can perform a demodulation of the RF signal, down-converting its effects to the DC-LF range. The demodulation can be anticipated from a preliminary analysis based on the quantum Zeeman-Stark model of equation (4). The results are also applicable to the classical Langevin-Lorentz model, i.e., to equations (2), because the quantum approach is more general and must consistently include the results of the classical one. On the other hand, demodulation cannot be seen from equations (2) at a glance, and, in order to become apparent, it requires the integration of the equations. In other words, demodulation is not a quantum effect per se, but is more easily pointed out by the quantum approach. As an example, we rely again on the five-state model (Moggia, Tommasi, Bianco, & Chiabrera, 1993) of a binding process, where the nonlinearity is provided by the endogenous Coulombic potential energy $(-\xi'/r)$. The four excited states above the ground state ε_1 are degenerate at the energy ε_2, where ε_1 and ε_2 are the first two eigenvalues of H_{th}. The corresponding energy gap

$$\varepsilon_2 - \varepsilon_1 = h/(2\pi)\omega_0 = (3/8)(2\pi)^2 M(\xi')^2/h^2 \qquad (28)$$

gives the order of magnitude of the energy depth of the protein potential well seen by the ion whose equivalent photon radian frequency is ω_0. The effective $\xi' < \xi$ to be used is analogous to the effective ω'_{end} discussed in the section "The Endogenous Field." If the matrix elements of the quantum operators are expressed in the orthonormal base of the eigenfunction of H_{th}, equation (4) gives a set of equations for the populations ρ_{ll} of the following type:

$$d\rho_{ll}/dt = \ldots + c\,^i_{lmn}\exp(\pm j(\omega_i - \omega_0)t)\lambda_{mn} + \ldots \tag{29a}$$

$$(m \neq n)$$

$$d\lambda_{mn}/dt = \ldots + d\,^i_{lmn}\exp(\pm j(\omega_i - \omega_0)t)\rho_{ll} + \ldots \tag{29b}$$

where c^i_{lmn}, d^i_{lmn} are constant coefficients, and $\omega_i = \omega_c$, or $\omega_i = \omega_+$, or $\omega_i = \omega_-$. The λ_{mn}s are related to the coherences ρ_{mn}. The resulting radian frequencies $\Omega_i = \omega_i - \omega_0$ of the exponential terms in equations (29) are

$$\Omega_c = \omega_c - \omega_0 \tag{30a}$$

$$\Omega_\pm = \omega_c - \omega_0 \pm \omega_m \tag{30b}$$

and Ω_i can assume any value from DC to LF if $\omega_0 \cong \omega_c$. Equations (29) are linear equations with time-varying periodic coefficients which form a quasi-periodic Floquet system. The equations (29) are quasi-periodic because some coefficients depend on the different radian frequencies Ω_i, and others depend on the radian frequencies $\omega_i + \omega_0$. More specifically, some of the coefficients are periodic with frequency $\Omega_i / (2\pi)$, as shown above. Thus, the solution of equations (29) for the populations ρ_{ll}, that are the only variables implied in the computation of $Tr(P\rho)$, contains terms related to the same frequencies. For example, if one considers the carrier only ($\omega_m = 0$), the condition $\omega_0 \cong \omega_c$ implies a down conversion of the carrier itself to DC, as discussed in the section "Numerical Results." Then, we have shown that demodulation can occur, so that the solution of equation (4) can contain LF components due to the down conversion of the RF signal. The situation becomes even more complex because resonance at ELF with the AC Larmor frequencies associated with the sine amplitudes of A_b, A_p, and with the DC Larmor frequencies associated with A_0, may be excited. Thus, any comprehensive attempt to evaluate the effects of the EM fields emitted by personal communication systems cannot be restricted to RF, but attention must be paid to the modulating frequencies per se, to the power line exposure and to the DC magnetic field.

Cooperativity and Synchronization

Two rather important topics should be carefully considered: cooperativity and synchronization. Both have been pointed out as potential enhancers of cell sensitivity to EM exposure. Unfortunately, these two topics so far have remained rather vague, in the sense that they have never reached the stage of a working biophysical model. Thus, more attention should be paid to these subjects. For instance, molecular biology and molecular biochemistry offer examples of molecular structures which exhibit allosteric cooperativity (Wyman & Gill, 1990). The best case is homotropic linkage, i.e., the case of proteins with two (or more) binding sites for the same ligand, and two (or more) allosteric conformations. The binding of the first ligand also induces an allosteric transition. In the new conformation, the association/dissociation constants of the second binding site can change considerably. Then, the structure determines ligand-binding properties, and ligand activities in turn determine bound populations. A small change in the binding conditions at the first site can have large consequences on the occupation of all the protein sites. We have tacitly assumed that the protein does not dissociate or aggregate. There are cases of polysteric linkage, in which ion binding controls the aggregation state of the protein, e.g. monomer/dimer, and each state can exhibit a different degree of allosteric cooperativity. We foresee that the area of generalized linkage phenomena is within the reach of theoretical scientists, opening new venues in understanding possible EM interaction mechanisms.

Another aspect of EM exposure is the fact that it provides the same input signal to a whole cell population so that cell synchronization can occur. Cell biology offers examples of biological effects enhanced by cell synchronization. Any further discussion is beyond the scope of this paper, as it is more related to the cell response, whereas we have restricted our analysis to the output of the first interaction step. Nevertheless, this subject also deserves further attention by researchers.

Frequency and Amplitude Windows

The analysis of the state of the science carried out in the previous sections clarifies that the so-called *frequency windows* in bioelectromagnetics are an obvious feature of the output of an ion-protein system as a consequence of the time derivatives in the state equations (2) or (4). On the contrary, any output insensitive to the frequency content of the EM input must be regarded as an exceptional situation. On the other hand, the low values of the collision frequencies (long lifetimes) which are necessary for the effectiveness of low-intensity EM inputs imply rather narrow bandwidths of the frequency windows so that a close matching between the EM exposure characteristics and an ion-protein system's characteristics is necessary. Accordingly, the occurence of any long-term matching is unrealistic in real life. In particular, this is true for the exposure of the human body (head) to EM fields generated by mobile telecommunication systems. An analogous argument applies to the so-called *amplitude windows*. The intrinsic nonlinearities of the protein-ion system imply, by default, that the output is affected in distinct ways depending on the specific amplitude range. The simplifications adopted in Bianco et al. (1988), Chiabrera et al. (1985), and Durney et al. (1988) allow obtaining in close form the resonance and antiresonance conditions discussed in the section "The Classical Langevin-Lorentz State Equations" that are the most clear-cut examples of amplitude and frequency windows so far available.

In conclusion, the input-output relationship of a typical ion-protein system must contain frequency and amplitude windows because it is nonlinear and the state equations [see equations (2), (4)] contain time-varying coefficients that depend on the signal waveform and intensity. These properties reduce the likeliness of biological effects on whole organisms exposed to EM fields generated by mobile telecommunication systems. On the other hand, a conclusive statement requires further extensive studies of equations (2) and (4) with *stochastic* exogenous EM signals that emulate the real situation. Of course, the opposite conclusion holds true if one deals with therapeutic applications, where exposure conditions are rather well controlled and reproducible.

Numerical Results

Some preliminary numerical results are discussed in this section. We consider the case of a TEM wave incident from the half space $y < 0$ (air) into a lossy semi-infinite medium, that fills the half space $y \geq 0$. The waveform is a sinusoid at $f_c = \omega_c / (2\pi) = 915$ MHz, and it emulates a continuous carrier. The medium conductivity is $\sigma = 1$ S/m, its relative dielectric permittivity is $\varepsilon_r = 80$, and its density is $\rho = 10^3$ kg/m^3. The process under consideration is the binding of a Ca^{++} ion to a receptor protein located at $x = z = 0$ and $y = 0^+$. The EM sinusoidal exposure is switched on at $t = 0^+$.

We adopt the five-state quantum model quoted in the previous sections, letting the lifetimes $\theta_{mn} = \theta = 10^{-7}$ s and $\tau_{mn} = \tau = 10^8$ s (m, n = 1 to 5 and m $\neq$ n). The output variable is $\rho_{11}(t)$, as representative of the occupancy of the ion-protein ground state and as an acceptable estimate of the binding probability. Finally, we choose $F_{bm} = F_{bm}\mathbf{i}_y$ and $F_{bm} / \beta = 2 \ 10^{-20}$ Ns at T = 300°K. By letting $\omega_0 / (2\pi) \simeq \omega_c / (2\pi) = 915$ MHz, the AC exposure should be optimally down-converted to DC, according to the discussion in the section "Cooperativity and Synchronization." In other words, the relative excess population $[\rho_{11}(0) - \rho_{11}(t)] / \rho_{11}(0)$ should evolve from the zero value at t = 0 to an average value different from zero for t→∞. Moreover, the effect should be negligible at thermodynamic equilibrium ($F_{bm} = 0$) because the exposure is at low intensity (1-10 mW/cm^2) so that it could become appreciable only if $F_{bm} \neq 0$.

The interesting preliminary results, that confirm our predictions, are summarized in Figure 6. For $F_{bm} = 0$ we find that $\rho_{11}(0) = \rho_{11,th} = 0.21$. Thus, at thermodynamic equilibrium, the ground state has small probability of being occupied because the binding site is shallow ($h\omega_0 / (2\pi) << kT$ at T = 300°K). An incident wave of 1 mW/cm^2 induces negligible changes in $\rho_{11}(t)$ compared with $\rho_{11,th}$, as anticipated. The corresponding SAR at the receptor location is 0.148 W/kg. If F_{bm} is increased up to 2 10^{-17} N, the first consequence is that $\rho_{11}(0) = 0.54$. Then, the effect of the basal metabolism force, per se, is to dramatically increase the probability of occupancy of the ground state. If the same EM exposure is switched on at t = 0$^+$, as before, $\rho_{11}(t)$ is *pumped* by the sinusoidal EM field to an asymptotic constant value that is appreciably lower than $\rho_{11}(0)$. If F_{bm} is further increased above 2 10^{-17} N, $\rho_{11}(0)$ does not change appreciably while the effectiveness of the EM exposure decreases. The effect becomes striking at 10 mW/cm^2 (SAR = 1.48 W/kg) and $F_{bm} = 2 \ 10^{-17}$ N, because the relative change of the asymptotic value of $\rho_{11}(t)$ becomes larger than 10%, a change that could have far-reaching biological consequences. Then, for *the first time in bioelectromagnetics* we have been able to show that a low-intensity RF exposure can affect an elementary biological process.

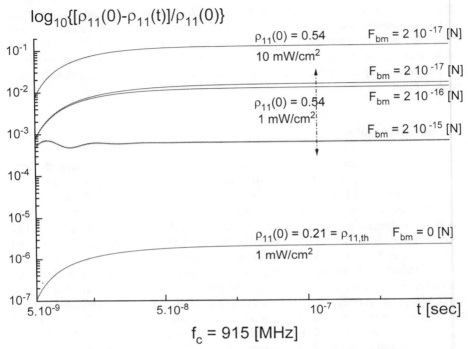

$$\log_{10}\{[\rho_{11}(0)-\rho_{11}(t)]/\rho_{11}(0)\}$$

$f_c = 915$ [MHz]

Figure 6. Plot of $[\rho_{11}(0) - \rho_{11}(t)] / \rho_{11}(0)$, chosen as output of a putative Ca^{++}-receptor system, in response to a 915 MHz TEM sinewave, switched at $t = 0^+$. The receptor is shallow, with a characteristic radian frequency $\omega_0 \cong 2\pi\ 915$ rad/s, in order to enhance the down-conversion of the sinewave to DC at large values of t. The effect is maximum for a basal metabolism force $F_{bm} \cong 2\ 10^{-17}$ N. At $t = 0$ (not shown), all the plots start from zero.

Conclusions

We have analyzed the state of the art concerning the existence of a biophysical basis for effects of low-intensity fields on cellular processes, with specific emphasis on a first interaction step and on modulated RF EM fields generated by personal telecommunication systems that represent one of the fastest growing segments of the telecommunications industry (Li & Qiu, 1995).

After providing a simple characterization of the input EM field of interest, we have discussed the classical and quantum modeling of an ion-protein system. The ion binding to a receptor protein is the process most widely studied, but results can be applied, by analogy, to ion transport through a protein channel.

Ion-protein interaction is a dynamic phenomenon that is very difficult to analyze theoretically, because it is complicated by the protein folding and unfolding, and by the reaction of the protein atoms to the ion transit under EM exposure. Atom oscillations, side chain/loop/arm displacement, helices/domains/subunits/opening fluctuations, folding and unfolding, collective many-body modes, solitons, and other nonlinear motions occur in amplitude ranges up to tens of nanometers, in time scales as long as hundreds of seconds (Karplus, 1985). The time scale of the exogenous EM field goes from 10^{-10} s to 1 s. Thus, molecular dynamics is the correct approach (D'Inzeo, Palombo, Tarricone, & Zago, 1995), but reliable and long simulations will need new, perhaps specialized, software and computers. For the time being, the modeling approach developed in this paper seems adequate to offer some predictive insight.

Six main issues have been analyzed:

1. The nonlinear endogenous field E_{th} inside a molecular structure has been characterized according to the Protein Data Bank. The reaction field E_r induced on the protein by the approaching ion has been evaluated, proving that the resulting actual endogenous field, $E_{end} = E_{th} + E_r$, experienced by the interacting ion can be lower than expected from the Protein Data Bank. The endogenous force provides a strong nonlinearity in the state equations for the ion-protein system. Its actual value inside the protein crevice is reduced in such a way that low-intensity exposure could affect dissociation constants and be able, in some cases, to drift the ion into a dynamic instability.

2. The ion collision frequency β in the hydrophobic interior of the protein is much less than that of bulk water so that viscous losses and thermal noise are small. The endogenous field at the protein boundaries is large enough and sufficiently nonuniform in space so that water molecules are rejected by the resulting dielectrophoretic force acting on their electric dipoles. Thus, any protein with a hydrophobic crevice or channel is a good candidate for hosting an effective interaction between low-intensity exposure and an ion.

3. Basal metabolism sustains the cell out of thermodynamic equilibrium. At the molecular level, such a situation is reflected in an additional field E_{bm} superimposed on E_{end}, which maintains the ion-protein system itself out of thermodynamic equilibrium. A well-known consequence of E_{bm} is the net voltage drop across the membrane of any living cell. The field E_{bm} supplies power to the system. This power can be converted, via the nonlinearity provided by E_{end}, into signaling power controlled by the low intensity EM exogenous field.

4. Thermal noise must always be considered in any theoretical attempt to evaluate potential EM bioeffects. Its characteristics and relationship with β are provided so that its contribution to the ion-protein output can be taken into account in the presence and in the absence of EM exposure, whose effectiveness must be judged from the comparison of the two situations. Some aspects related to stochastic resonance have been briefly addressed (Bezrukov & Vodyanoy, 1995; Chiabrera et al., 1995; Poponin, 1995), which could be relevant for RF interactions.

5. The possibility of a down-conversion of the RF signal due to the demodulation caused by the nonlinearity of $\mathbf{E}_{end}$ has been demonstrated. Thus, modulation aspects of RF fields are important, as LF resonances also may occur.

6. Some aspects related to frequency and amplitude windows, allosteric cooperativity, and cell synchronization have been discussed and need further consideration.

These results seem in contrast with those reported in Astumian, Weaver, and Adair (1995) and Weaver and Astumian (1994), irrespective of the similar physical approach adopted. The differences can be better understood by resuming the electronic jargon used at the end of the section "Basal Metabolism Field." In this paper we deal with a *transistor* analog of processes in *living* cells ($\mathbf{F}_{bm} \neq 0$), whereas the approach developed in Weaver and Astumian and Astumian, Weaver, and Adair deals with a *diode* analog of processes in *dead* cells ($\mathbf{F}_{bm} = 0$). In fact, if the exogenous EM exposure is switched off, the systems considered in those papers return to thermodynamic equilibrium, so that "it is difficult to make consistent biological effects with low fields strengths" in this case (Astumian, Weaver, & Adair, 1995).

In conclusion, we offer a plausible biophysical basis for potential effects of EM fields generated by mobile communication systems. Such a conclusion is presently limited to the analysis of the first interaction step. Caution must be used in analyzing full biological processes and in drawing conclusions on the end steps, which are very far from the first one. Nevertheless, on this established basis, some guidelines can already be referred to for in vitro experiments, in terms of characterization of biochemical processes and exposure parameters.

The reciprocal approach should also be advocated, i.e., a continuous update of the theoretical analysis in accordance with experimental findings and with the advances in the Protein Data Bank.

As far as in vivo experiments and epidemiological studies are concerned, any theoretical attempt to predict biological effects would be premature because of the highly complex (cascade, feedback, and feedforward aspects) processes involved and of the gaps in the related knowledge. The biophysical basis presented in this paper can, however, provide some guidelines for the specification of EM exposure parameters that are scientifically reasonable and practically affordable.

Acknowledgment

This work has been partially supported by the Italian MURST, by the University of Genoa, and by CyberLogic, Inc.

References

Adey, W. R. (1980). Frequency and power windowing in tissue interactions with weak electromagnetic fields. Proceedings of the IEEE, 68, 119-125.

Astumian, R. D., Weaver, J. C., & Adair, R. K. (1995). Rectification and signal averaging of weak electric fields by biological cells. Proceedings of the National Academy of Sciences of the United States, 92, 3740-3743.

Andersen, J. B., Johansen, C., Pedersen, G. F., & Raskmark, P. (1995). On the possible health effects related to GSM and DECT transmissions: A tutorial study for the European Commission. Aalborg, Denmark: Aalborg University.

Bawin, S. M., & Adey, W. R. (1976). Sensitivity of calcium binding in central tissue to weak environmental electric fields oscillating at low frequency. Proceedings of the National Academy of Sciences of the United States, 73, 1999-2003.

Bezrukov, S. M. & Vodyanoy, I. (1995). Noise-induced enhancement of signal transduction across voltage-dependent ion channels. Nature, 378, 362-364.

Bianco, B. (1994). Technical Report, DIBE. Genoa, Italy: University of Genoa.

Bianco, B., & Chiabrera, A. (1992). From the Langevin-Lorentz to the Zeeman model of electromagnetic effects on ligand-receptor binding. Bioelectrochemistry and Bioenergetics, 28, 355-365.

Bianco, B., Chiabrera, A., D'Inzeo, G., Galli, A., & Palombo, A. (1993). Comparison between classical and quantum modeling of bioelectromagnetic interaction mechanisms. In M. Blank (Ed.), Electricity and magnetism in biology and medicine (pp. 537-539). San Francisco: San Francisco Press.

Bianco, B., Chiabrera, A., & Kaufman, J. J. (1995, June). A new paradigm for studying the interaction of electromagnetic fields with living systems: An out-of-equilibrium characterization. Paper presented at the BEMS 7th Annual Meeting, Boston, MA.

Bianco, B., Chiabrera, A., Moggia, E., & Tommasi, T. (1993, October). Interaction mechanisms between electromagnetic fields and biological samples under a TEM exposure system. Paper presented at the 2nd International IEEE-URSI Scientific Meeting, Microwaves in Medicine, Rome, Italy.

Bianco, B., Chiabrera, A., Morro, A., & Parodi, M. (1988). Effects of magnetic exposure on ions in electric fields. Ferroelectrics, 83, 355-365.

Blackman, C. F., Benane, S. G., Robinovitz, J. R., House, D. E., & Joines, W. T. (1985). A role for the magnetic field in the radiation-induced efflux of calcium ions from brain tissue in vitro. Bioelectromagnetics, 6, 327-337.

Blackman, C. F., Blanchard, J. P., Benane, S. G., & House, D. E. (1995). The ion parametric resonance model predicts magnetic field parameters that affect nerve cells. FASEB Journal, 9, 547-551.

162

Blanchard, J. P., & Blackman, C. F. (1994). Clarification and application of an ion parametric resonance model for magnetic field interactions with biological systems. Bioelectromagnetics, 15, 217-238.

Carpenter, D. O., & Ayrapetyan, S. (Eds.). (1994). Papers in biological effects of electric and magnetic fields (Vol. I, II). Englewood Cliffs, NJ: Academic Press.

Chiabrera, A. (1987, June). Comments on the dynamic characteristics of membrane ions in multifield configurations of low-frequency electromagnetic radiation. Paper presented at the BEMS Annual Meeting, Portland, OR.

Chiabrera, A. & Bianco, B. (1987). The role of the magnetic field in the EM interaction with ligand binding. In M. Blank and E. Findl (Eds.), Mechanistic approaches to interactions of electric and electromagnetic fields with living systems (pp. 79-95). New York and London: Plenum.

Chiabrera, A., Bianco, B., Caratozzolo, F., Giannetti, G., Grattarola, M., & Viviani, R. (1985). Electric and magnetic field effects on ligand binding to cell membrane. In A. Chiabrera, C. Nicolini, & H. P. Schwan (Eds.), Interaction between electromagnetic fields and cells (pp 253-280). New York and London: Plenum.

Chiabrera, A., Bianco, B., & Kaufman, J. J. (1995, March). Biological effectiveness of low intensity electromagnetic exposure: Nonlinearity, out-of-equilibrium state and noise. Paper presented at the Electromagnetic Compatibility EMC 95, URSI Open Meeting, Commission K, Zurich, Switzerland.

Chiabrera, A., Bianco, B., Kaufman, J. J., & Pilla, A. A. (1992). Bioelectromagnetic resonance interactions: Endogenous field and noise. In B. Norden & C. Ramel (Eds.), Interaction mechanisms of low-level electromagnetic fields in living systems (pp. 164-179). Oxford, UK: Oxford Science Publications.

Chiabrera, A., Bianco, B., Kaufman, J. J., & Pilla, A. A. (1991). Quantum dynamics of ion in molecular crevices under electromagnetic exposure. In C. T. Brighton and S. R. Pollak (Eds.), Electromagnetics in biology and medicine (pp. 21-26). San Francisco: San Francisco Press.

Chiabrera, A., Bianco, B., Liebman, M. N., Kaufman, J. J., & Pilla, A. A. (1990, October). Movement of ions near macromolecules in the presence of electromagnetic exposure. Paper presented at the BRAGS 10th Annual Meeting, Philadelphia, PA.

Chiabrera, A., Bianco, B., & Moggia, E. (1993). Effects of lifetimes on ligand binding modeled by the density operator. Bioelectrochemistry and Bioenergetics, 30, 35-42.

Chiabrera, A., Bianco, B., Moggia, E., & Tommasi, T. (1994a). The interaction mechanism between EM fields and ion adsorption: Endogenous forces and collision frequency. Bioelectrochemistry and Bioenergetics, 35, 33-37.

Chiabrera, A., Bianco, B., Moggia, E., & Tommasi, T. (1994b, June). The out-of-equilibrium steady state of a cell as reference for evaluating bioelectromagnetic effects. Paper presented at the BEMS 16th Annual Meeting, Copenhagen, Denmark.

Chiabrera, A., Bianco, B., Parodi, M., Morro, A., & Liebman, M. N. (1991, June). Hydrophobicity of ion binding sites in proteins. Paper presented at the BEMS 13th Annual

Meeting, Salt Lake City, UT.

Chiabrera, A., Bianco, B., Tommasi, T., & Moggia, E. (1992). Langevin-Lorentz and Zeeman-Stark models of bioelectromagnetic effects. ACTA Pharmaceutica, 42, 315-322.

Chiabrera, A., Morro, A., & Parodi, M. (1989). Water concentration and dielectric permittivity in molecular crevices. Il Nuovo Cimento, 7, 981-992.

Chiabrera, A., & Rodan, G. A. (1984). The effect of electromagnetic fields on receptor-ligand interaction: A theoretical analysis. Journal of Bioelectricity, 3, 509-521.

D'Inzeo, G., Galli, A., & Palombo, A. (1993). Further investigations on nonthermal effects referring to the interaction between ELF fields and transmembrane ionic fluxes. Bioelectrochemistry and Bioenergetics, 30, 93-102.

D'Inzeo, G., Palombo, A., Tarricone, L., & Zago, M. (1995, June). Molecular simulation studies to understand non-thermal bioelectromagnetic interaction. Paper presented at the BEMS 17th Annual Meeting, Boston, MA.

Durney, C. H., Rushforth, C. K., & Anderson, A. A. (1988). Resonant DC-AC magnetic fields: Calculated response. Bioelectromagnetics, 9, 315-336.

Edmonds, D. T. (1993). Larmor precession as a mechanism for the detection of static and alternating magnetic fields. Bioelectrochemistry and Bioenergetics, 30, 3-12.

Galt, S., Sandblom, J., & Hamnerius, Y. (1993). Theoretical study of the resonance behaviour of an ion confined to a potential well in a combination of A.C. and D.C. magnetic fields. Bioelectromagnetics, 14, 299-314.

Halle, B. (1988). On the ciclotron resonance mechanism for magnetic field effects on trans-membrane ion conductivity. Bioelectromagnetics, 9, 381-385.

Honig, B., & Nicholls, A. (1995). Classical electrostatics in biology and chemistry. Science, 268, 1144-1149.

Karplus, M. (1985). Dynamic aspects of protein structure. Annals of the New York Academy of Sciences, 439, 107-123.

Kaufman, J. J., Chiabrera, A., Hatem, M., Bianco, B., & Pilla, A. (1990, October). Numerical stochastic analysis of Lorentz force ion binding kinetics in electromagnetic bioeffects. Paper presented at the BRAGS 10th Annual Meeting, Philadelphia, PA.

Lay, H., Horita, A., & Guy, A. W. (1994). Microwave irradiation affects radial-arm maze performance in the rat. Bioelectromagnetics, 15, 95-104.

Lednev, V. V. (1995). Comments on "Clarification and application of an ion parametric resonance model for magnetic field interactions with biological systems." Bioelectromagnetics, 16(4), 268-275.

Lednev, V. V. (1991). Possible mechanism for the influence of weak magnetic fields on biological systems. Bioelectromagnetics, 12, 71-75.

164

Li, V. O. K. & Qiu, X. (1995). Personal communication systems (PCS). Proceedings of the IEEE, 83, 1210-1243.

Liboff, A. R. (1985). Ciclotron resonance in membrane transport. In A. Chiabrera, C. Nicolini, & H. P. Schwan (Eds.), Interaction between electromagnetic fields and cells (pp.281-296). New York and London: Plenum Press.

Mcleod, B. R., & Liboff, A. R. (1986). Dynamic characteristics of membrane ions in multifield configurations of low-frequency electromagnetic radiation. Bioelectromagnetics, 7, 177-189.

Miklavcic, D., Karba, R., Vodovnik, L., & Chiabrera, A. (Eds.). (1994). Proceedings of the 2nd EBEA Congress: Advances in bioelectromagnetics. In Bioelectrochemistry and Bioenergetics, 35, 1-131.

Moggia, E., Tommasi, T., Bianco, B., & Chiabrera, A. (1993). Comparison of five-state vs. three-state coulombic Zeeman model of EMF effects on ligand binding. In M. Blank (Ed.), Electricity and magnetism in biology and medicine (pp. 556-558). San Francisco: San Francisco Press.

Pilla, A. A., Nasser, P. R., & Kaufman, J. J. (1994). Gap junction impedance, tissue dielectrics and thermal noise limits for electromagnetic field bioeffects. Bioelectrochemistry and Bioenergetics, 35, 63-69.

Poponin, V. (1995). Nonlinear stochastic resonance in weak emf interactions with diamagnetic ions bound within proteins. In Charge and field effects in biosystems-4 (pp. 306-319). Singapore: World Scientific.

Simunic, D. (Ed.). (1995). Papers of the Proceedings of the COST 244 Workshop on Biomedical Effects Relevant to Amplitude Modulated RF Fields, European Commission, DGXIII, Kuopio, Finland, Sept. 3-4, 1995.

Simunic, D. (Ed.). (1993). Papers of the Proceedings of the COST 244 Workshop on Mobile Communications and Extremely Low Frequency Fields, European Commission, DGXIII, Bled, Slovenia, Dec. 10-12, 1993.

Tarricone, L., Cito, C., & D'Inzeo, G. (1993). ACh receptor channel's interaction with MW fields. Bioelectrochemistry and Bioenergetics, 30, 275-285.

Tsong, T. Y. & Gross, C. J. (1994). Electric activation of membrane enzymes: Cellular transduction of high- and low-level periodic signals. In D. O. Carpenter & S. Ayrapetyan (Eds.), Biological effects of electric and magnetic fields, Vol. I. (pp. 143-164). Englewood Cliffs, NJ: Academic Press.

Wax, N. (Ed.). (1954). Selected papers on noise and stochastic processes. New York: Dover.

Weaver, J. C., & Astumian, R. D. (1994). The thermal noise limit for threshold effects of electric and magnetic fields. In D. O. Carpenter & S. Ayrapetyan (Eds.), Biological systems (pp 83-104). Mill Valley, CA: Plenum Press.

Wyman, J., & Gill, S. J. (1990). Binding and linkage. University Science Books.

12

WHERE DOES THE ENERGY GO? MICROWAVE ABSORPTION IN BIOLOGICAL OBJECTS ON THE MICROSCOPIC AND MOLECULAR SCALES

Asher R. Sheppard

Abstract

For many purposes of microwave dosimetry, it is sufficient to describe organisms in terms of bulk dielectric properties. However, biological systems reveal structural complexity at several scales. Microwave energy absorption occurs at the whole-body, tissue, cell, and molecular levels, although energy absorption by bulk water is the dominant factor for net energy absorption by an entire organism. Ultimately, energy is absorbed in biological molecules at the atomic scale and any biological effects would be related to the effect of changes in temperature and/or direct energy transfers. The frequency-dependence of dielectric responses establishes water, proteins, and cell membranes as the important features of biological responses to electromagnetic fields, but cell membranes are not important at microwave frequencies.

Introduction

The term "dosimetry" has several meanings in research on biological effects of exposure to radiofrequency fields. Topics in dosimetry include determinations of whole body average exposures far from a source, whole body and partial body exposures close to a source, and exposures to specific tissues and organs for both near- and far-field conditions. There also has been interest in evaluating exposure to specific portions of a biological cell or to its molecular components. In this paper, I focus on but two of many topics in dosimetry: dielectric properties of water in biological systems—the major mechanism for transduction of electromagnetic energy into heat—and interactions peculiar to large protein molecules. The focus of attention is mostly on interactions important at frequencies of 1 to 2 GHz, the frequency range used for cellular telephony.

There is now a considerable effort in getting quantitative information on the distribution of energy to the head of a user of a handheld cellular telephone transceiver. Principles and models needed for determination of energy distributions in the body for plane waves incident with a particular polarization have been known for years (for review, Johnson & Guy, 1972). For both far-field exposures and near-field exposures from hand-held devices, simple models for homogeneous objects such as a sphere have been succeeded by more realistic models that take into account anatomical shapes and the distinctive dielectric properties of various body tissues.

Regardless of the details of the energy distribution in the body, head, or other region, the biological effects on an exposed organism ultimately depend on how the applied energy affects the microscopic and molecular components of biological cells. It is widely recognized that water is the most important absorber of energy at the frequencies of interest. The dielectric properties of water—a feature of its unique molecular properties—define the main features of energy absorption in biologic systems. For purposes of accounting for the conversion of a given quantity of microwave energy, as measured by the specific absorption rate (SAR), it is necessary to assess the dielectric properties of the absorber. In the main, this is equivalent to assessing tissue water content.

When tissues are exposed to microwave fields strong enough to raise the temperature by one or more degrees, the mechanism is said to be thermal. Changes in temperature are significant because of the chemical and physiological systems which underlie biological functions. Enzymatically regulated biochemical reactions can be very strongly temperature-dependent, thereby giving rise to the same effects known with other sources of heat, such as exercise, fever, and the environment. In living organisms, the thermal mechanisms of interest are often physiological responses that help maintain normal body temperature rather than any of the underlying biochemical changes. For many purposes, dosimetry need go no further than establishing the net heat load to the whole body or regions of concentrated heat input.

Because radiofrequency waves at the frequency of cellular telephone systems have wavelengths of many centimeters (for example, 35 cm at 850 MHz), it would seem there are no readily apparent reasons to consider interactions with structures as small as a cell (10^{-3} cm). Specific effects on molecules (dimensions in the range of 10^{-7} cm) might seem to be of even less interest. For many years, there has been an interest in a more fine-grained analysis that focuses on energy absorption and transfer to particular biological structures, such as the cell's plasma membrane, or to biological molecules themselves. Molecules such as DNA, intrinsic membrane proteins (ion channels and ligand receptors), structural proteins of the cytoskeleton, and the many biochemically active enzymes and proteins have been scrutinized for unique microwave interactions. Although the amount of any one of these components in a cell is overwhelmed by the volume of water, distinctive microwave interactions, if established, could be important for the associated biochemical and biological changes despite the fact that the overall energy balance is determined by ubiquitous water.

In this paper, I discuss two aspects of interactions at the molecular level: direct microwave interactions at the molecular level and molecular-level localization of energy absorption. Although there are still interesting questions to be answered, all the known effects at molecular levels contribute to a picture in which microwave energy is rapidly and effectively transformed to heat. Heating is the only recognized way by which microwave energy acts on biological molecules for field strengths of interest in human exposures to the electromagnetic fields of telecommunications devices. Biological effects specific to extremely low frequency amplitude modulation of a microwave carrier indicate the existence of another mechanism that does not require significant temperature changes or energy transfer, but this topic is not treated here.

Where Does the Energy Go?

Oscillating electric and magnetic fields in biological objects set electric charges into motion. This happens whether the exposure is to tissues of a living animal or cells in a liquid medium in a laboratory experiment. In biological materials, these charges may be either ions that are free to move as an electric current or charges bound to molecules. Metals, in which electrons are abundant and free to move, have different characteristics when exposed to microwaves and are not discussed here. At microwave frequencies, the amount of energy lost in biological objects by collisions of the moving ions—that is, resistive loss—is smaller than loss from the movement of bound charges—that is, dielectric loss. Despite an abundance of mobile ions, the character of biological objects at high frequencies is dominated by the behavior of bound charges, of which the most important are the highly polarizable charges of water molecules.

The electrical properties of biological tissues are complicated because there are many ways in which charges bound to molecules or cells can respond to the surrounding electromagnetic field. Dielectric theory and measurements treat the electrical properties of nonmetal materials exposed to electromagnetic fields. An excellent review by Foster and Schwan (1995) treats dielectric phenomena of biological materials over the entire radiofrequency range and provides a concise historical overview of research spanning more than one hundred years. Although most molecules have some charged groups that respond to the field, water is important for the strength of its response. The association of two hydrogen atoms with an oxygen atom produces a solvent because of the resulting very strong electrical asymmetry of the H^+ and OH^- ion pair. This asymmetry also causes the strong interaction of water with microwave fields. The interaction strength is characterized by the relative dielectric permittivity of water which, at 1 GHz and a temperature of 37°C, is about 73 times the permittivity of free space (Hasted, 1973). The electric-field-driven movement of charge adds energy to the collisions between particles and thereby acts to transfer energy from the field to water molecules and other molecular sites of bound charge. Successive collisions lead to rapid diffusion of the energy among neighboring molecular constituents and to a generalized heating of the exposed tissue. This energy transfer constitutes "dielectric loss" and provides the major means by which energy is transformed from a microwave frequency electromagnetic wave to biologic tissue. Because water is so abundant and contributes so strongly to this energy transfer, the bulk properties of biological tissues and organisms are dominated by electromagnetic effects on water alone. Solutes, proteins, and cellular structure have significant effects in altering the dielectric property of pure water. There is an extensive literature from experimental observations and theoretical analyses for various dielectric phenomena over the spectrum from zero frequency to hundreds of gigahertz.

The presence of mobile ions, particularly Na^+, Cl^-, and K^+, results in resistive losses from the flow of current through tissue. In water at 1 GHz, resistive losses are about one-fourth the total dielectric loss (Hasted, 1973, Table 8.6).

At very low frequencies, the plasma membrane of a biological cell acts to insulate the cytoplasmic interior, but at microwave frequencies the membrane does not pose a barrier to the transmission of the electromagnetic field and it is as if the membrane were transparent. Therefore, there is equal exposure to all cell elements: the plasma membrane, membrane-bound proteins, structural proteins (including those of the cytoskeleton or those involved in motility), cytoplasmic organelles and cytoplasmic molecules (including many enzymes), and nuclear proteins (including nuclear enzymes and DNA). In terms of dielectric theory, the fact that charges of the cell membrane do not follow the rapid oscillations at microwave frequencies shows that the membrane is "fully relaxed" at these frequencies. In physical terms, the charged molecules of the membrane cannot vibrate fast enough to stay in step with the oscillating field. Likewise, ions cannot cross the membrane fast enough to follow the rapidly changing field and therefore cannot establish a voltage across the plasma membrane. Elsewhere, ions can respond to the field influence up to a maximum frequency, the "relaxation frequency." Water molecules can execute rotational motions that follow the applied field frequency up to about 25 GHz at 37°C. As a result, the relative dielectric permittivity falls from a value of 76 at 1 GHz (20°C), to approximately 30 at 25 GHz, until it reaches the asymptotic value of about 4.2, typical of water in the infrared or visible light regions.

Electric fields also act directly on protein molecules by exerting forces on side groups which have permanent electric dipole moments. Just as is true for water, charge asymmetry leads to charge motion and a coupling of electric energy to the molecule. Some molecular dipole moments are larger than the dipole moment for water. For example, proline has a dipole moment of 20 Debye units as compared to 1.8 Debye units for water (Hasted, 1973). However, the overall contribution to heating by such polar groups is dwarfed by the quantity of water. As a result, the losses from charges on proteins is a minor contribution to the total loss at 1-2 GHz. However, it is conceivable that the localized absorption of energy at proteins could have significant structural and biochemical effects. See below for additional discussion.

Some charged groups found on proteins are free to rotate. When exposed to microwaves in the range of 1 GHz, rotationally free groups can absorb somewhat more energy than other charge groups and overall contribute a small, but not insignificant, amount to the total energy transfer.

Water immediately adjacent to a protein molecule is, unlike other water, bound to the protein and not surrounded on all sides by other water molecules. Such "bound water" makes an additional contribution to energy absorption in biological systems at or below 1 GHz. At the molecular scale, the energy absorbed by bound water is immediately available to the adjacent proteins with the possibility of an effect on the protein.

Dielectric Properties of Cells, Tissues, and Biological Molecules

H.P. Schwan, whose theoretical and experimental work helped develop a large body of dielectric information for biological tissues, described the following dielectric hierarchy (Schwan, 1974; see Figure 1). The main dielectric phenomena are identified by the frequency regions in which dielectric properties change rapidly with frequency—regions of "dielectric dispersion." The changing dielectric responses correspond to interactions that involve the complex structures at low frequency and less complex elements at several gigahertz where the properties of pure water dominate. Going from low frequencies to high, the phenomena are:

α-dispersion -- For electrical purposes at low frequencies, biological cells have but three components: water, proteins, and a cell membrane. Cells have an extraordinarily large relative dielectric permittivity (up to several million times the free space permittivity) at frequencies of up to several thousand hertz to about one hertz or less. One mechanism for this large permittivity involves a population of mobile ions ("counterions") at the highly charged interface between the plasma membrane and the extracellular medium. Counterions can move freely along the cell surface at low frequency. For certain cells, such as muscle, a second low frequency mechanism is enhancement of transmembrane ion fluxes. At frequencies of several hundred to several thousand hertz, ions can no longer follow the applied field. The very large permittivities decline sharply with frequency in this range, thereby defining a relaxation known as the "α-dispersion."

β-dispersion -- At frequencies above the α-dispersion, a model cell consisting of only water and a plasma membrane still exhibits strong polarization because of the presence of the membrane. The increment in dielectric constant from membrane charging is large, for example, in the range from one- to ten-thousand-fold (Foster & Schwan, 1995)—not as strong as the α-dispersion. The decline in cell membrane charging (β-dispersion) usually takes place in the range from 500 kHz to several megahertz.

δ-dispersion -- A solution of water plus protein (without membranes) characterizes the responses at higher frequencies (~100 MHz to ~3 GHz) where the membrane is electrically transparent. The dielectric increment identified as the δ-dispersion results from interactions of water and proteins. Numerically, the δ-dispersion is relatively small, about 10 to 20 times the free space permittivity.

γ-dispersion -- At frequencies above about 3 GHz, only water can absorb significant amounts of energy from the electromagnetic field; the cell can be modeled in terms of its water content alone. The typical increment in relative dielectric permittivity over that of free space is by a factor of 50. The frequency regime where this interaction starts to fall off identifies the "γ-dispersion." The γ-dispersion region, which is centered at 25 GHz (37° C), extends from about 3 GHz to 100 GHz. At the latter frequency, the relative dielectric permittivity approaches the value at infrared or light frequencies, where it is 4.2.

How Much Heat IsTransferred?

The amount of heat transferred to a biological system is important for the purpose of distinguishing the cases where the biological system may be affected by a change in temperature from those where the energy is too little or too dispersed to cause any noticeable change in temperature. For laboratory experiments, exposure conditions can be classified in three categories: nonthermal, athermal, and thermal. Each category has slightly different meaning for studies conducted in vivo and in vitro. Table 1 provides definitions that, while not universal, capture common usage and suggest specific absorption rates (SARs) that typify each regime for common experimental conditions. The SARs listed should not be interpreted as boundaries for the different exposure regimes because factors such as animal species, environmental temperature, air flow and humidity, coolant medium, coolant flow, and exposed volume and surface may have a large influence on the character of a particular exposure.

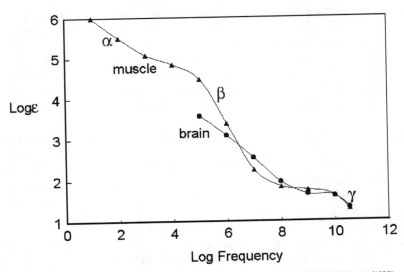

Data from Table 6, Foster and Schwan (1995)

Figure 1. Relative permittivity. The relative permittivity (ε) is shown for muscle tissue (triangles) over the range from 100 Hz to 35 GHz. The α-, β- and γ-dispersions are evident as the broad ranges in frequency over which the permittivity decreases from a value of 10^6 at 100 Hz, to about 2.5×10^3 at 1 MHz, and to about 60 at 1 GHz. Relative permittivity of brain gray matter is shown (circles) over the range 100 kHz to 35 GHz, including the β- and γ-dispersions. The relatively small δ-dispersion is not clearly evident.

Category	Type of experiment	Characteristics	Approximate SAR range (W/kg)
Nonthermal	in vivo	• no challenge to thermoregulation; • temperature unaffected	< 0.1 W/kg
	in vitro	• temperature is unchanged	< 0.1 W/kg
Athermal	in vivo	• challenges thermoregulation, but temperature is unaffected	0.1-1 W/kg
	in vitro	• without cooling, temperature may rise; • heat flow to coolant keeps temperature unchanged	0.1-50 W/kg
Thermal	in vivo	• thermoregulation is challenged • body temperature rises (e.g., > 2-5°C)	≥ 4 W/kg
	in vitro	• temperature rises "significantly" (e.g., >0.2, 1, 2, or 5°C)	≥ 1 W/kg

Table 1. Characteristics of experimental microwave exposures at various incident power levels for in vivo and in vitro experiments.

How Rapidly Does the Heat Travel?

At the molecular level, heat energy propagates by collisions among the mobile ions, collisions between ions and large molecules, and vibrational motions of molecules. Once again, the abundance of water permits the simplifying assumption that, for the purpose of estimating heat flow, the biological tissue can be treated as if it were all water. Since there are about 4×10^{11} collisions per second among water molecules at 37° C, it should not be surprising that the characteristic time for diffusion of heat over a distance of cellular dimensions (10 μm) is less than 10 milliseconds (Hille, 1984). Hence, a cell comes to equilibrium rapidly. If there were a localized pulse of heat at any microscopic structure, it would be dissipated within this time. Heat transfer over molecular dimensions is even faster.

The Effect of Temperature Change

According to the Eyring rate theory of chemical reactions, chemical reactions occur when the reacting molecules collide with sufficient energy to overcome the energy barrier keeping them separate (Volkenshtein, 1981). As a result, the reaction rate, k, depends on the Gibbs free energy of the reactants and the temperature,

$$k = v\exp(-\Delta G^{\ddagger}/RT)$$
$$= v\exp[(-\Delta H^{\ddagger} + T\Delta S^{\ddagger})/RT]$$
$$= v\exp(-\Delta H^{\ddagger}/RT)\ \exp(\Delta S^{\ddagger}/R),$$

where the double dagger symbol ($\ddagger$) indicates that the various thermodynamic quantities (G, Gibbs free energy, H, enthalpy, and S, entropy) are associated with the activation energy for the reaction. R is the universal gas constant, T is the thermodynamic temperature, and v is a constant. The equilibrium thermodynamic relation, G = H - TS, was used above to show that the temperature dependence of chemical reactions is related to the change in enthalpy, ΔH, whereas the entropy change, ΔS, is not temperature dependent. The enthalpy is essentially the energy barrier ("activation energy"). The above relation shows that chemical reaction rates rise exponentially with increasing temperature.

Tyazhelov and Alekseyev (1978) considered the possibility of differential microwave heating of integral membrane proteins, particularly the heating of ion channel proteins above the temperature of the surrounding electrolyte medium. According to the model, there is almost no channel cooling because the channel proteins are not in contact with the electrolyte medium and the only remaining mechanism for channel heat loss is radiation. Heat transfer from the channel protein to the lipid membrane was ignored. The model was applied to the results of experimental tests at 900 MHz on the ionic conductivity of alamethicin, amphotericin B, and valinomycin in artificial membranes exposed to strong microwave fields incident with the electric field perpendicular to the plane of the test membrane (Alekseyev & Tyazhelov, 1978; Tyazhelov, Alekseyev, & Grigor'ev, 1979). The time for changes in conductance was in the range from less than one second to three seconds.

Ultimately, for all the mechanisms considered, energy is absorbed in biological molecules at the atomic scale. From this perspective, the distinction between "thermal" and "athermal" conditions blurs and can be reinterpreted as a question of whether the energy density at critical microscopic or molecular sites is sufficient to alter the physicochemical functions of dynamic molecular structures.

Some Proposed Mechanisms That Do Not Depend on Changing Temperature

Illinger proposed that bound water—which contributes to the δ-dispersion—may transfer energy to proteins and thereby affect cooperatively determined structures (Illinger, 1970, 1981). Although structural water is at equilibrium, it may have a specific biochemical effect by providing energy that, in a cooperative fashion, permits conformational changes in an associated protein. Changes in protein conformation could, as is well known, have significant effects on physiologic functions of proteins. A similar consideration was proposed for the interaction of microwaves with cell membranes near a membrane phase transition. Illinger (1981) noted that changes in molecular order suggestive of a phase change occurred near 2 GHz for certain lipid-based hydrocarbon chains. The presence in biological systems of dissipative subsystems which utilize metabolic energy for anti-entropic processes implies another possible route by which the small energy from a microwave photon might have a significant influence on biological functions. Rabinowitz (1973) suggested that when microwave energy was absorbed, there may be changes in molecular stereochemistry that require very little energy, yet produce significant structural and functional changes. Rabinowitz and Weil (1984) point out that microwave interactions of this type would not result in novel configurations because there is, at normal biological temperature, abundant thermal energy to drive a system to the same states. These latter authors also review other proposed nonthermal mechanisms.

Barnes and Hu (1977) presented a model for microwave bioeffects that depended on shifts in ion concentration across a cell membrane. The nonlinear shift in ion concentrations is a direct result of an oscillating transmembrane potential. Although the model is evaluated for frequencies near 1 GHz, it is unclear if the model correctly predicts a concentration change in view of the near-zero transmembrane potentials at this frequency.

Effects of 9.14 GHz microwaves on Na^+/K^+ ATPase activity at various temperatures (Brown & Chattopadhyay, 1991) provide evidence for direct microwave effects on the enzyme's protein molecule. Previously, similar effects on enzyme activity were found for the same enzyme when it was studied at 2.45 GHz by Allis and Sinha-Robinson (1987) and by Fisher, Poznansky, and Voss (1982).

Cleary (1993) reviewed a number of other proposed nonthermal microwave effects involving free radical chemistry in melanin-containing cells, rates of gramicidin ion channel formation in a lipid bilayer system, altered frequency of acetylcholine ion channel openings, and altered rates of neuronal pacemaker firing.

The proposals noted in this section remain speculative and require further specification and experimental proof, such as those suggested by Illinger (1981), to see if there are indeed interactions of greater specificity than the well-understood thermalization of microwave energy absorbed by rotational modes in water molecules.

Conclusions

At frequencies of about 1-2 GHz, microwave energy incident on biological tissues is transformed into heat by interactions with water and other polarized molecules. Because of its strong polarizability and abundance, most of the direct energy transfer is to water. Interactions with water bound to proteins, cell membranes, and polar portions of proteins have been identified. Direct interactions with proteins contribute in minor ways to total energy absorption, but the direct transfer of energy to local molecular sites may be significant. In all cases, collisions rapidly transfer the heat energy over microscopic and macroscopic distances so that all lipids, proteins (including enzymes), and cell structures rapidly come to the same temperature.

References

Alekseyev, S. I., & Tyazhelov, V. V. (1978). Microwave effect on modified lipid bilayer conductance. Puschino, USSR: Institute of Biological Physics, Academy of Sciences of the USSR.

Allis, J. W., & Sinha-Robinson, B. L. (1987). Temperature-specific inhibition of human red cell Na^+/K^+ ATPase by 2,450-MHz microwave radiation. Bioelectromagnetics, 8(2), 203-212.

Barnes, F. S., & Hu, C.-L. J. (1977). Model for some nonthermal effects of radio and microwave fields on biological membranes. IEEE Transactions on Microwave Theory and Technique, 25(9), 742-746.

Brown, H. D., & Chattopadhyay, S. K. (1991). Ouabain inhibition of kidney ATPase is altered by 9.14 GHz radiation. Bioelectromagnetics, 12(3), 137-143.

Cleary, S. F. (1993). Biophysical mechanisms of interaction. In W. R. Stone & G. Hyde (Eds.), Review of radio science 1990-1992 (pp. 717-735). New York: Oxford University Press.

Fisher, P. D., Poznansky, M. J., & Voss, W. A. G. (1982). Effect of microwave radiation (2,450 MHz) on the active and passive components of $^{24}Na^+$ efflux from human erythrocytes. Radiation Research, 92(2), 411-422.

Foster, K. R., & Schwan, H. P. (1995). Dielectric properties of tissues. In C. Polk & E. Postow (Eds.), Handbook of biological effects of electromagnetic fields (2nd ed., pp.25-102). Boca Raton, FL: CRC Press.

Hasted, J. B. (1973). Aqueous dielectrics. London: Chapman and Hall.

Hille, B. (1984). Ionic channels of excitable membranes. Sunderland, MA: Sinauer Associates Inc.

Illinger, K. H. (1970). Molecular mechanisms for microwave absorption in biological systems. In S. F. Cleary (Ed.), Biological effects and health implications of microwave radiation (BRH/DBE 70-2, pp. 112-115). Rockville, MD: Bureau of Radiological Health, Food and Drug Administration.

Illinger, K. H. (1981). Electromagnetic-field interaction with biological systems in the microwave and far-infrared region: Physical basis. American Chemical Society Symposium Series, 157, 1-43.

Johnson, C. C., & Guy, A. W. (1972). Nonionizing electromagnetic wave effects in biological materials and systems. Proceedings of the IEEE, 60, 692-718.

Rabinowitz, J. R. (1973). Possible mechanisms for the biomolecular absorption of microwave radiation with functional implications [letter]. IEEE Transactions on Microwave Theory and Technique, 21(12), 850.

Schwan, H. P. (1974). Effects of microwave radiation at the cellular and molecular level. In Biological effects and health hazards of microwave radiation (pp. 152-159). Warsaw, Poland: Polish Medical Publishers.

Tyazhelov, V. V., Alekseyev, S. I., & Grigor'ev, P. A. (1979). Change in the conductivity of phospholipid membranes modified by alamethicin on exposure to a high frequency electromagnetic field. Biophysics [translation of Biofizika], 23, 750-751.

Tyazhelov, V. V., & Alekseyev, S. I. (1978). Possible model of microwave conductivity effect for lipid bilayer channels. Puschino, USSR: Institute of Biological Physics, Academy of Sciences of the USSR.

Volkenshtein, M. V. (1983). Biophysics. Moscow: Mir Publishers.

Weil, C. M., & Rabinowitz, J. R. (1984). RF-field interactions with biological systems. In J.A. Elder & D.F. Cahill (Eds.), Biological effects of radiofrequency radiation (pp. 3-6 to 3-24). Research Triangle Park, NC: U.S. Environmental Protection Agency.

13
BIOLOGICAL EFFECTS AND MECHANISMS
Bernard Veyret

Abstract

There is a need for a careful distinction between the various levels at which microwaves can act on living matter: (i) bio-interaction (macroscopic level), (ii) bioeffects (biochemical or physiological changes within the cell, tissue, or organism), and (iii) human health aspects. A brief review of European research projects on bioeffects will be given, together with a discussion of the various types of bioeffects and corresponding mechanisms. The link between animal cancer models and real-life health situations will also be addressed.

Introduction

In view of the current concern about possible biological effects of microwaves used in mobile communications, it is important to assess the body of knowledge on microwave-induced bioeffects and to determine proper research strategies. This short paper addresses the basic definitions of types of effects, the status of European research, and some considerations on mechanisms and health impacts.

There are three aspects to consider: (i) the interaction of electromagnetic fields with living matter at macroscopic and microscopic levels (biointeraction); (ii) changes in biochemical and/or physiological parameters (bioeffects); and (iii) the effect on health of such changes.

Biointeraction of Microwaves

Theoretical and experimental dosimetry deals with the evaluation of the interaction of electromagnetic fields with living organisms: values of $E(t)$ and $H(t)$ inside the organism are measured or calculated. However, this is usually only a macroscopic evaluation, while analysis of possible bioeffects often has to be carried out at the cellular or the molecular level. There is thus a need for a better understanding and evaluation of the actual field values at these levels. This problem is addressed in the papers by C. Gabriel, A. Chiabrera, and A. Sheppard.

Moreover, when people speak about thermal bioeffects, they usually refer to an increase in the core temperature of the organism, and they assume that this increase is either due to the interaction of the radiofrequency (RF) field with water in the tissues or to induced electric currents. In contrast, athermal effects may occur while the thermoregulation system stabilizes the temperature. However, it has been suggested that there are specific bioeffects that correspond to a negligible increase in macroscopic temperature. If these exist, they must be thought of as originating from interaction of the electromagnetic field at a level that does not involve bulk water heating. Since the thermal load corresponding to the use of a mobile telephone is clearly in the lower range of the scale, the question of the existence of specific bioeffects—which are not taken into account in the current definition of exposure limits—is thus of central importance.

In order to address these issues, one approach should be to compare results obtained with extremely low frequency (ELF) and ELF-modulated RF fields using the same biological model. Such evaluations or investigations should provide insight on demodulation mechanisms, as everyone emphasizes the role of ELF modulation in the elicitation of specific bioeffects. However, such an approach has rarely been put forward, mainly because of a paucity of well-documented experiments performed simultaneously with both types of fields on the same biological model.

Biological Effects

In view of the small number of experimental investigations on bioeffects performed at RF wavelengths and power levels of current interest, a major research effort has been launched in the past few years. This renewed interest in RF research is not yet fully coordinated worldwide.

Laboratory Research in Europe

The last two years have seen a rapid increase in the number of research projects conducted in this field in Europe. An overview of this research effort will be published soon (Veyret & Semm, in press). Some of the completed and on-going projects are described briefly below.

Human Models.
Since legislation makes it easier in Europe than in the USA to experiment on humans, projects have been started on volunteers exposed to actual mobile phones. Some results have already been obtained. In Nîmes, France, human volunteers were exposed to Global System for Mobile Communications (GSM) signals (2 hours/day, 5

days/week, for 4 weeks) and the levels of the hypothalamo-pituitary hormones were assessed (project sponsored by France Télécom). There was no detectable influence of exposure on these hormone levels. A continuation of this study (sponsored by Motorola) will look at the circadian level of hormones (including melatonin). Two other studies on melatonin levels in response to mobile phone exposure are in progress in Mainz, Germany, under the sponsorship of Deutsche Telekom.

An EEG study is being conducted at the Institute of Occupational Health in Helsinki, Finland on human volunteers exposed to GSM signals. In a similar study performed in Giessen, Germany, EEG changes were observed that were comparable to changes induced by a minor analgesic activation of the opioid system (Reiser, Dimpfel, & Schober, 1995).

Animal Models.

Many studies on cancer are being conducted or are planned in Europe. In our study on tumor growth in rats (sponsored by France Télécom), no influence of exposure to GSM-like microwaves (900 MHz, 50 or 200 $\mu W/cm^2$, 2 hours/day, 5 days/week, for 2 weeks) was observed on the timing of the appearance of the chemically-induced tumors, survival, lymphocyte subpopulations, or tumor marker levels (Chagnaud, Veyret, & Després, 1995a). In a study performed at ENEA, Rome, Italy, mice bearing grafted tumors were exposed at 900 MHz (whole-body specific absorption rate [SAR] of 0.4 W/kg), and there was no difference in the rate of tumor growth between exposed and sham-exposed groups (Marino, Antonini, Avella, Galloni, & Scacchi, 1995). The development of DMBA-induced tumors will be investigated in rats under GSM exposure in Tübingen, Germany (sponsored by Deutsche Telekom). Since brain tumors are obviously an important cancer model relevant to mobile phone studies, a rat brain glioma model was studied in Lund, Sweden. Animals were exposed to 915 MHz microwaves either continuous or modulated at various frequencies including 200 Hz (7 hours/day, 5 days/week, for 2-3 weeks). There was no influence of exposure on the growth of tumors under any of the conditions studied (Salford, Brun, Persson, & Eberhardt, 1993).

Specific effects on the nervous system of RF exposure are also being investigated in Europe. In Frankfurt, Germany, cells from the central nervous system of birds were found to respond to GSM-pulsed microwave exposure (Semm, Dombek, Hollmann, & Beason, 1995). Continuous waves did not elicit the effect (project sponsored by Deutsche Telekom). A study, sponsored by Motorola, is in progress in Köln, Germany and Zürich, Switzerland to investigate possible acute reaction and injury to the central nervous system (CNS) of rats exposed to GSM signals. The level of neurotransmitters in rats exposed to GSM-microwaves is being assessed in Nîmes, France (sponsored by France Télécom).

Following studies on the permeability of the blood-brain-barrier in rats exposed to the fields of magnetic resonance imaging, a group in Lund, Sweden (Salford, Brun, Sturesson, Eberhardt, & Persson, 1994) has carried out experiments in transverse electromagnetic (TEM) cells at 915 MHz (whole-body SAR between 0.016 and 5 W/kg) and reported a significant increase in albumin leakage under both pulsed-modulated and continuous microwave exposures.

Animal studies on the level of melatonin in rats exposed to low-level, pulsed microwaves is in progress in Mainz, Germany under the sponsorship of Deutsche Telekom, which is also funding an investigation in Frankfurt, Germany on melatonin levels in birds. Preliminary evidence seems to indicate that there is a shift in the melatonin peak at night due to exposure to the microwaves.

As regards genotoxicity, a series of studies sponsored by Belgacom has been performed on rats by a group in Mol, Belgium (Maes, Collier, Slaets, & Verschaeve, in press). Preliminary results showed genetic alterations only when animals were placed almost in contact with base station antennas.

Cellular Models.

Experiments involving exposure of cells in vitro have not yet been numerous in Europe. Our experiments in Bordeaux on three types of tumor cells yielded negative results: cells were exposed for 4 h to GSM-modulated microwaves at 900 MHz and 200 μW/cm^2, plane-wave, and proliferation was assessed 24 and 48 h later (Chagnaud, Veyret & Despres, 1995b). In Aalborg, Denmark, cells were exposed in a TEM cell to GSM-modulated microwaves and there was preliminary evidence for changes in proliferation at certain exposure levels (Kwee & Raskmark, 1995).

Mechanisms

In order to progress toward the understanding of mechanisms of possible specific bioeffects, it is necessary to make the distinction between mechanisms at the biological level (animal tissue, cultured cells) and at the physical or biochemical level. Moreover, in order to suggest theoretical hypotheses, one must evaluate the validity of results obtained with RF exposures, such as the results obtained by Lai and coworkers over the years on the neuroendocrine system (Lai, 1994). There is still a need for replication of experiments that have been reported to show specific bioeffects, such as changes in neuroendocrine parameters, blood-brain-barrier permeability, etc.

In addition, possible synergies between physical or chemical factors and microwaves may be occurring under certain experimental exposure conditions. For example, in our laboratory we have evidence that some ELF effects occur only when cells have been submitted previously to stimuli that "prepare" the action of the magnetic field. Analysis of published results and new experiments could be planned to assess the validity of the hypothesis.

As regards basic physical mechanisms, there is still a lack of valid theoretical hypotheses at ELF and even more so at RF or ELF-modulated RF. Only when robust data are available will there be a real incentive for such theoretical effort.

Health Relevance

Extrapolation of results obtained in vitro to animal models has always been criticized for obvious reasons. However, in vitro experiments, which are sometimes easier to conduct and to interpret than in vivo experiments, are needed and especially so when they correspond to standard toxicology assays. They are most useful when the influence of one variable must be assessed independently of the homeostatic environment of the organism. Our own negative results on the proliferation of cells under exposure to GSM-modulated microwaves is a good example of such a case.

The question regarding extrapolation of animal experiments to human health is addressed in the paper by A. Sivak. In principle, most animal tumor-promotion experiments performed so far have been to help evaluate human health risk. Our own negative results on rats bearing chemically-induced tumors and exposed to pulsed microwaves only demonstrate that there is no gross effect to fear. Such investigations are also being carried out to show to the public that experiments are being done under "real life" exposure conditions on "real life" biological models, since cancer promotion is the major concern for most telephone users. This type of nonscientific justification cannot be rejected totally, but must be taken into account in the planning of research programmes. This is also obviously true for long-term studies, since telephone usage is seen as a "chronic" type of exposure.

Moreover, we have learned from ELF studies that the possibility that some individuals may be particularly susceptible to magnetic field exposure as regards their health cannot be ruled out.

Conclusion

With regard to RF-induced bioeffects, it is most useful to examine in detail the knowledge on bioeffects of ELF fields, because of: (i) the vast number of studies; (ii) the analogies between some of the effects; and (iii) the role of ELF modulation in mobile communications. It will thus be necessary to compare effects of pulsed-modulated and continuous microwaves.

European studies have given preliminary results that show no effect on cancer models but some on the nervous system. Since most investigations concerning the nervous system are being performed in Europe, collaboration between the various laboratories involved should provide some answers in the near future.

Research in Europe has been very active in the last few years, but there has been a lack of coordination between projects in spite of the creation and action of the COST 244 programme. The DG XIII-programme that is being set up by the European Commission (DG XIII) should help improve that situation.

References

Chagnaud, J.-L., Veyret, B., & Després, B. (1995a). Effects of pulsed microwaves on chemically-induced tumors [abstract]. 17th Annual Meeting of the Bioelectromagnetics Society, Abstract Book, 28.

182

Chagnaud, J.-L., Veyret, B., & Després, B. (1995b). No effect of exposure to GSM-modulated microwaves on the proliferation of GH3, MolT4 and C6 tumor cells. Manuscript in preparation.

Kwee, S., & Raskmark, P. (1995, September). The effects of microwave radiation on cell proliferation. Paper presented at the COST 244 Workshop on Biological Effects of Modulated RF Radiation, Kuopio, Finland.

Lai, H. (1994). Neurological effects of radiofrequency electromagnetic radiation. In J. C. Lin (Ed.), Advances in electromagnetic fields in living systems: Vol. 1 (pp. 27-80). New York: Plenum Press.

Maes, A., Collier, M., Slaets, D., & Verschaeve, L. (In press). Cytogenetic effects of microwaves from mobile communication frequencies (GSM). Electromagnetobiology.

Marino, C., Antonini, F., Avella, B., Galloni, L., & Scacchi, P. (1995). 900-MHz effects on tumoral growth in in vivo systems. 17th Annual Meeting of the Bioelectromagnetics Society, 191-193.

Reiser, H.-P., Dimpfel, W., & Schober, F. (1995). The influence of electromagnetic fields on human brain activity. European Journal of Medical Research, 1, 27-32.

Salford, L. G., Brun, A., Persson, B. R., & Eberhardt, J. L. (1993). Experimental studies of brain tumor development during exposure to continuous and pulsed 915 MHz radiofrequency radiation. Bioelectrochemical Bioenergetics, 30, 313-318.

Salford, L. G., Brun, A., Sturesson, K., Eberhardt, J. L., & Persson, B. R. (1994). Permeability of the blood brain barrier induced by 915-MHz electromagnetic radiation, continuous wave and modulated at 8, 16, 50 and 200 Hz. Microscopy Research and Technique, 27, 535-542.

Semm, P., Dombek, P., Hollmann, H., & Beason, R. C. (1995). Neuronal responses to high frequency low intensity electromagnetic fields in the avian brain. Manuscript in preparation.

Veyret, B., & Semm, P. (1996). European research on the effects of RF fields on biological systems. In N. Kuster, Q. Balzano, & J. C. Lin (Eds.), Progress in safety assessments of mobile communications. Chapman & Hall.

14

ELECTROMAGNETIC FIELDS AND CARCINOGENESIS—AN ANALYSIS OF BIOLOGICAL MECHANISMS
Thomas S. Tenforde

Abstract

A summary is presented of laboratory research relevant to the possible biological mechanisms through which electromagnetic fields could exert carcinogenic effects. A focus of this discussion is the potential influence of electromagnetic fields on the initiation, promotion, and progression of cancer cells. In addition to summarizing and critically evaluating published studies related to electromagnetic fields and carcinogenesis, recommendations are made for future research on this subject, with an emphasis on modulated radiofrequency fields such as those emitted by wireless communication systems.

One of the most controversial issues related to the possible health effects of exposure to nonionizing electromagnetic fields is the question of whether these fields exert carcinogenic effects. A large number of laboratory studies and epidemiological surveys have provided conflicting evidence on this subject for electromagnetic fields (EMF) ranging in frequency from radiofrequency (RF) to extremely low-frequency (ELF). The amplitude- and pulse-modulated RF fields emitted by wireless communication systems pose a particular challenge in terms of assessing their influence on carcinogenic processes. The Fourier components of fields from wireless communication systems encompass a broad spectral range as a consequence of their modulation properties. Assessing the biological interactions and possible carcinogenic effects of these fields therefore requires an analysis of relevant information acquired on fields that encompass a broad segment of the nonionizing radiation spectrum (Chiabrera, Bianco, Moggia, Tommasi, & Kaufman, 1995). The primary objective of this paper is to analyze the evidence obtained from studies with both in vitro cellular systems and in vivo animal models for possible carcinogenic effects of EMF at frequencies ranging from ELF to RF.

The framework that will be used for the analysis of possible relationships between EMF exposures and cancer risk is the multistage model of tumor development depicted in Figure 1. It is now widely accepted that carcinogenesis proceeds through

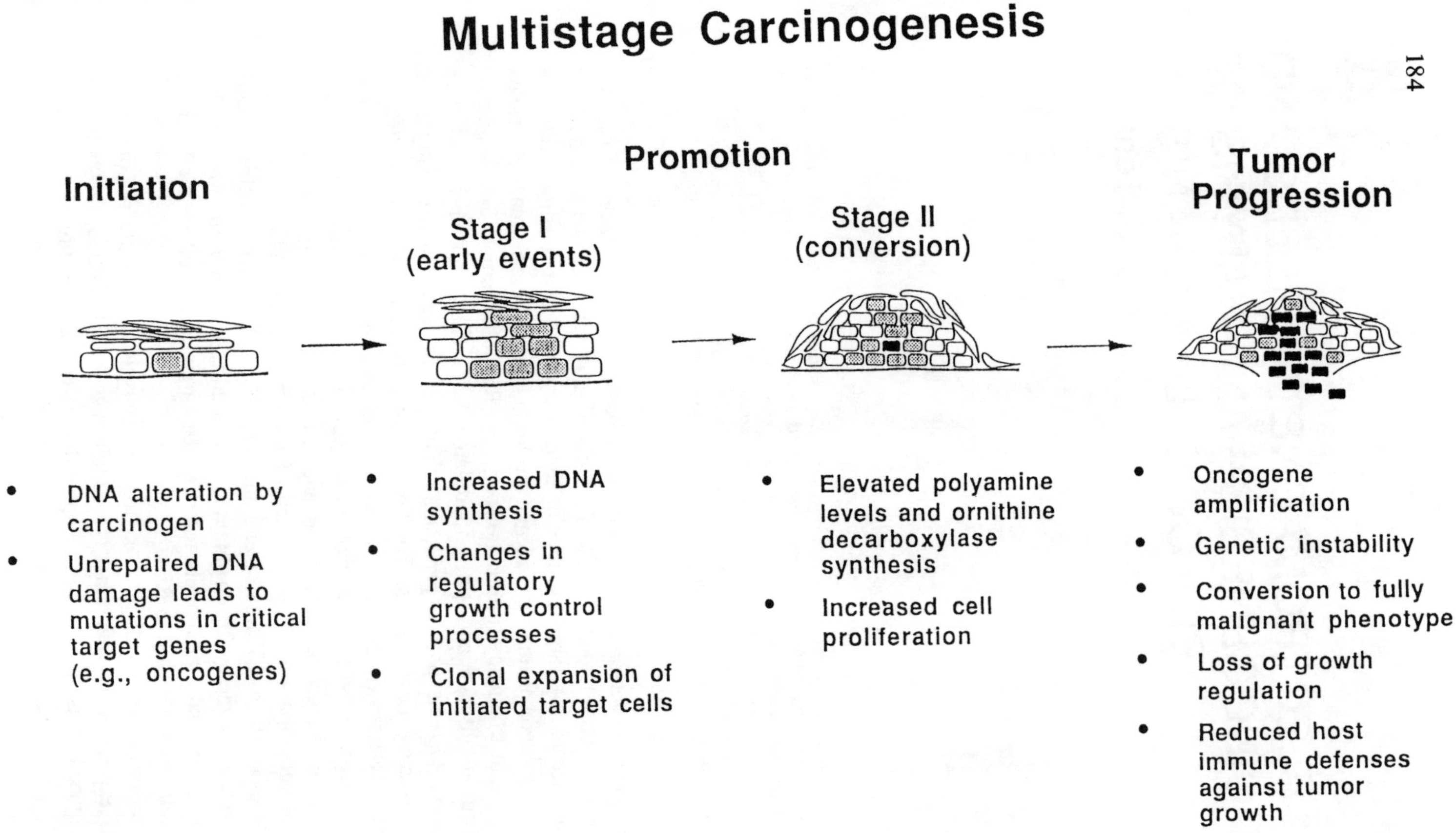

Multistage Carcinogenesis

Initiation

Promotion

Tumor Progression

Stage I (early events)

Stage II (conversion)

- DNA alteration by carcinogen
- Unrepaired DNA damage leads to mutations in critical target genes (e.g., oncogenes)

- Increased DNA synthesis
- Changes in regulatory growth control processes
- Clonal expansion of initiated target cells

- Elevated polyamine levels and ornithine decarboxylase synthesis
- Increased cell proliferation

- Oncogene amplification
- Genetic instability
- Conversion to fully malignant phenotype
- Loss of growth regulation
- Reduced host immune defenses against tumor growth

Figure 1. Depiction of major events in the initiation, promotion, and progression of tumor growth.

a series of events that can be represented by three primary stages: (a) <u>initiation</u>, involving mutations in critical genes as a result of unrepaired DNA damage by either physical or chemical carcinogens; (b) <u>promotion</u>, which involves an increase in the rate of DNA synthesis and proliferation of the mutated cells; and (c) <u>progression</u>, during which the tumor cells exhibit increased genetic abnormalities and conversion to a fully malignant phenotype. In several classes of tumors, such as skin carcinomas, there are at least two relatively distinct stages of tumor promotion, with a significant elevation in polyamine biosynthesis and clonal cell proliferation in the later stage. At this point in the carcinogenic process, the initial clones of neoplastically transformed cells are undergoing conversion to a fully malignant state.

In the following sections of this paper, the evidence for effects of EMF on each of the major stages of cancer development are described for both fields at low frequencies (primarily ELF) and RF fields. The reader should bear in mind, however, that the interactions of ELF and RF fields with tissue differ in significant ways that can profoundly influence their effects on the structure and functions of biological systems. Although both low-frequency and high-frequency fields applied to the body through air induce electric fields and currents in tissue, at microwave frequencies above 300 MHz in the RF band, the fields can significantly influence the energy states of water and other molecules through dielectric loss phenomena. At these higher frequencies, exposure to intense RF fields can induce significant tissue heating and resultant thermal effects on the structural and functional properties of molecular, cellular, and tissue systems. In contrast, at frequencies in the lower part of the RF band down to ELF frequencies, the inductive coupling of fields applied to the body through air is sufficiently weak that no measurable tissue heating occurs even with a prolonged period of exposure.

The primary objective of the following discussion is to provide an overview and general conclusions on the possible carcinogenic effects of EMF. In addition, gaps in the existing body of information are identified that need to be filled by carefully planned research programs in the near future. The literature citations are limited primarily to recent publications of particular relevance to the possible influence of EMF on carcinogenic processes.

Cancer Initiation

The initial events that can ultimately lead to the loss of growth regulation typical of cancer cells involve damage to DNA and chromatin structures caused by a chemical or physical agent. As a consequence of unrepaired or misrepaired damage to the genetic material of cells, mutations occur that are the basis of neoplastic cell transformation. These early events that can ultimately lead to a malignant tumor have been studied primarily with in vitro cellular systems exposed to either ELF or RF fields.

For ELF fields there is strong evidence that exposure of cells to these fields does not alter DNA or chromatin structure, as evidenced by a lack of field-induced DNA strand breaks, chromosome aberrations, or sister chromatid exchanges (reviews are presented in Cridland, 1993; McCann, Dietrich, Rafferty, & Martin, 1993;

Sienkiewicz, Cridland, Kowalczuk, & Saunders, 1993; Tenforde, 1996). Using 10T1/2 cells grown in vitro, no evidence was obtained for an increase in neoplastic transformation by ELF fields applied alone or in combination with X-rays (Frazier, Reese, & Morris, 1990). These findings are not surprising in view of the extremely small amount of energy imparted to living tissues by externally applied ELF fields, which is orders of magnitude below the level that would disrupt chemical bonds in DNA or chromatin structures. To date there have been no major in vivo laboratory studies to examine tumor initiation in animals exposed to ELF fields. However, a large study on carcinogenesis in rodents exposed to 60 Hz magnetic fields is currently underway at the IIT Research Institute in Chicago, Illinois.

A large number of in vitro studies have been conducted to detect effects of RF fields on DNA and chromosome structures (Cridland, 1993; Michaelson & Lin, 1987; National Research Council [NRC], 1987). As discussed in summaries of the published literature by Brusick (1995) and Meltz (1995), many of the positive findings of RF-induced DNA strand breaks, sister chromatid exchanges, or chromosome aberrations occurred under conditions in which the temperature of the cell culture was elevated as a result of exposure to RF fields. In some cases, reports of damage to DNA or chromosome structures from RF exposures have been attributable to secondary experimental factors, such as the leaching of copper ions from an RF antenna (Sagripanti, Swicord, & Davis, 1987) or the use of a metal thermistor placed directly into the cell sample that could cause localized heating ("hotspots") during RF field exposure (Maes, Vershaeve, Arroyo, DeWagter, & Vercruyssen, 1993).

In vivo studies of damage by RF fields to DNA and chromatin have also led to mixed positive and negative findings. No elevation in the rate of sister chromatid exchanges or chromosome aberrations has been observed following exposure of animal tissues to nonthermal levels of RF radiation. However, two recent studies have provided evidence for DNA structural damage in brain and testis tissues isolated from rodents following nonthermal RF exposures (Lai & Singh, 1995; Sarkar, Ali, & Behari, 1994). The results presented in these studies, however, may be attributable to factors other than direct DNA structural damage by RF fields. For example, in the study by Lai and Singh, the increase in DNA strand breaks in the exposed tissue was as large, or larger, at 4 hours following termination of the RF exposure than immediately after the exposure was ended. Various alternative hypotheses can be proposed to explain this observation. One possible explanation is that the elevated level of DNA strand breaks could be attributable to an effect of RF radiation on DNA structure that does not involve a direct disruption of covalent bonds. For example, an effect of the RF field on DNA helix conformation could facilitate strand breakage by endogenous oxygen radical species produced during normal aerobic metabolism. An effect on helix conformation may be slowly repaired, so that enhanced DNA strand breakage by endogenous oxygen radicals could continue for a significant period of time following termination of the RF exposure. A second alternative hypothesis is that the RF radiation in some unknown manner inhibits the cellular enzymatic mechanisms that normally repair DNA strand breaks caused by endogenous radical species in a rapid and efficient manner.

Studies of cellular mutation and neoplastic transformation resulting from RF exposures have led to similarly conflicting findings. In vivo studies of RF-induced mutation and cancer initiation have, in general, not led to strong positive findings under conditions in which no significant tissue heating occurred (Berman, Carter, & House, 1980; Kunz et al., 1985). However, in spite of the fact that Kunz et al. did not observe an increase in overall tumor incidence in rodents chronically exposed to a 2450 MHz field, a small, but statistically significant, increase in primary malignancies was observed. An extensive series of in vitro studies provided evidence for an elevated rate of neoplastic transformation of 10T1/2 cells exposed to 2450 MHz microwaves pulse-modulated at 120 Hz (Balcer-Kubiczek & Harrison, 1985, 1989, 1991). This effect was field-strength dependent, and the RF enhancement of cell transformation was observed only when a chemical tumor promoter, 12-O-tetradecanoylphorbol-13-acetate (TPA), was added to the culture medium.

Cancer Promotion and Progression—In Vitro Studies

A large number of studies with in vitro cell lines exposed to ELF and RF fields have been carried out to detect field-induced changes in cellular functional properties such as ion transport, second messenger signaling, DNA synthesis, gene expression, protein biosynthesis, and the rate of cell proliferation. All of these interrelated aspects of cellular physiology are relevant to the types of field-induced changes that could underlie a loss of growth regulation and the promotion and progression of tumor development. Unfortunately, in spite of the very large database available in the published literature, there are numerous examples of inconsistencies and inability to replicate studies conducted in different laboratories using similar cell lines and field exposure conditions (Cridland, 1993; Michaelson & Elson, 1996; Sienkiewicz et al., 1993; Tenforde, 1996). For example, as reviewed in detail by Cridland, reports of increases, decreases, and no effects have been published in studies on the effects of ELF and RF fields on the rates of DNA synthesis, protein synthesis, and cell proliferation in eukaryotic cells. A particularly striking example of this variability in experimental results is provided by the effects of EMF at various frequencies on mitogen responses in lymphoid cells.

Despite this lack of consistency among observations in different laboratories, several reported effects of ELF and RF fields are noteworthy because of their potential implications relative to field-induced changes in cellular growth states and tumor promotion and progression. Three specific examples of such studies are the following:

- Protein Kinases. Several studies have examined the effects of ELF fields and RF fields with ELF amplitude modulation on protein kinase activity in eukaryotic cells (Byus, Lundak, Fletcher, and Adey, 1984; Luben, in press; Monti et al., 1991). Because these enzymes, especially phosphokinase C, are known to be key components in the cellular signaling pathways activated by tumor promoters such as TPA, an effect of EMF on kinase activity could promote the growth of transformed cells in a similar manner. None of the studies conducted to date, however, have shown a clear relationship between the observation of EMF effects on kinase activity and an elevated rate of cellular proliferation.

• <u>Gene Expression</u>. It has been reported that transient elevations in the expression of several oncogenes (e.g., c-*myc* and c-*fos*) occur in response to exposure of eukaryotic cells to low-intensity ELF magnetic fields. These studies have been conducted primarily with transformed cell lines, such as HL-60 leukemic cells (Goodman & Henderson, 1991) and CEM-CM3 T-lymphoblastoid cells (Phillips, Haggren, Thomas, Ishida-Jones, & Adey, 1992), but the results nonetheless have implications for possible alterations in cellular growth states and carcinogenic effects of EMF. Recently, two independent series of experiments with HL-60 cells failed to replicate the original observations of Goodman and Henderson on the increased expression of c-*myc* and other genes such as ß-actin following exposure to ELF fields (Lacy-Hulbert, Wilkins, Hesketh, & Metcalfe, 1995; Saffer & Thurston, 1995). The basis for this lack of reproducibility is not well understood, but the possibility that EMF can modulate the expression of oncogenes is of sufficient importance to merit further careful study.

• <u>Ornithine Decarboxylase (ODC)</u>. Both ELF and RF fields with ELF amplitude modulation have been observed to produce transient elevations in the intracellular activity of the growth-related enzyme ODC (Byus, Kartun, Pieper, & Adey, 1988; Byus, Pieper, & Adey, 1987; Litovitz, Krause, & Mullins, 1991; Litovitz, Krause, Penafiel, Elson, & Mullins, 1993). This enzyme, which controls the rate-limiting step in the biosynthesis of polyamines, is consistently elevated in cells that are stimulated to proliferate by exposure to tumor-promoting agents such as TPA. However, in studies with several cell lines, the ODC response to EMF has been found to be weaker than that observed following exposure to TPA. Furthermore, no evidence has been obtained for an elevation in the rate of DNA synthesis in cells exhibiting elevated levels of ODC following EMF exposure, as contrasted with the response observed following treatment of the cells with TPA. These findings suggest that the field-induced transient elevation in ODC activity may reflect a release of this enzyme from nascent cellular binding sites rather than *de novo* synthesis of new ODC transcripts. Because of the importance of this enzyme in the biosynthesis of DNA, RNA, and proteins, and its well established relationship to increased states of cell proliferation during tumor promotion, further studies on the effects of EMF on ODC activity are warranted.

Cancer Promotion and Progression—In Vivo Studies

Experiments have been conducted with several types of rodent tumors to determine whether ELF magnetic fields exert tumor-promoting effects or influence the progression of established tumor nodules. As recently reviewed by the author (Tenforde, 1996), the results of these experiments have generally been negative, with the exception of several findings of a promoting effect of ELF fields on the development of chemically-induced mammary carcinomas in rats. With both nitrosomethylurea-induced mammary tumors (Beniashvili, Bilanishvili, & Menabde, 1991) and 7,12-dimethylbenzanthracene-induced mammary tumors (Baum, Mevissen, Kamino, Mohr, & Löscher, 1995; Löscher, Mevissen, Lehmacher, & Stamm, 1993; Mevissen et al., 1993), ELF magnetic fields have been observed to significantly increase the rate of tumor development without affecting tumor incidence. The fact that mammary tumors, but not other types of cancer such as skin, liver, and brain tumors, are promoted by ELF fields may be related to a secondary effect of these fields on hormonal factors that influence the growth of mammary carcinomas. The experimental basis for this hypothesis is discussed in a later section of this paper.

A number of studies have also been performed to detect effects of RF fields on tumor promotion and progression. As reviewed in an NRC report (1993), many of the early studies used microwave fields with high power densities that led to tissue heating, and several reports on transplanted and chemically-induced rodent tumors actually demonstrated an inhibition of tumor growth as a result of hyperthermic exposure conditions. In more recent studies with athermal levels of RF radiation, no effects of the exposure were found on the development of B16 melanoma tumors in mice, brain glioma tumors in rats, or colon tumors in mice (Santini, Hosni, Deschaux, & Pacheco, 1988; Salford, Brun, & Eberhardt, J., 1993; Wu, Chiang, Shao, Li, & Fu, 1994). In one study, the development of spontaneous breast cancer in C3H/HeA mice was accelerated by exposure to both thermal and athermal levels of 2450 MHz radiation, which the authors attributed to a reduced host immune defense against the developing tumors (Szmigielski et al., 1982). The observation of an apparent tumor-promoting effect of RF fields on the development of mammary cancer in rodents is similar to effects of ELF fields observed in other studies discussed above. The possible effects of EMF on breast tumor promotion and progression clearly merits further investigation.

Tumor-Host Interactions in Carcinogenic Processes

An important, but poorly understood, aspect of possible EMF effects on cancer development is the influence of these fields on endocrine and immune system functions of the tumor host. Alterations in the physiological state of either or both of these systems could have important implications for tumor-host interactions that are known to play a role in carcinogenesis. For that reason, a brief review is provided here of endocrine and immune system effects of electromagnetic field exposure, with an emphasis on aspects of these interactions that could lead to the promotion and progression of tumor growth.

• Endocrine Interactions. Exposure of mammals to ELF and RF fields has been observed to alter the functions of specific components of the endocrine system. In the case of ELF fields, the most extensively studied endocrine response is the suppression of nocturnal melatonin synthesis by the pineal gland that has been observed in several species of mammals, including humans (Graham, in press; Kato, Honma, Shigemitsu, & Shiga, 1993; Tenforde, 1996; Wilson, Anderson, Hilton, & Phillips, 1981, 1983; Wilson et al., 1990). It was first suggested by Stevens that the decrease in concentration of melatonin in the circulation as a result of ELF field exposure leads to an increased concentration of estrogen, which in turn, can stimulate the proliferation of breast tissue (Stevens, 1987). Through this mechanism, foci of breast cancer cells with high levels of estrogen receptors could enter a rapid growth state characteristic of tumor promotion. Other mechanisms through which a field-induced decrease in melatonin levels could affect tumor promotion and progression exist as well. First, because of the neuroimmunomodulatory functions of melatonin, a decreased immune system response to tumor-specific antigens could occur under conditions in which melatonin production is suppressed (Maestroni, Conti, & Pierpaoli, 1986). Second, a reduced scavenging by melatonin of free radicals that damage DNA would also be anticipated to occur when the circulating levels of this hormone are depressed (Reiter, 1995). Third, data have recently been obtained which suggest that ELF magnetic fields can directly interfere with the oncostatic effect of melatonin on estrogen-receptor-positive breast cancer cells (Liburdy, Stoma, Sokolic, & Yaswen, 1993). All of these diverse mechanisms through which the influence of ELF fields on melatonin could facilitate tumor development deserve further investigation.

Tissue heating by RF fields has been shown in studies on several species of mammals to elicit neuroendocrine responses that alter the activity and the complex interactions of the hypothalmic, pituitary, adrenal, and thyroid systems (Michaelson & Lin, 1987). At thermal levels of RF exposure, plasma corticosterone levels are elevated, and this endocrine response is dependent upon ACTH secretion by the pituitary. Depressed thyroid hormone levels are also observed at thermalizing levels of RF exposure, and this response has been linked to an inhibition of secretion of thyrotropin by the pituitary gland. Because of the neuroimmunomodulatory effects of steroid hormones, the endocrine effects of RF fields could reduce immune surveillance against tumor development. In addition, the alterations in endocrine functions in response to high-intensity RF fields could lead to growth promotion in certain types of hormone-dependent tumors. An interesting question in regard to RF field effects on the endocrine system that has not as yet been addressed is the potential influence of these fields on nocturnal melatonin synthesis by the pineal gland. In view of the implications of altered melatonin levels on the development of breast tumors and other forms of cancer, the possible effects of RF fields on this important component of the endocrine system should be investigated.

- Immune System Interactions. Although direct in vivo studies on the effects of ELF and RF fields on immune responsiveness have been limited in both number and scope, the majority of these investigations have provided no indication of immune suppression (deSeze et al., 1993; Graham, Cook, & Cohen, 1990; Kunz et al., 1985; McLean et al., 1991; Morris, Sasser, Buschbom, & Anderson, 1990). Exceptions to this general pattern of experimental findings in animals and humans are the results of several studies in which thermal levels of RF fields were found to exert an immunosuppressive effect (Liburdy, 1979; Michaelson & Lin, 1987; NRC,

1993; Rama Rao, Cain, Lockwood, & Tompkins, 1983; Yang, Cain, Lockwood, & Tompkins, 1983). These changes are consistent with the cytotoxic effects on lymphocytes that are expected to occur as a result of the increased release of steroid hormones into the circulation at RF power densities that produce tissue heating.

A number of in vitro studies on the effects of EMF on cell-mediated immune responses have led to both positive and negative findings (Cridland, 1993; Lyle, Ayotte, Sheppard, & Adey, 1988; NRC, 1993; Roberts, Lu, & Michaelson, 1983; Roberts, Michaelson, & Lu, 1984). In general, suppression of lymphocyte responses to mitogens and target-cell antigens has been observed either as a result of high current densities induced in the cell suspension by ELF fields, or as a result of thermal effects of RF radiation at high power densities. However, amplitude- and pulse-modulated RF fields at athermal levels have been reported to suppress immune responses mediated by T-lymphocytes and cytotoxic antibodies (Lyle, Schechter, Adey, & Lundak, 1983; Veyret et al., 1991). These findings merit further investigation in the context of modulated RF fields associated with wireless communication systems.

Conclusions and Recommendations for Additional Research

As described in this review, several reported molecular, cellular, and tissue responses to EMF require additional studies in the context of possible effects on carcinogenic processes. In general, biological effects of relevance to carcinogenesis have been observed primarily in response to high-intensity fields at either ELF or RF frequencies. However, there are examples of biological responses to fields of moderate to low intensity, such as reduced pineal melatonin synthesis resulting from exposure to low-intensity ELF fields, that could influence tumor promotion and progression. As evidenced by the summary of experimental results presented above, there is a clear rationale for further research to clarify the possible role in carcinogenic processes of exposure to EMF at both low and high frequencies and over a broad range of intensities. The following specific biological targets of EMF interactions have been identified as those for which replication efforts, extensions of ongoing investigations, and new research activities are needed: (a) DNA damage, (b) neoplastic cell transformation, (c) oncogene expression, (d) ornithine decarboxylase synthesis and cell proliferation, (e) endocrine system effects, especially on the circulating levels of melatonin and steroid hormones, (f) immune system effects, and (g) tumor promotion and progression, especially in breast tissue. In each of these areas, highly focused research will be required to clarify the potential linkages between EMF exposure and carcinogenesis, with an emphasis on the effects of modulated RF fields that closely mimic those of wireless communication systems.

192

References

Balcer-Kubiczek, E. K., & Harrison, G. H. (1985). Evidence for microwave carcinogenesis in vitro. Carcinogenesis, 6, 859-864.

Balcer-Kubiczek, E. K., & Harrison, G. H. (1989). Induction of neoplastic transformation in C3H10T1/2 cells by 2.45-GHz microwaves and phorbol ester. Radiation Research, 117, 531-537.

Balcer-Kubiczek, E. K., & Harrison, G. H. (1991). Neoplastic transformation of C3H10T1/2 cells following exposure to 120-Hz modulated 2.45-GHz microwaves and phorbol ester tumor promoter. Radiation Research, 126, 65-72.

Baum, A., Mevissen, M., Kamino, K., Mohr, U., & Löscher, W. (1995). A histopathological study on alterations in DMBA-induced mammary carcinogenesis in rats with 50-Hz, 100-μT magnetic field exposure. Carcinogenesis, 16, 119-125.

Beniashvili, D. S., Bilanishvili, V. G., & Menabde, M. Z. (1991). Low-frequency electromagnetic radiation enhances the induction of rat mammary tumors by nitrosomethylurea. Cancer Letters, 61, 75-79.

Berman, E., Carter, H. B., & House, D. (1980). Tests of mutagenesis and reproduction in male rats exposed to 2450-MHz (CW) microwaves. Bioelectromagnetics, 1, 65-76.

Brusick, D. (1998). Genotoxicity of radiofrequency radiation. In G.L. Carlo (Ed.), Wireless phones and health: Scientific progress (pp. 91-98). Norwell, MA: Kluwer Academic Press.

Byus, C. V., Kartun, K., Pieper, S., & Adey, W. R. (1988). Increased ornithine decarboxylase activity in cultured cells exposed to low-energy modulated microwave fields and phorbol ester tumor promoters. Cancer Research, 48, 4222-4228.

Byus, C. V., Lundak, R. L., Fletcher, R. M., & Adey, W. R. (1984). Alterations in protein kinase activity following exposure of cultured human lymphocytes to modulated microwave fields. Bioelectromagnetics, 5, 341-351.

Byus, C. V., Pieper, S. E., & Adey, W. R. (1987). The effects of low-energy 60-Hz environmental electromagnetic fields upon the growth-related enzyme ornithine decarboxylase. Carcinogenesis, 8, 1385-1389.

Chiabrera, A., Bianco, B., Moggia, E., Tommasi, T., & Kaufman, J. J. (1998). Recent advances in the biophysical modeling of radiofrequency electromagnetic field interactions with living systems. In G.L. Carlo (Ed.), Wireless phones and health: Scientific progress (pp. 135-164). Norwell, MA: Kluwer Academic Press.

Cridland, N. A. (1993). Electromagnetic fields and cancer: A review of relevant cellular studies (Rep. No. NRPB-R256). Chilton, United Kingdom: National Radiological Protection Board.

deSeze, R., Bouthet, C., Tuffet, S., Deschaux, P., Caristan, A., & Moreau, J. (1993). Effects of time-varying uniform magnetic fields on natural killer cell activity and antibody response in mice. Bioelectromagnetics, 14, 405-412.

Frazier, M. E., Reese, J. A., & Morris, J. E. (1990, June). Effect of 60-Hz electromagnetic fields on growth rates and transformation frequencies of C3H10T1/2 cells. In Bioelectromagnetics Society 12th Annual Meeting Abstracts, 9.

Goodman, R., & Henderson, A. S. (1991). Transcription and translation in cells exposed to extremely-low-frequency electromagnetic fields. Bioeletrochemistry and Bioenergetics, 25, 335-355.

Graham, C. (In press). General physiological effects of ELF fields. In Extremely-low-frequency electromagnetic fields: Issues in biological effects and public health (NCRP Report No. 16). Proceedings of the 1994 Annual Meeting of the National Council on Radiation Protection and Measurements, Bethesda, MD.

Kato, M., Honma, K., Shigemitsu, T., & Shiga, Y. (1993). Effects of exposure to circularly polarized 50-Hz magnetic field on plasma and pineal melatonin levels in rats. Bioelectromagnetics, 14, 97-106.

Kunz, L. L., Johnson, R. B., Thompson, D., Crowley, J., Chou, C.K., & Guy, A. W. (1985). Effects of long-term low-level radiofrequency radiation exposure on rats: Vol. 8. Longevity, cause of death, and histopathological findings (Report No. USAFSAM-TR-85-11). Seattle, WA: University of Washington.

Lacy-Hulbert, A., Wilkins, R. C., Hesketh, T. R., & Metcalfe, J. C. (1995). No effect of 60-Hz electromagnetic fields on *myc* or ß-actin expression in human leukemic cells. Radiation Research, 144, 9-17.

Lai, H., & Singh, N. P. (1995). Acute low-intensity microwave exposure increases DNA single-strand breaks in rat brain cells. Bioelectromagnetics, 16, 207-210.

Liburdy, R. P. (1979). Radiofrequency radiation alters the immune system: Modification of T- and B-lymphocyte levels and cell-mediated immunocompetence by hyperthermic radiation. Radiation Research, 77, 34-46.

Liburdy, R.P., Stoma, T.R., Sokolic, R., & Yaswen, P. (1993). ELF magnetic fields, breast cancer, and melatonin: 60-Hz fields block melatonin's oncostatic action on ER$^+$ breast cancer cell proliferation. Journal of Pineal Research, 14, 89-97.

Litovitz, R., Krause, D., & Mullins, J.M. (1991). Effect of coherence time of the applied magnetic field on ornithine decarboxylase activity. Biochemical and Biophysical Research Communications. 178, 862-865.

Litovitz, T. A., Krause, D., Penafiel, M., Elson, E. C., & Mullins, J. M. (1993). The role of coherence time in the effect of microwaves on ornithine decarboxylase activity. Bioelectromagnetics, 14, 395-403.

Löscher, W., Mevissen, M., Lehmacher, W., & Stamm, A. (1993). Tumor promotion in a breast cancer model by exposure to a weak alternating magnetic field. Cancer Letters, 71, 75-81.

Luben, R. A. (In press). Membrane signal transduction and the cellular effects of nonionizing electromagnetic fields. In Extremely-Low-Frequency Electromagnetic Fields: Issues in Biological Effects and Public Health (NCRP Report No. 16). Proceedings of the 1994 Annual Meeting of the National Council on Radiation Protection and Measurements, Bethesda, MD.

194

Lyle, D. B., Ayotte, R. D., Sheppard, A. R., & Adey, W. R. (1988). Suppression of T-lymphocyte cytotoxicity following exposure to 60-Hz sinusoidal electric fields. Bioelectromagnetics, 9, 303-313.

Lyle, D. B., Schechter, P., Adey, W. R., & Lundak, R. L. (1983). Suppression of T-lymphocyte cytotoxicity following exposure to sinusoidally amplitude-modulated fields. Bioelectromagnetics, 4, 281-292.

Maes, A., Vershaeve, L., Arroyo, A., DeWagter, C., & Vercruyssen, L. (1993). In vitro cytogenetic effects of 2450-MHz waves on human peripheral blood lymphocytes. Bioelectromagnetics, 14, 495-501.

Maestroni, G. J. M., Conti, A., & Pierpaoli, W. (1986). Role of the pineal gland in immunity: Circadian synthesis and release of melatonin modulates the antibody response and antagonizes immunosuppressive effect of corticosterone. Journal of Neuroimmunology, 13, 19-30.

McCann, J., Dietrich, F., Rafferty, C., & Martin, A. O. (1993). A critical review of the genotoxic potential of electric and magnetic fields. Mutation Research, 297, 61-95.

McLean, J. R. N., Stuchly, M. A., Mitchell, R. E. J., Wilkinson, D., Yang, H., & Goddard, M. (1991). Cancer promotion in a mouse skin model by a 60-Hz magnetic field: II. Tumor development and immune response. Bioelectromagnetics, 12, 273-287.

Meltz, M. L. (1998). Studies on microwave induction of genotoxicity: A laboratory report. In G. L. Carlo (Ed.), Wireless phones and health: Scientific progress (pp. 105-112). Norwell, MA: Kluwer Academic Press.

Mevissen, M., Stamm, A., Buntenkötter, S., Zwingelbert, R., Wahnschaffe, U., & Löscher, W. (1993). Effects of magnetic fields on mammary tumor development induced by 7,12-dimethylbenz(a)anthracene in rats. Bioelectromagnetics, 14, 131-143.

Michaelson, S. M., & Elson, E. C. (1996). Interaction of nonmodulated and pulse-modulated radiofrequency fields with living matter: Experimental results. In C. Polk & E. Postow (Eds.), Handbook of biological effects of electromagnetic fields (2nd ed., pp. 435-533). Boca Raton, FL: CRC Press.

Michaelson, S. M., & Lin, J. C. (1987). Biological effects and health implications of radiofrequency radiation. New York: Plenum.

Monti, M. G., Pernecco, L., Moruzzi, M. S., Battini, R., Zaniol, P., & Barbiroli, B. (1991). Effect of ELF pulsed electromagnetic fields on protein kinase C activation process in HL-60 leukemia cells. Journal of Bioelectricity, 10, 119-130.

Morris, J. E., Sasser, L. B., Buschbom, R. L., & Anderson, L. E. (1990, November). Natural immunity in rats exposed to 60-Hz magnetic fields. In Abstracts of the DOE Annual Review of Research on Biological Effects of 50 and 60 Hz Electric and Magnetic Fields, A-23.

National Research Council. (1993). Assessment of the possible health effects of ground wave emergency network. Washington, DC: National Academy Press.

Phillips, J. L., Haggren, W., Thomas, W. J., Ishida-Jones, T., & Adey, W. R. (1992). Magnetic field-induced changes in specific gene transcription. Biochimica et Biophysica Acta, 1132, 140-144.

Rama Rao, G., Cain, C. A., Lockwood, J., & Tompkins, W. A. F. (1983). Effects of microwave exposure on the hamster immune system. II. Peritoneal macrophage function. Bioelectromagnetics, 4, 141-155.

Reiter, R. J. (1995). Melatonin suppression by time-varying and time-invariant electromagnetic fields. In M. Blank (Ed.), Electromagnetic fields: Biological interactions and mechanisms (pp. 451-465). Washington, DC: American Chemical Society Books.

Roberts, Jr., N. J., Lu, S.-T., & Michaelson, S. M. (1983). Human leukocyte functions and the U.S. safety standard for exposure to radiofrequency radiation. Science, 220, 318-320.

Roberts, Jr., N. J., Michaelson, S. M., & Lu, S.-T. (1984). Exposure of human mononuclear leukocytes to microwave energy pulse-modulated at 16 or 60 Hz. IEEE Transactions on Microwave Theory and Technique, 32, 803-807.

Saffer, J. D., & Thurston, S. J. (1995). Short exposures to 60-Hz magnetic fields do not alter myc expression in HL-60 or Daudi cells. Radiation Research, 144, 18-25.

Sagripanti, J.-L., Swicord, M. L., & Davis, C. C. (1987). Microwave effects on plasmid DNA. Radiation Research, 110, 219-231.

Salford, L. G., Brun, A., & Eberhardt, J. (1993). Experimental studies of brain tumor development during exposure to continuous and pulsed 915-MHz radiofrequency radiation. In M. Blank (Ed.), Electricity and magnetism in biology and medicine (pp. 379-381). San Francisco, CA: San Francisco Press.

Santini, R., Hosni, M., Deschaux, P., & Pacheco, H. (1988). B16 melanoma development in black mice exposed to low-level microwave radiation. Bioelectromagnetics, 9, 105-107.

Sarkar, S., Ali, S., & Behari, J. (1994). Effect of low-power microwaves on the mouse genome: A direct DNA analysis. Mutation Research, 320, 141-147.

Sienkiewicz, Z. J., Cridland, N. A., Kowalczuk, C. L., & Saunders, R. D. (1993). Biological effects of electromagnetic fields and radiation. In W. R. Stone & G. Hyde (Eds.), The review of radio science: 1990-1992 (pp.737-770). Oxford, UK: Oxford University Press.

Stevens, R. G. (1987). Electric power use and breast cancer: A hypothesis. American Journal of Epidemiology, 125, 556-561.

Szmigielski, S., Szudzinski, A., Pietraszek, A., Bielec, M., Janiak, M., & Wrembel, J. K. (1982). Accelerated development of spontaneous and benzopyrene-induced skin cancer in mice exposed to 2450-MHz microwave radiation. Bioelectromagnetics, 3, 179-191.

Tenforde, T. S. (1996). Interaction of ELF magnetic fields with living systems. In C. Polk & E. Postow (Eds.), Handbook of biological effects of electromagnetic fields (2nd ed., pp. 185-

196

230). Boca Raton, FL: CRC Press.

U.S. Department of Energy, Office of Scientific and Technical Information. (1990). Immunological and biochemical effects of 60-Hz electric and magnetic fields in humans. Midwest Research Institute Final Report [Contract No. DE-FC01-84-CE-76246 (Order No. DE90006671)]. Oak Ridge, TN: Graham, C., Cook, M.R., & Cohen, H.D.

Veyret, B., Bouthet, C., Deschaux, P., deSeze, R., Geffard, M., & Joussot-Dubien, J. (1991). Antibody responses of mice exposed to low-power microwaves under combined pulse- and amplitude-modulation. Bioelectromagnetics, 12, 47-56.

Wilson, B. W., Anderson, L. E., Hilton, D. I., & Phillips, R. D. (1981). Chronic exposure to 60-Hz electric fields: Effects on pineal function in the rat. Bioelectromagnetics, 2, 371-380.

Wilson, B. W., Anderson, L. E., Hilton, D. I., & Phillips, R. D. (1983). Chronic exposure to 60-Hz electric fields: Effects on pineal function in the rat [erratum]. Bioelectromagnetics, 4, 293.

Wilson, B. W., Wright, C. W., Morris, J. E., Buschbom, R. L., Brown, D. P., & Miller, D. L. (1990). Evidence for an effect of ELF electromagnetic fields on human pineal gland function. Journal of Pineal Research, 9, 259-269.

Wu, R. Y., Chiang, H., Shao, B. J., Li, N. G., & Fu, Y. D. (1994). Effects of 2.45 GHz microwave radiation and phorbol ester 12-0-tetradecanoylphorbol acetate on dimethylhydrazine-included colon cancer in mice. Bioelectromagnetics, 15, 531-538.

Yang, H. K., Cain, C. A., Lockwood, J., & Tompkins, W. A. F. (1983). Effects of microwave exposure on the hamster immune system. I. Natural killer cell activity. Bioelectromagnetics, 4, 123-139.

15
HUMAN EXPOSURE TO RADIOFREQUENCY RADIATION— PUBLIC HEALTH ISSUES
Andrew Sivak

This paper will deal largely with issues completely at the other end of the spectrum from the other papers in this set describing in eloquent biophysical terms some theories about interactions of radiofrequency radiation (RFR) with biological systems. This paper will attempt to address some public health issues relating to cancer. The primary reason for this is the public concern that has been generated about cancer and the use of wireless communication devices driven largely by litigation rather than science. The model that will be used stems from the kinds of information that have been used to examine the consequence of exposure to chemical agents in the environment. There are three kinds of information that have been utilized to assess risks to humans from exposure to chemicals in the environment, and these information types are directly applicable to the situation with RFR. These three kinds of information are: (1) epidemiology studies; (2) chronic animal bioassay studies; and (3) mechanistic studies, the evaluation of the effects of chemicals on processes and events in cells and in the body.

Epidemiology is clearly the strongest kind of evidence that we have. The basic reason for this is that epidemiology involves direct evidence on the species of most importance to us—*Homo sapiens*. Notwithstanding its difficulties, when one has associations between exposures and health outcomes that are reasonable and strong in epidemiology, one really does not need animal bioassays and studies on mechanisms to address public health issues. At this point, there are no published epidemiological studies on wavelengths of concern for wireless communication instruments. Although the available data are not extensive as yet, the information Dr. Rothman shared with us from his large cohort study do not suggest any immediate concerns (Rothman, 1995).

Another way to determine whether there may be a risk for humans is to expose animals for a long time—generally most of their life span—to the agents of concern at a range of doses, including the highest that is biologically feasible. It is quite interesting that there are five studies already completed, considering that wireless communication is such a relatively new technology. There are three carcinogenesis studies: one in Sprague-Dawley rats and two in C3H mice. There are two other chronic studies that were done where the end point was not cancer or pathological changes in tissues. A summary of the cancer bioassays is shown in Table 1. The first one was done by Chou et al. (1992) from the University of Washington. They exposed Sprague-Dawley rats at 2450 MHz for a little over two years. Shelton, Banks, and Toler (1994), at Georgia Tech, ran a study with C3H mice, and Frei, Berger, Jauchem, and Merritt (1995), at Trinity University in San Antonio, Texas, have just completed a study with C3H mice. In none of the studies was any statistically significant increase in cancer noted at any specific organ site. In the Chou study, a small increase in the total number of tumors was observed in treated as compared to control animals. However, in the Frei study, the opposite effect occurred, with a reduction in the total number of tumors in animals exposed to RFR as compared to controls. An interesting finding was that the level of reduction of breast tumors in the microwave-exposed animals almost reached significance. There were two other long-term RFR exposure studies reported (Table 2). In the one done by Spalding, Freyman, and Holland in 1971, body weight, some hematological parameters, and behavior were evaluated, and no effects resulting from the exposure were found. Unlike most of the studies which were done using 2450 MHz exposures, this study used 800 MHz, which is quite close to the radiation band that is of primary interest to us. The study by Liddle, Putnam, and Huey (1994), done at the U.S. Environmental Protection Agency, evaluated only life span. At the lower power density of 2 W/kg, no change in life span was found. At the higher power density of 6.8 W/kg, a 30% decrease in life span was found. However, their measurements indicated that there was significant core-body temperature heating at the upper level, which is a likely explanation for the reduced life span in the high exposure group.

Investigator	Frequency	Animal	Exposure
Chou et al. (1992)	2450 MHz	Sprague-Dawley rats male	0.2-0.4 W/kg 20 hours/day 25 months
Shelton et al. (1994)	435 MHz	C3H/HeJ mice female	0.32 W/kg 20 hours/day 94 weeks
Frei et al. (1995)	2450 MHz	C3H/HeJ mice female	0.3 W/kg 20 hours/day 18 months

Table 1. Summary of Chronic Animal Carcinogenicity RFR Studies

Investigator	Frequency	Animal	Exposure
Spalding et al. (1971)	800 MHz	RFM mice female	12 mW/cm² 2 hours/day 35 weeks
Liddle et al. (1994)	2450 MHz	CD1 mice female	2 or 6.8 W/kg 1 hour/day 2 years

Table 2. Summary of Other Chronic Animal RFR Studies

One of the critical factors in assessing environmental risks and extrapolating from animal studies to humans is comparative exposures. If one examines the exposures in the chronic animal studies (about 7300 hours per year), one finds that they are orders of magnitude above typical human exposures (about 28 hours per year). The third area of interest in the assessment of environmental risk from external exposures involves the mechanistic studies. There are very few data in this area. In the area of induction of cell proliferation by exposure to RFR, there are only a few studies: one done by Dr. Veyret, a member of this panel (Chagnaud, Veyret, and Despres, 1995); one done by Dr. Adey from Loma Linda, California (Stagg, Thomas, Jones, & Adey, 1995); and one from Dr. R. Fitzner from Germany (Fitzner, Langer, Zeman, Niebig, & Brinkmann, 1995). None of these studies showed any effect of microwave radiation on cell proliferation.

As with the studies on cell proliferation, there are only a few studies on tumor cell growth, where tumors are inoculated into animals, and the animals are exposed to microwave radiation. In these studies, no increase in the numbers of animals succumbing from the tumors was found with RFR exposure (Marino, Antonini, Avella, Galloni, & Scacchi, 1995; Prausnitz & Susskind, 1962; Preskorn, Edwards, & Justesen, 1978).

There was only one study found that dealt with calcium transport. These experiments by Wolke, Niebig, Eisner, Gollnick, and Meyer (1995) from Bonn, Germany found no effect on calcium transport in the heart myocyte cell culture system with RFR exposure.

Finally, there is the issue of tumor promotion. Why is tumor promotion important? One of the main reasons that it is important is that RFR cannot induce genetic change. Therefore, if RFR affects the cancer process—and there is no evidence available at the present time that it does—then it must be the nongenetic, post-initiation processes, the promotion-progression phases, that are critical. Because of these factors, Wireless Technology Research (WTR), LLC felt that a consideration of tumor promotion was a very important aspect to try to understand, and they asked me to put together a panel of people to consider this issue. When we started the process, WTR laid out three questions and issues for the panel to address. The first was: evaluate in vitro and in vivo studies involving RFR and tumor promotion. The second: determine the relevance of animal promotion models to humans. And third: examine possible mechanisms of tumor promotion by radiofrequency radiation.

With respect to the first issue, of the studies that are available, there are essentially no reliable ones that indicate any tumor promoting effect of RFR in a variety of cell culture and experimental animal systems. In one cell culture system, a modest enhancement (20-30%) of phorbol ester promotion of x-ray induced transformation was observed, but these studies were done at power levels that likely increased the temperature of the target cells. There is only one true promotion study using a mouse colon cancer system, and the results with RFR exposure were negative.

The issue of the relevance to humans of tumor promotion as found in experimental animal systems is a key issue in addressing cancer risk in humans. Promotion has an interesting history. Tumor promotion was first defined by Friedewald and Rous (1944), and the first studies were then done by Shubik and Berenblum (1947) at the University of London. The basic procedures for doing those studies have not largely changed in 50 years. Promotion studies are uniquely animal studies, however, in that promotion studies involve a single exposure to a carcinogen, followed by repeated doses of a noncarcinogenic promoter, and that model is simply not applicable to humans. We are generally exposed to low levels of environmental carcinogens every day of our lives, and if one wants to have an animal model that might be relevant to humans, it should be co-carcinogenesis. The panel determined that direct inferences from promotion studies with respect to making public health decisions about humans are not appropriate. The one thing we can learn from promotion studies relates to an understanding of the steps in the carcinogenic process. The key question to address is whether RFR affects any processes that are known to be important for the advancement of the cancer process and thereby examine possible mechanisms.

To address the third question posed by WTR, the panel determined that it really is premature to try to think about mechanisms at the biological level from exposure to RFR. We know very little, if anything, about how a biological system senses RFR radiation and responds to it, and, although we have had some elegant models proposed from the biophysical point of view, there are no data available to aid in the understanding of a possible biological mechanism related to RFR exposure. Until we gain this kind of information and/or find some markers or some measures for understanding how molecules, cells, or tissues respond to RFR, any construct of a mechanism is very premature.

Based on all of the information available to date—the epidemiology, the long-term carcinogenesis studies that have been completed, and the absence of any positive effects in a few of the studies that look at mechanistic effects—there seems to be no reason to raise a large concern about cancer from exposure to RFR at this time. The available scientific data do not indicate a significant concern for carcinogenesis from exposure to RFR from wireless communication devices.

Certainly other health end points are quite important to pursue. Indeed, if the only organ that receives any exposure from use of wireless communication devices is the brain, then certainly behavior and other neural functions deserve attention.

The great frustration to a toxicologist and a risk assessor is that the very meager information on the effects of RFR in biological systems will not even allow the proposal of an experimental model to test. When one deals with chemical exposures, one can get quantitative information on the amounts that enter and leave the body and the tissues and organs of the body. One can measure interactions with DNA and other macromolecules.

With RFR, we have none of that. We are really just at the threshold, biologically, of trying to find out what, if anything, RFR may be doing in biological systems and if, in fact, we need to be concerned about a health effect.

Another issue that merits consideration is safety standards. It would be nice to have some sort of a biological anchor on which to base the standard. Although much effort is expended by some very hard-working and competent scientists, they do not have the necessary information at their disposal to develop a more biologically relevant standard. The significant challenge over the coming years will be to provide this information.

References

Chagnaud, J. L., Veyret, B., & Despres, B. (1995). No effect of exposure to GSM-modulated microwaves on the proliferation of GH3, MolT4 and C6 tumor cells. Manuscript in preparation.

Chou, C. K., Guy, A. W., Kunz, L. L., Johnson, R. B., Crowley, J. J., & Krupp, J. H. (1992). Long-term, low-level microwave irradiation of rats. Bioelectromagnetics, 13, 469-496.

Frei, M. R., Berger, R. E., Jauchem, J. R., & Merritt, J. H. (1995). Chronic exposure of cancer prone mice to low-level 2450-MHz radiofrequency radiation [abstract]. Proceedings of the 1995 Annual Meeting of the Bioelectromagnetics Society, (#P64-A).

Friedewald, W. F., & Rous, P. (1944). The initiating and promoting elements in tumor production. Journal of Experimental Medicine, 80, 101-126.

Fitzner, R., Langer, E., Zeman, E., Niebig, U., & Brinkmann, K. (1995). Growth behaviour of human leucemic cells (promyelozyt) influenced by high-frequency electro-magnetic fields (1.8 GHz pulsed and 900 MHz pulsed) for the investigation of cancer promoting effects [abstract]. Proceedings of the 1995 Annual Meeting of the Bioelectromagnetics Society, (#8-6).

Liddle, C. G., Putnam, J. P., & Huey, O. P. (1994). Alteration of life span of mice chronically exposed to 2.45 GHz CW microwaves. Bioelectromagnetics, 15(3), 177-181.

Marino, C., Antonini, F., Avella, B., Galloni, L., & Scacchi, P. (1995). 900 MHz effects on tumoral growth in in vivo systems [abstract]. Proceedings of the 1995 Annual Meeting of the Bioelectromagnetics Society, (#P48-C).

Prausnitz, S., & Süsskind, C. (1962). Effects of chronic microwave radiation on mice. Biomedical Electronics, 9, 104-108.

Preskorn, S. H., Edwards, W. D., & Justesen, D. R. (1978). Retarded tumor growth and augmented longevity in mice after fetal irradiation by 2450-MHz microwaves. Journal of Surgical Oncology, 10, 483-492.

Rothman, K. J. (1998). State of the science in RF epidemiology. In G. L. Carlo (Ed.), Wireless phones and health: Scientific progress (pp. 205-223). Norwell, MA: Kluwer Academic Press.

Shelton, W., Banks, D., & Toler, J. (1994). Bioeffects of radiofrequency radiation on cell growth and differentiation. (U.S. Air Force Report AL-TR-1992-0106). San Antonio, TX: Brooks Air Force Base.

Shubik, P., & Berenblum, I. (1947). A new quantitative approach to the study of stages of chemical carcinogenesis in the mouse's skin. British Journal of Cancer, 1, 383-391.

Spalding, J. F., Freyman, R. W., & Holland, L. M. (1971). Effects of 800-MHz electromagnetic radiation on body weight, activity, hematopoeisis and life span in mice. Health Physics, 20(4), 421-424.

Stagg, R. B., Thomas, W. J., Jones, R. A., & Adey, W. R. (1995). Cell proliferation in C_6 glioma cells exposed to 836.55 MHz frequency modulated radiofrequency field [abstract]. In Proceedings of the 1995 Annual Meeting of the Bioelectromagnetics Society, (#8-3).

Wolke, S., Niebig, U., Eisner, R., Gollnick, F., & Meyer, R. (1995). Intracellular calcium in heart muscle cells is not changed by pulsed highfrequent electromagnetic fields [abstract]. In Proceedings of the 1995 Annual Meeting of the Bioelectromagnetics Society (#P 119-B).

IV

EPIDEMIOLOGY AND RADIO FREQUENCY RADIATION RESEARCH

Editor's Note:

Epidemiology is the cornerstone of post-market surveillance, and as such, will be determinative in assessing the health impact of wireless technology over time. Results from epidemiological studies provide the only direct evidence of effect on humans, and are the clearest pathway toward public health intervention. In the long term, rigorous epidemiological surveillance is the best method for protecting public health with respect to wireless instruments. However, because epidemiology is time-dependent, in the near term in vitro studies and in vivo bioassays must be relied upon for early indications of public health risk.

The papers by Drs. Rothman, Morgan, Goldsmith and Wynder set the stage for the interpretation of forthcoming epidemiological studies. Dr. Rothman's work, in particular, includes pilot studies to assist epidemiologists in defining exposure and in implementing in-field methods.

In addition, ongoing review of epidemiological studies relevant to radio frequency is being done by Dr. Elisa Bandera at the State University of New York at Buffalo (Bandera, E. V., Vena, J. E., Steffens, R. A., & Carlo, G. L. [1998, June]. Monitoring the possible health effects of cellular telephone use. The epidemiology surveillance program of Wireless Technology Research. Poster session presented at the annual meeting of the Bioelectromagnetics Society, St. Pete's Beach, FL.).

G. L. C.

16

STATE OF THE SCIENCE IN RF EPIDEMIOLOGY

Kenneth J. Rothman

Abstract

RF exposure is now prominently in the public eye as a result of the rapid growth of cellular communication devices. The scientific and public debate over electromagnetic field (EMF) exposure from power lines and household sources has led to increased public concern, and skepticism among some scientists that research on RF exposures may be unable to provide clear answers. But the epidemiologic study of RF exposures differs from the epidemiologic study of EMF in several important respects. For hand-held portable cellular telephone users in particular, these differences are crucial: the exposure is concentrated at one side of the head, and the user's exposure is recorded by both billing companies and in the user's memory. These differences favor reaching a clearer answer with regard to possible effects of RF exposure, and especially exposure from cellular telephones, than has been reached in EMF research.

RF exposure has, until recently, largely been an occupational or avocational exposure; those sustaining the highest levels of exposure have been those manufacturing or repairing RF devices, police and emergency workers, military personnel or ham radio operators. Although some population exposure comes from radio and television broadcast signals, the major source of population exposure today and in the future seems to be from cellular telephones. To date, there are no published results from studies of cellular telephone exposure, but several studies have been published describing morbidity and mortality of occupationally exposed groups. These studies have suffered from inadequate control of confounding factors, lack of specific biologic hypotheses, poor exposure information, and small numbers. Research currently underway or being planned should provide more definitive data regarding RF exposure in general, and especially exposure to the head from portable hand-held cellular telephones.

Epidemiology may be somewhat unfamiliar to many of you. Epidemiology is also handicapped by a bad image because it often provides a nagging reminder of what we need to do. Cynics say that the findings from epidemiology will not make your life any longer, it will just make it seem longer. Seriously, though, the fact is that epidemiology in the end will provide the clearest answers to the questions that we raise about health concerns and health risks.

Growth in the number of subscribers of cellular telephone service in the United States has been substantial, and the growth has been equally dramatic in Europe. This phenomenal growth, if it continues as many predict, will lead to a technology that will become highly prevalent in a very short time. There is intense interest therefore, not only on the part of industry, but also governments and the population in general, as to what the possible health effects of this new technology might be.

Recent news coverage about cellular telephones has focused on lawsuits, and recent stories in the *Wall Street Journal*, *Time Magazine*, and other publications have questioned whether cellular telephones are safe (Elmer-DeWitt, 1993; Morrison & Cummins, 1994). Such coverage indicates the general concern of the business community and the public about this technology. In general, the public tends to be skeptical about health risks, just as they are skeptical about the latest findings from research studies. The public tends to be slow to worry about problems like this. Eventually, though, the public too will want answers to the kinds of questions that we might be able to address through epidemiology.

Now, what is epidemiology going to do about it? What have we learned from epidemiology and RF exposure in general up to now? What is the current state of research? And what is the future?

Science is measurement; measurement is what we do in all of the natural sciences. Lord Kelvin said that we do not really understand the nature of anything until we can measure it. In epidemiology our goal is likewise to measure, but measurement is not always easy. There is a story about an epidemiologist, an engineer, and a physicist who were standing around on the university campus trying to determine the height of a flagpole. While they were talking, an English professor walked up to them and said, "What are you doing?" After they explained he said, "Well, let me borrow that yardstick over there." He grabbed the flagpole, put it down on the ground, and measured it. He said, "Eight meters." As he walked away, the engineer turned to the epidemiologist and said, "Well, isn't that just like an English professor? We're trying to measure the height and he gives us the length."

Let's introduce a couple of basic concepts. First, what do we mean by "causation" in epidemiology? We use the term "cause" in two different ways. One way we use it is to refer to "sufficient cause." For some diseases, there might be several different sufficient causes or causal mechanisms; this implies that there is more than one mechanism that might lead to a particular disease. For example, looking at brain cancer, or cardiovascular disease, or diabetes, there are theoretically various mechanisms that could give rise to the disease. When we talk about a cause in epidemiology, however, we don't typically speak about the entire causal mechanism—what we are speaking about is one of the components. We might talk about, for example, component C of sufficient cause 1, and that might be what we would think of as a potential cause of disease. When we speak about smoking as a cause of lung cancer, for example, we do not mean that it is a sufficient cause—that it is the whole causal mechanism. Smoking is only one component in one or more causal mechanisms that lead to disease. One implication of this is that not everybody who experiences a cause will get disease, since there are always complementary factors that need to be present for a given case of disease to occur. Another implication is that some people who do not experience a cause of disease could still get the disease through different mechanisms that do not involve that specific cause.

A factor we have not discussed so far is how different components of a given causal mechanism work together to end up producing disease. In particular, it may be that a given component cause might play some biological role that will lead to disease, but that ultimate action may not be apparent for many years. During the time period before disease occurs, various things are happening. One thing that might be happening is that the other component causes that need to act will play their role. So a given cause might act, and then a period of time goes by, which we call the induction period, and at the end of the induction period, disease occurs. Then the sufficient cause is complete. Even at the time disease occurs, however, we sometimes do not detect it. There may be no symptoms, or there might not be a lab test that could detect disease at this point. Only after a further interval, during which the disease is present but still latent, or hidden, can we detect the disease. The time that we have to wait might ultimately be a very long interval.

Perhaps the clearest example of a very long induction period in epidemiology is that of diethylstilbestrol (DES) exposure. DES is a hormonal drug that was given to women during pregnancy in order to prevent miscarriage. Women born to mothers who had taken DES were at risk for developing a cancer that was otherwise not seen—adenocarcinoma of the vagina—when they reached the age range 15 to 30. The median age of occurrence was in the early 20s. Here we have disease resulting from an exposure that occurred at a very well-delineated point in time, with a cancer occurring approximately two decades later. Obviously, that cause was insufficient and obviously, there were other things that had to happen, other component causes that acted during the long induction period, before the cancer occurred. That is a useful model for us to have in mind when we think about the factors that we study having health effects even decades later.

Having laid out what we mean by cause and the importance of the induction period, I want to mention at least one more important issue in epidemiology. Unlike some other sciences, we seldom have the opportunity to do experimental studies. Typically, when we study the effects of environmental agents, we have to do what we call "nonexperimental studies," or what some people call "observational studies." In nonexperimental studies, we do not have the luxury of assigning the agent to comparable groups. Instead, we have to design a study by selecting people who are comparable, and controlling for confounding factors in the handling of the data. If we go to Costa Rica and look at the death rate, we will find that it is lower than the death rate in Sweden, but that does not mean living in Costa Rica is necessarily better for your health. The difference is explained by understanding that the population age distribution in Costa Rica is different than in Sweden—it is much lower in Costa Rica, and people who are younger have lower death rates. If we make adjustments for the differences in the age distributions, then, in fact, the death rates are higher in Costa Rica than in Sweden. This is an example of the problem epidemiologists describe as confounding, a problem that we worry about in essentially every epidemiologic study.

What can we look for as the end product of an epidemiologic study? Like other sciences, we do not express ourselves in simply yes or no terms. We might use a graph

208

to display the results of a study. The effect measure might be displayed on the vertical axis, showing the actual mortality rate, or the number of deaths among 1,000 people in one year. Dose might be displayed on the horizontal axis. You would want to be assured in reading the methods of the paper that the groups that were compared at the different dose levels were indeed comparable with respect to factors that might affect their disease rate or their death rate, either in the way they were selected or in the way the data were handled. At each dose level, there are confidence intervals to indicate the amount of variability in the effect; in some cases, there might be a fair amount of uncertainty at each level. There are other ways that you might describe these data. You might fit trend lines, for example, to describe the trend, or you might fit a confidence interval for the trend line as a somewhat more elaborate way of describing it. This is the kind of end product that we look forward to in epidemiology.

We are fortunate to have on our panel today a man who was a pioneer in the study of the health effects of cigarette smoking, especially with regard to lung cancer—Dr. Ernst Wynder. We have known for quite a long time that cigarette smoking has a dramatic effect on lung cancer and on many other health outcomes. This is solid knowledge that has come from nicely designed epidemiologic studies that have given clear answers. For example, cancer of the larynx has an even stronger relation to cigarette smoking than cancer of the lung. In fact, I do not think there are too many biologists who have ever found a relation as close to linear as this one. The ultimate result that we might hope for in epidemiology is to come out with an answer as clear as this one.

Epidemiology has made clear progress in the study of certain exposures such as cigarettes, but the range of topics that epidemiologists have been addressing of late has naturally shifted to other environmental problems. Some of the effects now under study are either nonexistent or subtle. It is very difficult to study these effects because it becomes quite problematic to distinguish between a small effect and no effect. This problem has led to some criticism of our profession, exemplified by an article published last summer in *Science*, "Epidemiology Faces its Limits" (Taubes, 1995). The writer of this article wrote a very good book about cold fusion called Bad Science. Gary Taubes, the author, is now very concerned about the study of electromagnetic fields (EMF). Quite a number of epidemiologic studies aimed at EMF have come up with diverse findings that cannot be reconciled with today's knowledge in physics and biology. These studies also have a fair amount of inconsistency with respect to the epidemiologic measures and the outcomes that have been studied. Nevertheless, there are a number of epidemiologists active in this field who are persuaded that there is a real health effect from exposure to magnetic fields. Gary Taubes thinks this is another illustration of bad science—like cold fusion—where the problem was essentially the study of measurement error. He thinks that epidemiologists studying EMF are looking at measurement error.

I mention the EMF controversy because many people who contemplate the epidemiologic study of cellular telephones think that the quagmire about EMF effects will simply expand to include the effects of RF exposures as well—in particular, the possible health effects of cellular telephones. I disagree. I think epidemiology will provide, much more quickly than it can for EMF, clear answers about the health effects of cellular telephone use in particular, and RF use in general.

With respect to cellular telephones specifically, there are some key differences between the EMF situation and cellular telephone exposure (Table 1). For EMF, the exposure is very often, although not always, to the whole body. Some appliances have more localized exposure, but a lot of exposure is to the magnetic fields from power lines, for example, or from other generating sources that encompass the entire body, so many target organs are potentially affected. In comparison, RF exposure from cellular telephones is usually very localized. It is unilateral to the head, basically, except in unusual circumstances.

EMF	RF
Whole Body	Unilateral, to Head
Affects Groups	Affects Individuals
Continuous	Occasional
Surreptitious	Obvious
Steady over Time	Sharply Increasing

Table 1. Differences of Epidemiologic Relevance Between EMF Exposure and RF Exposure from Cellular Telephones

EMF exposure, because the fields are widespread, tends to affect groups of people at the same time, whereas RF exposure from cellular telephones tends to affect one person at a time—the person using the telephone. EMF exposure also tends to be continuous. Power lines are sending power constantly; it does vary from time to time, perhaps, but the RF exposure from cellular telephone use is intermittent and occasional. It is not continuous. EMF exposure is surreptitious in that the people who are exposed do not ordinarily know that they are exposed at the time that the exposure is occurring. This is not true with users of cellular telephones. They know when they are using the telephone.

Finally, EMF exposure has been gradually increasing, maybe doubling, tripling or more over the past decades, but there has been an explosive, dramatic, exponential increase in population exposure to RF over a very short time. If there really were a strong health effect, it would even likely show up in health registry statistics eventually because of the dramatic time trend.

Portable cellular telephones top the list of possible sources of RF exposure for the general population, because if they are not yet, they will soon be, the major source of population exposure (see Table 2). Radio and TV broadcast are low-level exposures, but they affect lots of people, so in a population sense, they are an important source of exposure. Radar is another, as are cellular base stations. It is debatable how many people are affected by this exposure, but it is certainly something to consider. There are also non-cellular mobile communication devices and automobile cellular telephones, although we do not believe there is significant exposure coming from this source.

- Portable Cellular Telephones
- Radio and TV Broadcast
- Radar
- Cellular Base Stations
- Non-cellular Mobile Communication Devices
- Automobile Cellular Telephones

Table 2. Sources of Possible RF Exposure

Next let us look at some of the epidemiologic markers of RF exposure that we might use in epidemiologic studies, some of which have already been used in completed studies. We have a range of options to consider in measuring exposure in epidemiologic studies. There is always an interest in occupational studies on the part of epidemiologists. In general, people in occupations tend to sustain heavier exposure than consumers, and it always makes sense to study people who are getting the highest level of exposure. How do we measure exposure? With occupations, we often have to use records to measure exposure, and often the only records we can take advantage of are records indicating the type of job a person had. Perhaps information on general exposures for that job are available, but seldom are they available on the individual level. Other possible markers depend on what kind of study you are conducting. If you are living near a transmitting tower, your residence might be important. Residence location is a theoretical marker of exposure that we are already using.

Telephone companies keep records of phone calls in order to send out bills. These records provide information on the amount of use that has occurred for a given telephone, and may provide a description of the amount of exposure an individual has had that can be used in epidemiology studies. We can also use self reports. In case-control studies that are now underway, interviews are being conducted to ask people about their cellular telephone use. In a study we hope to conduct, we plan to interview large populations of cellular telephone users to get information directly from them about their telephone use, and then follow them up for health effects.

The type of cellular telephone makes a big difference in the amount of exposure. An automobile telephone with the antenna in a different location from the handset should provide essentially no exposure to the individual, whereas a hand-held portable cellular telephone provides the exposure with which we are most concerned. So, type of telephone is an important marker of exposure. The level of the cellular power output is another potential marker, if we can get it. Cellular telephones change their power output depending on the transmission needs for completing a connection between the telephone and the tower. In areas where a telephone is shielded or the phone is remote from the cellular base station it is using, the power output will be comparatively high. In areas where a base station is close and there is little shielding, the power output will be comparatively low. Power output therefore affects the exposure that an individual sustains. If power output can be determined, it would be a useful epidemiologic marker. We do not have any convenient way of determining it for an individual telephone call or even for an individual user, but we might be able to determine it for populations. In some areas the average power output for the telephones might characteristically be high, perhaps because there are few towers, whereas other areas might have a dense array of towers, so the average power output for each call might be low. Geographic location might actually serve as a surrogate for the level of power output.

The position of the cellular telephone antenna is certainly a potential marker; however, it is hard to measure for epidemiologic purposes. Laterality of exposure is also potentially a very important measure. If a user always holds the telephone to the right side of the head, it would be the right side of the head that would sustain the exposure. If RF exposure causes brain cancer and the brain cancer occurs on the left side of the head, we would not think that it would be connected to that particular exposure. To take advantage of the laterality information, however, there must be a good way of assessing laterality. We can always ask people on which side of the head they hold the telephone. We had hoped that handedness—left-handedness or right-handedness—might be an indicator of laterality; that data will be presented in a moment. Finally, other factors hard to assess include metal implants, jewelry, eyeglasses and so forth. These factors could be addressed in case-control studies.

There are some groups that might be studied in order to provide answers to the question of risk from RF exposure. Some of these groups have already been studied: ham radio operators, a group that has been studied by Sam Milham; workers manufacturing RF appliances are another occupational group of interest; military personnel have been studied a couple of times, radar workers in particular and others in the military sustain RF exposures. Police are another study group of potential interest, as well as CB radio operators, cellular telephone users, of course, and potentially diathermy patients, since they sustain very high RF exposures.

Results from a few epidemiologic studies that have been published are summarized in Tables 3-7. They are provided for some familiarity with the literature, but study designs will not be discussed here. Table 3 illustrates the Milham study of amateur radio operators. In this study, as in many of the others, a population of people, in this case ham radio operators, were identified and their mortality rate determined by linking identifying information with mortality data from the entire U.S.. One concern about this study is that amateur radio operators might not be expected to have the same mortality rate as the rest of the U.S. population. There is evidence either that that is true, or that the linkage of mortality data was not as good as it could have been. The standardized mortality ratio (SMR) is a measure of the mortality rate in the studied population compared with the U.S. population. The SMR would be 1.0 if there were no difference in the mortality rates. The overall SMR was 0.7 for all causes of death, and probably indicates either that there was insufficient identification of deaths or that this population is healthier than the general population. This is a common epidemiologic problem and it does not necessarily invalidate the study, but it reflects on the methodology of this study and is an important feature to consider

We often see results such as this among working populations. This bias is called the "healthy worker" effect. It comes about because people who are too ill to work will not be found in working populations. As a result, when we study working populations, we find that they inevitably have a lower mortality rate than the general population, which includes people who are too ill to work. Some people say this should be called the "sick population" effect, rather than the "healthy worker" effect. Either way, it is the kind of issue to keep in mind when looking at results from studies like this.

Author:	Milham, 1988	
Population:	67,829 men from CA & WA with FCC licences obtained 1979-1984	
Cause of Death	Observed/ Expected	SMR (95% CI)
All Causes	2485/3478.9	0.71 (0.69-0.74)
Cancer	741/836.9	0.89 (0.82-0.95)
Brain/CNS	29/20.8	1.39 (0.95-1.98)
Lung	209/315.6	0.66 (0.58-0.76)
Leukemia	36/29	1.24 (0.88-1.70)
Lymphatic/Hematopoietic	89/72.1	1.23 (1.00-1.51)

Table 3. Amateur radio operators

This SMR is also low enough that we probably need to be concerned about the linkage of data in this particular study, although it is a little hard to say because it depends upon the health characteristics of radio operators. Looking down the list, you can see the findings for the specific categories of outcomes in this study. One that is worth noting—because it is an exposure of interest for cellular telephone studies—is the brain finding at 1.4. This is a relatively modest increase and there is a fair amount of statistical uncertainty in the findings.

Table 4 summarizes a study of U.S. Embassy Workers (Lilienfeld et al., 1978). The overall SMR here is a very low 0.47, very likely indicating that this is an exceptionally healthy population. The reason U.S. embassy workers were studied is that the embassy in Moscow was bombarded with microwaves from the surrounding buildings. This particular population was not very large, so the outcomes that reported the effect measures are not very stable statistically.

A study of U.S. Navy personnel (Robinette, Silverman, & Jablon, 1980; Table 5) compared soldiers with high levels of exposure to soldiers with low levels of exposure. The reported mortality ratio for all causes of death was 0.96, very close to 1.0. In any case, the numbers are small. In all of these studies, it is important to point out that the investigators had very little ability to control for particular confounding factors that might affect the results. These are record-based studies and the investigators did not have access to all the information that they might have used if they were controlling for all the risk factors that they might have been interested in.

Author:	Lillienfeld, 1978
Exposure Level:	Maximum of $18\mu W/cm^2$ for up to 18 hours/day
Population:	4388 embassy workers, 8283 dependents from 1953 through mid 1970s

Cause of Death	Observed/ Expected	SMR (95% CI)
All Causes	49/105.3	0.47 (0.4-0.6)
Cancer	17/19.0	0.89 (.05-1.4)
Brain/CNS	0/0.9	0.00 (0.0-3.3)
Lung	5/5.8	0.86 (0.3-2.0)
Leukemia	2/0.8	2.5 (0.3-9.0)

Table 4. U.S. Moscow Embassy

Author:	Robinette et al., 1980
Exposure:	Exposure to microwaves at about 1-10 mW/cm²
Population:	20,109 men with "high" exposure and 20,781 men with "low" exposure

Cause of Death	Number of Deaths	Mortality Ratio
All Causes	310	0.96
Cancer	96	1.04
Lung	24	1.14
Lymphopoietic	26	1.18

Table 5. U.S. Navy personnel 1950-1974

Table 6 summarizes the MIT radiation laboratory study. The study found no serious increases, based on very small numbers. The 1.7 on the bottom row is lymphatic and hematopoietic cancers. For leukemia, which is elevated in some of these other reports, there was a small deficit. These are extremely small numbers, so we can't really make much out of them. For overall cancer, there was no elevation to speak of, and the same for brain cancer.

Table 7 is a new report from Poland on Polish military personnel by Szmigielski (1996). There are large numbers in this study. The methodology is not reported in great detail, so it is hard to know exactly what was done. For example, there is no report of exactly how the follow-up occurred. A curious finding is a relative risk of 2.1 for all cancers, which, for me, raises a doubt about how to interpret any of the results from this study. It seems too far-fetched that there could be a doubling in all cancers in a population exposed to RF—not impossible, but the fact that we see it makes me think more of methodological explanations than biological ones for this particular study.

Author:	Hill, 1988	
Exposure:	Radar up to 2-5 mW/cm^2	
Population:	1,492 men from MIT employed 1940-1946 and followed through 1986	
Cause of Death	Observed/ Expected	SMR (95% CI)
All Causes	213/246.0	0.87 (0.78-1.02)
Cancer	47/43.0	1.09 (0.80-1.45)
Brain/CNS	3/2.8	1.07 (.022-3.13)
Leukemia	2/3.1	0.64 (0.08-2.30)
Lymphatic/Hematopoietic	9/5.2	1.72 (0.84-3.15)

Table 6. MIT radiation laboratory

Author:	Szmigielski, 1995	
Exposure:	RF and microwave exposures of about 0.2 mW/cm^2	
Population:	Approximately 130,000 men followed during 1971-1985	
Site of Cancer	Relative Risk	(95% CI)
All Sites	2.1	1.1-3.6
Respiratory	1.1	0.7-1.6
Brain/CNS	1.9	1.1-3.5
Lymphatic/Hematopoietic	6.3	3.1-14.3

Table 7. Cancer incidence among Polish military personnel

Table 8 is intended to emphasize a distinction between the hand-held portable telephones and mobile phones. Hand-held portable phones have the antenna in the handset, operate at comparatively lower power (maximum of 0.6 watts), and the RF exposure is unilaterally to the head. Mobile telephones, what we call car phones, are usually installed in a car. The same kind of telephone can be installed in a bag that you carry around, but the antenna is not in the handset. It operates at up to 3 watts of power in the U.S. and there is little or no RF exposure to the head. If you hold the portable bag phone close to the body, there can be some corporal exposure, but for the car phone, there tends to be none.

Hand-held Portable
• self-contained until with antenna in handset
• operates at ≤ 0.6 watts radiofrequency (RF) energy
• RF exposure to head during use
Mobile
• installed in car or transportable bag; no antenna in handset
• operates at ≤ 3 watts RF
• little or no RF exposure to the head

Table 8. Types of cellular phones

Epidemiology Resources Inc. (ERI) is currently conducting a series of studies on cellular telephone effects. One study is attempting to link mortality records to billing records of cellular telephone use. We first conducted a preliminary study, a type of validation study if you will, to find out whether it made sense to use billing records as an index of exposure to RF from cellular telephones. The main objective was to measure the proportion of time that a person who owned the account was actually using the phone. This item was of interest because the account could be billed when the phone was in use by someone other than the account holder. We wanted to know the proportion of time that the account holder used the phone and the overall correlation between use of the phone by the individual and the amount of use reported on the bill.

While we were doing the survey, we thought this would be an opportunity to assess the question of laterality. First, how often do people switch the phone from one side to the other? Is there consistency in using the left or right side, that is, holding the telephone to the left ear or the right ear, or do people tend to switch? Secondly, if people tend to use one side rather than the other, to what extent is that preference associated with their handedness—that is, do left-handed people tend to use the left ear or vice versa? If laterality were related to handedness, we would have a convenient surrogate for this crucial component of measuring risk. If we could identify laterality of use, we would have a powerful test of the hypothesis in any study showing a positive relation between RF exposure and brain cancer.

We conducted the survey with the help of a cellular telephone provider that had data for four cities: Boston, Chicago, Dallas, and Washington, DC (Table 9). We mailed survey questionnaires to more than 5,000 people and received responses from about 4,000 people—a little better than a 70 percent response rate. The characteristics of respondents are shown in Table 10. The median age was 41 years and about 60 percent were male. Eighty-nine percent were right-handed, which corresponds very well with population levels. Table 11 shows the distribution of phone types among these cellular telephone users. Twenty-six percent used mobile telephones, 34 percent used hand-held telephones, 34 percent used bag phones, and 6 percent had multiple phones. This distribution is changing rapidly, so this is just a snapshot in time for this particular population. We also found out something about respondents' phone use. The median call length was about 2 minutes, and the median number of calls per week by these respondents was 8 calls. The survey was mailed to a random sample of all subscribers to this particular telephone company, so these can be considered good descriptions of the typical phone users in this population.

Geographic Areas:	Boston, Chicago, Dallas, Washington, DC
Number Contacted:	5550
Number Responding:	3949 (71%)

Table 9. Survey sample

Age:	Median = 41 years
Gender:	61% male
Handed:	89% right-handed

Table 10. Respondent characteristics

Phone:	26% Mobile
Type:	34% Hand-held, 34% Transportable Bag, 6% Multiple types
Phone Call Length and Frequency	
Median Length:	2 minutes
Median No./Week:	8 calls

Table 11. Phone type and use

Table 12 shows the key results from the survey, which is what we have termed the level of telephone monopolization—that is, the extent to which the account holder monopolized the use of the telephone. The first column is the proportion of respondents who claim that they, as the account holders, use the telephone 100 percent of the time. These numbers were surprisingly high and encouraging to us. The right column represents a somewhat more relaxed definition of monopolization—the proportion of users reporting that they use the phone at least three quarters of the time that it is in use. So we have 70 percent or better for the two categories of greatest interest—encouraging findings. Billing records, although not perfect indicators of exposure, are apparently highly correlated with the actual amount of use for an individual.

Phone Type	Level of Phone Monopolization	
	100% of time	≥75% of time
Mobile in car	49%	73%
Hand-held	46%	70%
Bag phone	53%	69%
Multiple phones	34%	54%

Table 12. Percentage of respondents who report that they are the main user of their cellular telephone

Table 13 shows actual correlation coefficients for the amount of billed minutes on the account and the amount of personal use reported by the respondent. These are Spearman correlations, which means that we assigned every value its rank in the distribution and looked at the correlation in ranks, which avoids the artificial inflation of the correlation coefficient from outliers that might have distorted the distribution. We found that the correlations were greater than 0.7, which was really quite encouraging. Correlation coefficients were 0.74 for hand-helds and 0.72 for mobile telephones. Table 14 shows similar findings for those who reported that they were the sole user of the telephone. The correlation coefficients here were even higher—0.8 for handhelds and 0.78 for mobile telephones. Bear in mind that these correlations are never expected to reach 100 percent, because the use reported by the respondent is something that had to be recalled. We asked, "How many minutes did you use the phone?" There is obviously built-in error in the individual's recall. Neither the billed amount of time nor the reported amount of time is a perfect measure of the actual time, and because of that, the correlations could not be 100 percent. The fact that they were as high as they were meant that billed use is a good predictor of the actual time spent by the individual on the telephone. In short, these correlations underestimate the actual correlation between the billed use and the real amount of exposure to the individual.

Findings related to switching the phone from ear to ear—our laterality interest—are found in Table 15. For mobile phone users, frequent switching occurred only in 5 percent. Those who basically do not switch from ear to ear were 72 percent—fairly high—but unfortunately, not as high for the hand-held telephone users. Car phone users are using the telephone in the car, which may account for a more regular pattern of laterality. Portable phone users may not be using the telephone in the car very often and they switch comparatively more often. Table 16 shows even worse news on laterality. There was only a modest correlation between handedness and laterality, so in order to get information on laterality, we have to find out directly on which side of the head the phone is used. We can not ask about handedness because it is not strongly correlated with the side of the head on which the phone is used. This finding puts an end to the idea of using handedness as a surrogate variable.

Type of Phone	Correlation Coefficient
Mobile in car	.72
Hand-held	.74
Bag phone	.76
Multiple phones	.61

Table 13. Spearman correlations of reported weekly minutes of personal use and billed minutes

Type of Phone	Correlation Coefficient
Mobile in car	.78
Hand-held	.80
Bag phone	.76
Multiple phones	.70

Table 14. Spearman correlations of reported weekly minutes of use and billed minutes (sole use only)

	Frequency of Switching		
Phone Type	Hardly Ever	Occasionally	Frequent or Often
Mobile	72%	23%	5%
Hand-held	55%	36%	9%
Bag phone	70%	24%	6%

Table 15. Frequency of reported switching of the phone from ear to ear, by phone type

	Ear Used by Respondent		
Handedness	Right Ear	Left Ear	Total
Right Handed	624 (63%)	371 (37%)	995 (100%)
Left Handed	52 (39%)	80 (61%)	132 (100%)
		r = 0.15	

Table 16. Handedness by ear preference (users of portable phones only)

Table 17 summarizes what we learned from the survey. The account holder is typically the primary phone user a large proportion of the time. The reported amount of personal use is strongly associated with the amount of billed use, strong enough that we feel confident conducting epidemiologic studies using billed use as a surrogate for exposure. Switching sides is comparatively uncommon, but, unfortunately, more common in hand-held users than in mobile phone users, and hand-held users are the group of greatest interest. Lastly, handedness was not strongly associated with the side of the head on which the phone was used.

- The account holder is typically the primary phone user a larger proportion of the time
- Reported amount of personal use is strongly associated with amount of billed use
- Switching is uncommon
- Handedness is weakly associated with ear used for phone

Table 17. Survey summary

Table 18 describes the goal, study design, and study focus of the mortality study ERI is conducting. The study goal is to evaluate risk of death, particularly from brain cancer, among a large cohort of portable cellular telephone users. We refer to the study as our mortality surveillance study, and it is entirely record-based. We are not actually contacting individuals. We are using telephone company records to get a roster of individuals, and from that roster the needed information. We have information on the amount of use, and information that helps us determine what kind of telephone is being used (hand-held or mobile), so that we can classify people by type of telephone. Finally, we get identifying information that enables us to link this information to mortality data.

Study Goal
- Evaluate the risk of death from brain cancer among a cohort of portable cellular telephone users.

Study Design
- Assemble a cohort of cellular telephone users from account and billing records of several cellular telephone companies
- Evaluate cause-specific mortality and continue with periodic surveillance

Study Focus
- Individuals with a single cellular telephone account who have used the phones for at least 2 months before entry into the study

Table 18. ERI cohort study of cellular telephone users

We want to assemble the cohort using account billing records. We already have a couple of telephone companies on board and we are attempting to enroll more. The study has some built-in weaknesses, but we hope that the main strength that will compensate for the weaknesses will be the very large study size. Ultimately, we will look at cause-specific mortality rates and continue with periodic surveillance so that we can find out what the effects might be over potentially long induction times. Our focus is on individuals who have just a singular cellular telephone account. These are intended to be consumer accounts and not business telephones. We are going to exclude business telephones, and we will include only those individuals who have had a telephone for at least two months prior to enrollment. Information we assemble from the records from the telephone company and from related sources are shown in Table 19. We get the name, address, and gender from the telephone company. We do not always get gender directly, but we can get it from the credit bureau if the telephone company doesn't have it. We also get the date of birth, which is essential in order to get age-specific mortality rates, and we get the social security number in order to link with mortality records.

Table 20 describes possible indices of amount of exposure that we will be able to construct. The most important one is to distinguish the hand-held telephone users from the mobile phone users. We will use the electronic serial number (ESN) to obtain this information with the cooperation of telephone manufacturers. Ultimately, we should also be able to distinguish analog from digital phones through the ESN. We will have information on the number of calls, the minutes of use, and the beginning date of service, so all of these could be put into one or more indices of the amount of RF exposure. The final marker that we might possibly use is the cell-site density for the markets that are served. The number of cells in a given geographic area have ramifications for the average distance between telephone and tower, which will affect the power output. We would like to be able to incorporate this variable into an index of exposure, but we are not sure that we will be able to.

- Name
- Address
- Gender*
- Date of Birth*
- Social Security Number*

  *   May be obtained from company's credit bureau if not available from telephone company

Table 19. Company customer records

- ESN — used to identify telephone as portable or mobile and analog or digital (through linkage with phone manufacturing data)
- Amount of telephone use
  - Number of calls
  - Minutes of use
  - Start of service date
- Cell site density for each market served

Table 20. Possible exposure indices

Based upon these indices, we intend to make a variety of comparisons (Table 21). The main comparison will be portable versus mobile phone users. We will also try to create subgroups by number and length of calls, length of service and possibly density of cell sites.

- Portable vs. Mobile Phone Users
- Subgroups Classified by Number and Length of Calls
- Subgroups Classified by Length of Service
- Subgroups Classified by Density of Cell Site in Home Area

Table 21. ERI cohort study of cellular telephone users: Key comparisons

Some of the steps involved in this project are outlined in Table 22. We first must develop a roster of study participants for each company for each year, take in the exposure data described above, and find record linkage information, which we might have to get from outside sources. We then have the big job of quality control because these data were not recorded originally for research purposes, so we have a series of checks that we put the data through in order to make sure that we can eliminate as many errors as possible. Ultimately, we are going to calculate exposure indices. We are going to link these account records to death records, using the National Death Index in the U.S. and, as a supplement, the Social Security Administration death master files. Ultimately, we have to go get the death certificate in order to get cause of death, although the National Death Index is working on a means of providing us directly with cause of death information. Right now, there are some administrative barriers to getting the information we need in a timely way. Because of these barriers, we have to write to each state that is involved in order to get the death certificates, and it can take many, many months to get a response. You have to pay to get a copy of each certificate, and it is a slow process. When we get the death certificates, we code each one and enter the cause of death. At this point, we are able to calculate the cause-specific mortality rates.

- Develop roster of study participants for each company for each year
- Acquire data on exposure (phone use, density of cell site, and phone type)
- Obtain record linkage information where needed (SSN, gender & dates of birth)
- Edit data and conduct quality control
- Calculate exposure indices
- Initiate record linkage to identify deaths
  - National Death Index
  - Social Security Administration Death Master Files
- Obtain death certificates
- Code & enter causes of death
- Analyze cause-specific mortality rate
- Obtain qualified reviews of preliminary results & draft reports
- Finalize reports, prepare abstracts and make presentations
- Maintain cohort rosters and periodically update information
- Continue surveillance

Table 22. Study tasks

We are also involved in some early planning discussions with people from a number of university groups in the U.S. to do a cohort study with direct contact of cellular telephone users. The initial interview would be conducted through a mailed questionnaire, and then users would be contacted periodically to get additional information, including information on health outcomes. We hope to be able to get funding for this project and to implement it in a geographic area that has a high average level of power output per telephone call. We will therefore go to small-size cities, where there are comparatively fewer towers, so that the power output would be comparatively high among those users. This population would be approached directly and report on their own telephone use, then they would be followed individually over a long period of time to study long induction time effects. This type of study would compensate for many of the difficulties that we have in a purely record-based study.

Table 23 shows the announcement of the request for proposals that was put out by WTR recently for studies related to cellular telephone use. Requests include new studies on general morbidity/mortality, analogue and digital technologies, U.S. studies, European studies, a prospective cohort study of high, medium, and low use, and case-control studies of glioma, meningioma, neuroma, salivary gland tumors and adult leukemia. Several case-control studies are also underway right now: one at the National Cancer Institute and one at the American Health Foundation.

•   General Morbidity/Mortality Studies
      •   Analog/Digital
      •   United States/Europe
•   Prospective Cohort Study of High, Medium, and Low Use
•   Case-control Studies of Glioma, Mengioma, Neuroma, Salivary Gland Tumor, Adult Leukemia

Table 23. WTR omnibus request for epidemiology proposals

Finally, although we are focusing on cancer as the main effects, there are other effects to think about. In fact, there are reports of some unusual affects alleged to result from RF exposure in a group of workers in Sweden. A recent cartoon also shows the highway lane for the cellular telephone users up here, which illustrates the possible problem of using a telephone while in the automobile, and the important implication for automobile accidents. That is another topic that is currently being studied and is one of the potential outcomes, in fact, that we will be able to look at in our mortality surveillance.

References

Elmer-DeWitt, P. (1993, February 8). Dialing "P" for panic, Can cellular phones cause brain cancer? There's scant evidence but lots of fear. Time, 141(6), 74.

Lilienfeld, A. M., Tonascia, J., Tonascia, S., Libauer, C. H., Cauthen, G. M., Markowitz, J. A., & Weida, S. (1978). Evaluation of health status of foreign service and other employees from selected Eastern European posts. Baltimore, MD: The Johns Hopkins University and Washington, DC: Department of State, Office of Medical Services. (NTIS No. PB-288-163)

Millham, S. Jr. (1998). Increased mortality in amateur radio operators due to lymphatic and hematopic malignancies. American Journal of Epidemiology, 127, 50-54.

Morrison, D., & Cummins, C. (1994, September 2). Questions remain about cellular phone-cancer link. The Seattle Times, F2.

Robinette, C. D., Silverman, C., & Jablon, S. (1980). Effects upon health of occupational exposure to microwave radiation (radar). American Journal of Epidemiology, 111(1), 39-53.

Szmigielski, S. (1996). Cancer morbidity in subjects occupationally exposed to high frequency (radiofrequency and microwave) electromagnetic radiation. Science of the Total Environment, 180, 9-17.

Taubes, G. (1995). Epidemiology faces its limits. Science, 269, 164-169.

17
OCCUPATIONAL HEALTH STUDIES
Robert W. Morgan

Abstract

Because occupational exposures are often greater in magnitude, more frequent, and better documented, the workplace provides a laboratory for epidemiologic studies, and has been called, "the sentinel for the community." Workers who design, manufacture, test, install, or use radiofrequency (RF)-emitting devices can be expected to have a greater probability of exposure than the general population, although modern manufacturing techniques, including use of robots, keeps most exposure to low levels. These workers form cohorts that can be followed for either incidence or mortality studies. Cohort studies have the advantage of being able to examine many diseases within a single study, and can be designed to be relatively free of bias in assessing RF exposure. The weaknesses of cohort studies include limited sample sizes, lack of actual exposure measurements (especially in the past), and problems in dealing with any potential confounders or RF exposure outside the workplace.

Within the cohort, there is the opportunity for case-control studies. Because exposure is more frequent than studies based within the general population, there is greater statistical power. There is also the ability to better quantify RF exposure and to validate those estimates. The major limitation of such studies is the small sample size expected without massive cohorts to generate enough cases for study. Fortunately, some very large cohorts do exist, and thus the case-control studies are more feasible.

Currently, we are completing a cohort mortality study of over 133,000 workers. Based on US vital statistics, this cohort is expected to generate about 70 cases of brain cancer and 175 cases of hematolymphopoietic malignancy for two nested case-control studies.

I was asked, originally, to comment on Dr. Rothman's paper. For those of you who have not done a lot of epidemiology, Dr. Rothman's differentiation between induction time and latency, although correct, is a differentiation that we can not make, because as he pointed out, you do not know when the disease was induced. So, when you see the term "latency" in most epidemiologic studies, it is usually defined as the interval from first exposure to the onset of the disease. It encompasses both of those.

We also have not paid enough attention, perhaps, to the difference between a cause and a risk factor. The classic example that we use in teaching medical students is that yellow fingers are a risk factor for lung cancer, but they are not the cause of lung cancer. Clearly, as Dr. Wynder showed us so many years ago, it was the cigarette-smoking that caused them both.

In looking at the need for studies of radiofrequency (RF) and RF effects, I think that we are now being driven not by a biologic imperative, if you like, but by a public health imperative. As a technology expands, there is a need and a desire to know whether or not there is any health effect, even though from a biologic point of view there may not be a lot of biologic credibility because the amount of energy actually delivered to any particular kind of tissue is relatively low. So, we are doing studies that, I think, are in the interest of the public, but I do not have a strong belief in the biology part of it.

We are faced with a vexing challenge, which may also be an epidemiologic opportunity, and that is the issue of changing technology. We have seen the move from the mobile telephone (that is, the car phone), to the transportable telephone (the telephone in a bag), to the portable telephone, which is the common cellular phone. We also have combinations. My particular car telephone I can unplug and put in my pocket or leave in my car. We are moving from analog to digital. We have pulse technologies. We have a change in frequencies. All the technology is changing very rapidly. When you combine the change in technology with the need for an adequate latency period—and for cancers, the latency is probably over 10 years for almost any type of malignancy—you are going to see that this is a problem for epidemiology.

I would also caution you in looking at epidemiology—although you have heard a lot of the negatives about it—that there are some problems. In the early part of my career in epidemiology, which was about 30 years ago, somebody said that epidemiology could be defined as the tedious pursuit of the obvious. I think it was true that people went to enormous lengths to prove relative risks of 10, 20 and things like that. That was the tedious pursuit of the obvious. As Dr. Wynder pointed out, he was able to show relationships without the use of elegant statistics or biostatistical methods. What we see today is the proliferation of studies and papers reporting relative risks not of 10, 12, 15, or 20, which most of us would agree are unlikely to be discovered ever again, but more and more research revolving around the risks from 1.2, 1.5, and 2. As every epidemiologist knows, this is the relative risk area where it's very difficult to tell the confounders from the cause. My colleague Richard Monson, writing about the problems of EMF, which is closely related to RF, pointed out that with a series of relative risks between 1.2 and 1.3, we are now in the area where EMF could never be satisfactorily proven or disproven to cause anything. Those who would say it is causing a disease or causing mortality can point to studies that show that, and people who do not believe it can point out many, many reasons for confounding, for example, that people who live near transformers also live near the street.

I thought it interesting, looking at the Honolulu study on base stations for phones, that maybe these antennae are put on the top of hills. Who lives on the top of the hill? Do the people on the top of the hill have the same socioeconomic factors, the same occupational factors, as the people at the bottom of the hill? It depends where you live, but it is the kind of confounder that will interfere with any ecologic studies that we do.

We must also be careful in going back over previous work that other people have done and indulging in what epidemiologists have somewhat ingloriously called "data-dredging," although it is a term that appears in the Dictionary of Epidemiology. That is going over old data to try to find answers to current problems. As I mentioned, with the changes in technology that are occurring, I am not sure that the older studies can give us much clue or any answers as to what to expect. Having commented on some of the previous speakers, I would like to tell you something of what we do. Looking at occupational studies, we have a principle that the workplace is the sentinel for the community. Typically, people who make or design equipment or materials are exposed to levels of that substance or levels of that energy, or whatever, that are considerably more than in the general population. I would submit to you that, for instance, people who use cellular telephones in the course of commercial transactions are probably getting more exposure because they make more calls. Their calls are probably more monitored in terms of one user, one telephone, than you will find in noncommercial use. So we have adopted the policy of looking at hazards in terms of the workplace.

Occupational studies have certain advantages (Table 1), the first of which is that you are usually dealing with a defined population. Most companies, especially large ones, know who worked there. Those people have employment records, in part because the people who pay workers are very unlikely to throw away records. Sometimes there are health and mortality records associated with a company, perhaps because of a health policy or a life insurance program that the company maintains. Exposure estimates are occasionally available. I think there is a misconception that industries know what their workers are exposed to; I would say that is true in perhaps semi-quantitative terms. Unfortunately, we rarely have specific exposure estimates or even exposure estimates for areas or groups in the workforce. In occupational studies, you can do both cohort and case control studies. For those of you not familiar with epidemiology, the term "cohort"—which, fittingly enough, I think began in Rome as a description of the Roman Legions—is a group of people with a common experience. We follow them over time to see what happened. In case-control studies, we compare the diseased and non-diseased populations and look backwards and see what their prior exposure was. I did not discuss ecologic studies here, because I do not feel ecologic studies are as important in occupational studies.

•   Defined population
•   Employment records
•   Health, mortality records
•   Exposure estimates
•   Both cohort and case-ontrol studies feasible

Table 1. Advantages of occupational studies

Occupational epidemiology is not without its problems (Table 2). The first of these is the issue of sample size. You do not have industries or groups that are exposed in the large numbers that might be true in the population. When Dr. Rothman talks about his cohort of telephone users, he's talking in terms of potentially millions of people. No company employs millions of people. As we search for smaller and

228

smaller relative risks, and as we get more and more confounders, and the power of our study declines, there is a need for larger and larger studies. So one of the difficulties in doing the occupational studies is just that—you may run out of power. There is also the issue of ascertainment bias. There are at least two papers in the literature describing what appears to be ascertainment bias, which may be especially true in the United States. For example, if a person who has good health insurance and is well covered by the company medical plan develops headaches, nausea, blurred vision, he or she will go to the doctor, have an examination of their eyes, perhaps go for X-rays, perhaps CAT scans or MRIs, and may have a brain tumor diagnosed. On the other hand, a person who does not have that kind of health insurance, or that accessibility to health care, may take some analgesics, some aspirin, or something like that for headaches, ignore the blurred vision until such a time as perhaps they bleed into the tumor. So, they bleed into the brain tumor, and they arrive in the emergency room. Their blood pressure might be up from the tumor itself or because they are African-American. A spinal tap is done. There is blood in the spinal fluid, showing there is a hemorrhage in the brain. The staff tends to write this off as a brain hemorrhage, and if the person dies before further investigation, the brain tumor may go unnoticed and undiagnosed, especially as autopsy rates are relatively low. What this means, then, is that the affluent or the employed or the insured may be more likely to get a brain tumor diagnosed than the person who is not this way. This gives a bias, and it may be responsible for some of the findings that brain tumors occur more frequently in more affluent people. The occupational group is not the general population.

•	Sample size restrictions
•	Ascertainment bias (e.g., brain cancer reporting)
•	Lack of exposure data
•	Not the general population

Table 2. Problems of occupational studies

I think you have heard allusion to the issue of the "healthy worker effect," in that people who work and who are able to work tend to be healthier than the general population. In epidemiology, we have known this for a long time; it still bedevils us. One of the things we sometimes try to do is, as they did in the Robinette studies of the military, to compare workers with workers on the issue of exposed versus unexposed (Robinette, Silverman, & Jablon, 1980). In that way, you get around some of the "healthy worker effect." Then the question is: how do you extrapolate this to the general population? That provides another set of problems. So although there are advantages to occupational studies, as I mentioned before, we still have some problems and some limitations.

If we are interested in radiofrequencies as an energy source and as a potential health hazard, who would we study? From the occupational end (Table 3), we look at device manufacturing, and in "manufacturing," we also get into the people testing the devices. In modern-day manufacturing, however, device testing is more and more often done by robots working inside a shielded box, where there is little or no exposure to any of the workers surrounding it. In looking at manufacturing groups, we found, actually, that the greatest exposure is probably among the security people. They are always running around using their cellular phones or radios. Then, we have the issue of important bystanders. This would be someone who is not actually using a phone, but is always there when it is used. The amount of power a cellular telephone puts out (a maximum of .6 watts) and the diminution in energy as you move away from the source, however, makes bystander exposure much less important. If there were higher elements of power, that might be more important.

• RF device manufacturing
• Device testing
• Device use
• Important bystanders

Table 3. Types of occupational groups for study

In doing an occupational cohort study (Table 4), one of the things we look at is the probability of exposure. When we look at dose, we have to look at the amount received, the intensity of the exposure, and the duration of the exposure. For example, given a certain job title, was this person likely to be exposed or not? We need good demographic data, such things as Social Security numbers. We always find that there are certain families where they share a Social Security number. We have problems in company records, no matter what the company is, with Social Security numbers being inaccurately recorded, etc. When we are doing a cohort study, we have the advantage that we can look at multiple outcomes, so we can look at 70 or 80 causes of death if we are doing a mortality study and not a just one. It is an advantage, but it's also a disadvantage, because now you are being given data for which you had no prior hypotheses, and you are having a multiple comparison problem with statistics. In an occupational cohort study, you can often get more latency, because the people were exposed to the technology before it became a common consumer exposure. For example, a company might have been in the telephone or radio business since the 1940s, first making military applications and then moving onward.

• Probability of exposure
• Good demographic data (SSNs, etc.)
• Multiple outcome measures
• More latency
• Case source for case-control studies
• Problems with potential confounders
• Data lacking regarding other RF exposure

Table 4. Occupational cohort studies

The occupational cohort is a very good source of cases and controls for case-control studies. These people have a higher probability of exposure, so the statistical power increases in the study, and you can get better data perhaps than you can by interviewing people in the general population. There still may be a problem with potential confounders, however. For example, people who are exposed to RF may also have had exposure to other things like solvents, etc. Confounders are what we have to deal with in epidemiology day in and day out. The other problem we have is missing data about other RF exposure. In one of the companies that we are studying at the moment, for instance, a very high proportion of the company happens to be ham radio operators. We have managed to get the CD-ROM from the Federal Communications Commission which has all the licenses so we can match people in the cohort to their ham radio status.

Occupational case-control studies (Table 5) can be nested or not within the cohort. In case-control studies, we have the advantage of gathering more specific data about the nature of the exposure, whether it was to certain wavelengths or certain powers of RF. We have better control over some of the potential confounders, but not all of them. For instance, we rarely have smoking history from occupational studies. Restricted sample size is still an issue.

• Nested or not-nested within cohort
• Advantage of gathering more specific data
• Better control over potential confounders
• Restricted sample size

Table 5. Occupational case-control studies

In our current studies, we are using several factors to measuring exposure (Table 6). We are looking at the intensity (that is measured in different ways, watts, etc.); the frequency, not frequency as physicists know it, but how often people are exposed; and whether they are exposed on an hourly daily, weekly, or monthly basis. The duration of that exposure usually reflects how long they worked in that particular job. Probability is an estimate, if you like, of the likelihood of that job having been exposed. From these four measures, we will create an index of exposure.

• Intensity
• Frequency (how often)
• Duration
• Probability

Table 6. RF exposure in occupational studies

In summary, occupational studies have many strong advantages for the issue of RF exposure. No single study design is best. We are going to employ the scientific method, which has been defined as "doing your best with whatever you've got." So, we use both case-control and cohort studies. There are certain problems, and they will not give a complete answer.

One of the troubling things we must deal with is the anticipation of results. If our studies show no significant increases, people will say that we did not study enough people for a long enough period of time with enough exposure, so therefore we have not proven safety. On the other hand, because of the multiple comparisons and the perhaps 70 outcomes, if we find something of what I would call mild significance—a relative risk of, say, 1.2 to 1.5—we will never be able to show that it was either confounding or an actual cause-and-effect relationship. We have to look forward to being interpreted and misinterpreted by various people in various ways. The epidemiology, though, in the final conclusion, is really the definitive answer as to whether this affects human health or not. So although the basic science research is important, the question at the end of the day is still whether anyone got hurt. Epidemiology will have to try to address that. The RF question is going to take many years of people examining it. Do not expect answers quickly. Remember that Dr. Rothman's study has another 20 or 30 years to go, and even when he is finished, it will be criticized as a study of the affluent, whatever that means.

Reference

Robinette, C. D., Silverman, C., & Jablon, S. (1980). Effects upon health of occupational exposure to microwave radiation (radar). American Journal of Epidemiology, 112(1), 39-53.

18
REVIEW AND DISCUSSION OF STATE OF THE ART, EPIDEMIOLOGY
John R. Goldsmith

Abstract

Two major and often cited studies (of Naval personnel in the Korean War, and of workers and families exposed at U.S. Embassy in Moscow) are reevaluated on the basis of their findings and on the documented statements of their leading investigators. The balanced interpretation of these studies at the time of publication may have been distorted by the Cold War. Findings suggested by these studies have been supported by independent research, even though the recommended follow-up has not been done.

Several types of occupational studies are also briefly reviewed. Two suggest increased malignant melanoma among workers making electronic equipment. Air traffic controllers show evidence of reversible lymphocyte mutation. Cancer of the testis is noted among military personnel and traffic police using hand-held radar.

Relevance of findings to regulation and balance of studies between those exposed as phone users and those potentially exposed near broadcast is urged. Five guidelines are offered.

Two Major Epidemiological Studies

There are two principal studies that provide some epidemiological evidence on the possible effects of radar exposure. One study reports on exposures sustained by Naval personnel during the Korean War (Robinette, Silverman, & Jablon, 1980). This study classifies more than 40,000 men into six occupational categories, according to presumed radar exposure, with follow-up reported through 1976. The data from this study are excerpted and reanalyzed in Appendix A. A second study evaluates outcomes among workers in the US Embassy in Moscow and their dependents (Lilienfeld et al., 1978); the embassy was exposed to microwave irradiation by the Soviets during the period 1953-1976. These workers were evaluated in 1976, and their experience compared to employees and their dependents from other Eastern European Embassies. Its findings and some of the other circumstances preceding the study are reported elsewhere (Goldsmith, 1995). Each of the reports recognizes the importance of additional follow-up and urges that it be conducted; however, no follow-up to either study has been done or is known to be underway.

It is essential to recall that each of these studies were done during the Cold War. In this context, publishing a clear interpretation that the Moscow signal—whatever its purpose may have been—was causing increases in cancer risk may not have been in the national interest. Similarly, to report a finding of positive, systematic associations between leukemia and increasing potential radar exposure of Naval personnel may have affected morale and could have been interpreted as giving aid and comfort to those hostile to the United States. Under today's circumstances, when wide use of communication systems by the public is forecast, these findings have a different relevance to the national interest. In light of this situation, it is necessary to note that no criticism is felt or implied as to how the data were initially interpreted. We now have, however, the obligation to re-interpret them.

The Authentic Voice of the Epidemiologists from These Studies

In the abstract of the first study (Robinette et al., 1980), the following conclusion is drawn: "No adverse effects were detected in these indices that could be attributed to potential microwave radiation exposure in 1950-1954." Dr. Charlotte Silverman, the second author of the study and an epidemiologist with the U.S. Food and Drug Administration, wrote elsewhere concerning the same set of data: "While some significant differences among the occupational groups classified by level of potential exposure have been found with respect to all the endpoints studied, the differences could not be interpreted as a direct result of microwave exposure. . . . Because no measures of actual as opposed to potential exposure were available, the so-called 'high exposure' rosters were made up of a mixture, in unknown proportions, of men whose actual exposure varied from high to negligible" (Silverman, 1979; emphasis added).

In short, significant elevations of endpoint rates for the potentially more exposed are consistently shown, but since the exposure was not measured, the endpoints cannot be attributed directly to microwave exposures. On the basis of Dr. Silverman's characterization, buried in her article, this is a suggestive study, not a negative one. Data derived from this study are excerpted and analyzed in Appendix A; this work reaches the same conclusion as did Dr. Silverman.

With regard to the second study, the Freedom of Information (FOI) Act has made it possible to read the minutes of the meeting in which Prof. Lilienfeld's opinions were changed by the State Department Contract Officer, Dr. Pollack. I do not know who obtained the data under the FOI Act, nor specifically from which files. Nor can I direct another interested person to the source of these files; they were provided to me by an attorney representing two former employees who served in the Moscow Embassy and died of cancer. Yet, having read them carefully in the context of the report prepared and distributed by the National Technical Information Service, Department of Commerce (Lilienfeld et al., 1978), I am convinced of their authenticity and relevance and am willing to put such previously secret information (now cleared) into the public record.

We have available some notes of a meeting on October 17, 1978 at which the research group from Johns Hopkins University was persuaded to alter Professor Lilienfeld's opinion as reflected in his Final Report of July 31, 1978 (Prof. Lilienfeld was in the hospital at the time). Selected pages of the Final Report were included in the FOI material. Specifically, the following issues are of interest.

1. With regard to page 240 of the draft, "Dr. Pollack pointed out, and it was agreed, that the reference to the microwave surveillance at one or more the Comparison embassies is really heresay [sic] and should be deleted." The assertion that workers were irradiated at other Eastern European Embassies was independently made by the President of the Foreign Service Worker's Association. Professor Lilienfeld had written in his Final Report of July 31, 1978 that "the possibility that one or more of the Comparison posts was exposed to microwave surveillance could compromise their use as a Comparison for the Moscow population. Unfortunately no access to the underlying data collected was possible. This was of concern, especially since several participants in the study informed us that there indeed was surveillance using microwave technology at some of the Comparison posts."

2. Professor Lilienfeld wrote in the July 31, 1978 Final Report: "During 1967-1971, the five female deaths were one each from breast cancer, uterine cancer, skin cancer (not melanoma), leukemia and senility (including other and ill-defined causes). For the period 1972-1976, the two deaths were from breast cancer and uterine cancer. Although, of these seven deaths, six were from cancer, they were from different types of cancer. Since these types of cancer have different epidemiological factors associated with them, such as later age a first pregnancy for breast cancer and early age at first coitus for cervical cancer, it is difficult if not impossible to determine whether they could have been caused by microwave exposure. At this point in the analysis one can regard this findings as being only suggestive." At the meeting with Dr. Pollock, the notes available read: "Dr. Pollock questioned the emphasis on the seven cancer deaths in women and whether the findings should be considered 'suggestive.' It was agreed after some discussion, that small numbers, latent periods for human cancer and the non-specificity of cancer sites all would argue against a microwave effect."

3. In his Final Report of July 31, Lilienfeld wrote: "There were no discernible differences in the Moscow and Comparison females in total mortality or mortality from specific causes. It was disturbing to note a relatively high proportion of cancer deaths in both female employee groups—8 out of 11 deaths among the Moscow and 15 out of 31 deaths among the Comparison group." When Dr. Pollock met with the group, "It was agreed that the characterization of 8 out of 11 deaths in Moscow women and 15 out of 31 in Comparison women due to cancer as 'disturbing' is too strong. However this high ratio of cancer deaths should be studied further—most appropriately with a surveillance of subsequent deaths in the Moscow group." (This

additional surveillance has not been done.)

4.	In the notes of the meeting with Dr. Pollack, we read: "In the third paragraph (page 101), Dr. Pollack noted that the reference to a 'potential infertility effect' may be quite inappropriate, because the experimental work was done at very high doses and there are no controlled human studies. This clause will be modified to reflect the very speculative nature of the reports, but the FSHSS [Foreign Service Health Status Study] data will be presented as is."

The notes also say two other things. First, that "many revisions had been anticipated and were discussed with Dr. Lilienfeld before his hospitalization. We will forward written responses to reviewer's comments to Dr. Pollack and make any revisions necessary. Dr. Lilienfeld will be kept informed in writing of all these matters." Secondly, Dr. Pollack offered to provide additional data on microwave exposure and on cancer cases at the meeting, but the staff replied that it was too late to incorporate any additional data into the study.

In summary, the view of the investigative team was that there were suggestive findings, and that some of the findings were disturbing. How specifically these findings could be related to microwave exposure was not clear. The need for further follow-up was strongly expressed. Prof. Lilienfeld noted that the apparent increase in exposure intensity in 1975 could hardly be reflected in any results of a study ending in 1976. It is not a negative report, as is often alleged. It is a suggestive one, the interpretation of which has been distorted in a negative direction by pressure from the Contract Officer.

Selected Occupational Studies

Author's Note:
> *The choice of the studies to be discussed is arbitrary and may not represent the universe of such studies. The decision to present these was taken late in the preparation of the this report, at a time when it was clear that only an outline of Dr. Rothman's State-of-the-Art Review would be available in advance. One set of studies was derived from the excellent review of epidemiological studies on long term effects of radiofrequency and microwave electromagnetic fields prepared by Paola Vecchia (1995).*

Mortality Study of Boeing Workers Exposed to Electromagnetic Pulses

Muhm (1992) reports on the mortality of 304 men exposed to electromagnetic pulses, with a follow-up of 3,362 person-years. Three deaths were identified where leukemia was listed among the causes of death; one was identified as a secondary cause and the other two as the primary cause. These findings were highly significant and not explained by other exposures.

Malignant Melanoma among Telecommunications Workers

In Montreal, DeGuire, Theriault, Iturra, Provencher, Cyr, and Case (1988) reported on an observation that seven patients with malignant melanoma had worked for a single large telecommunications company. All 9590 employees of the company were surveyed and compared to new cases diagnosed between 1 January 1976 and 31 December 1983 among metropolitan residents 15 years of age or older (852 cases). Ten of the cases were employees of the company; all were men. The standardized incidence ratio was 2.71 (95% C.I.= 1.31-5.02). It is not at all clear whether radiation was causally linked to these cases, since five cases were office workers.

Cancer morbidity was checked for 2918 workers in the Swedish telecommunications industry by Vagero, Ahlbom, Olin, and Sahlsten (1985). Twelve workers had melanoma of the skin, with a standardized mortality ratio of 2.6. No specific exposures could account for the increase in the authors' view.

In none of the three studies is there any proof that radiation is involved, but at the same time in none can it be excluded.

Radar Exposures and Mutation in Air Traffic Controllers

The specificity of microwave exposure among air traffic controllers is not contested. Most of the occupational health studies in this group have focused on the tension of the work rather than on the radiation exposure. Among the scientists who have attended to the possible radiation risk, those in Zagreb, Croatia are prominent. The hematological studies of Goldoni (1990) were mentioned in my review (Goldsmith, 1995).

A series of studies have also demonstrated that radar exposures are mutagenic, both in vivo and in vitro. The initial paper of the series was "The effect of microwave radiation on the cell genome" (Garaj-Vrhovac, Horvat, & Koren, 1990). The investigators used cultured Chinese hamster cells and exposed them to 7.7 GHz radiation, at power densities of 30 mW/cm^2, for 15, 30, and 60 minutes. The incorporation of thymidine into DNA after four hours incubation was decreased stepwise according to the length of exposure and recovered nearly completely in 24 hours. In addition, chromosomal aberrations increased stepwise according to the duration of exposure. The background metaphase percentage was 1.7%, increasing to 4.8% with 15 minute exposure, 6.3% with 30 minute exposure, and 8.9% with 60 exposure.

In their second report, the same authors report on "T] ·elationship between colony-forming ability, chromosome aberrations, incidence of micronuclei in V79 Chinese hamster cells exposed to microwave radiation" (Garaj-Vrhovac, Horvat, & Koren, 1991). They were able to show damage to the genome of the cells and changes in chromosome structure based on observations of structural chromosomal aberrations and micronuclei tests. The exposure was to 7.7 GHz radiation at 30 mW/cm^2, for 15, 30, and 60 minutes. The structural changes replicated the changes found in the initial paper. The micronuclei / 1000 cells were: background 0.016, 0.043 with 15 minute exposure, 0.050 with 30 minute exposure, and 0.073 with 60 minute exposure. The authors believe the result cannot be explained on the basis of cell heating.

In the third paper (Garaj-Vrhovac, Fucic, & Horvat, 1992), human lymphocytes were used instead of Chinese hamster cells, and a correlation was shown between micronuclei percents and specific chromosomal aberrations (acentric fragments and dicentric chromosomes). Temperature was held constant, and an additional level of power density at 0.5 mW/cm^2 was added. Its use led to a 2.7% aberration and 1.4% micronuclei, compared to control levels of 1.5% and 0.9%.

The final paper in the set traces the occurrence and repair of chromosomal aberrations in personnel repairing aircraft traffic control radar (Garaj-Vrhovac, Fucic, & Pevelak-Kozlina, 1993). The signal was 1250-1350 MHz in a field of 10 to 20 mW/cm^2. No long term trend in chromosomal aberrations was found, but short term increases of as great as 33% of the 200 metaphases studied occurred. The apparent half-time to recovery was about 12 weeks.

These findings are epidemiologically important because of the need for biological indicators of exposure, and because of the theory that somatic cell mutations lead to increased risk of cancer. That any one of the three tests could be useful as a biological monitor seems clear from the data and from the findings of excess numbers of mutations among chromosomes in the blood of the group exposed at the US Embassy in Moscow (Lilienfeld, et al., 1978).

In a prospective study of persons with stable mutations, an increase in lymphoreticular cancer was found, but no such effect was seen in persons with transient changes or changes of a chromatid type (Hagmar, Brugger, Hansteen, Heims, & Hogstedt, 1994). A recent review by Akiyama et al. (1995) summarizes the present understanding of the prognostic importance of somatic cell mutation.

Evidence That Radar (Microwaves) Exposure Is Related to Cancer of the Testis

With regard to microwave exposure and cancer of the testis, the following facts have been developed.

1. Traffic policemen using radar for traffic monitoring seem to have an unusual frequency of testicular cancer (Davis & Mostofi, 1993; Volkers, 1992).

2. Among U.S. Veterans, in an effort to relate Agent Orange to testicular cancer, the results only showed that testicular cancer was more frequent in naval personnel (Bullman, Watanabe, & Kang, 1994).

3. In another study, radar exposure seemed to be related to self-reported exposure to microwaves or other radio waves with an Odds Ratio of 3.5, when the subjects were restricted to those from military hospitals (Hayes et al., 1990). The association was not found when industrial hygienists made the exposure estimates.

4. Finally, admitting that radar has the effect of relatively deep tissue heating, it has been shown through comparison of 250 cases and 250 matched

referents for age and residence that occupational exposures to extreme temperatures are associated with a risk ratio of 1.71 (significant) and to high temperature alone (RR = 1.20; non-significant) (Zhang, et al., 1995).

It would follow that short term, high exposures to radar may be associated with testicular cancer on the basis of such exposures having effects on tissue heating. The incidence of testicular cancer has been steadily increasing in many countries since World War II, when radar was first introduced.

In a report prepared for the Commission of the European Communities, Leonard, Berteaud, and Bruyere (1983) concluded ". . . the testes must be considered as much more critical organs in the assessment of microwave genetical hazard, as shown by the existence of testicular damage after mammalian exposures to microwaves, which is due to the fact that these organs do not have an adequate vascular system for the exchange of temperature."

These data are consistent with, but do not establish, that increased testicular cancer risk may be associated with increased exposure to radar (microwave) radiation. Exposures in the vicinity of the head and neck seem less likely to be harmful than whole body exposures or exposures in the area of the groin.

Contribution of Epidemiology to Microwave Regulation

Whether dealing with regulations of air or water pollution, noise, occupational exposures, heat or cold, food contamination, or radiation, we have come to realize the need for a balanced input and evaluation of three types of scientific information: toxicological information based on animal and, where ethical, human experimentation; epidemiological analyses of the experiences of human populations exposed to various levels of the contaminants or agents; and various types of environmental sciences, including exposure estimation. As I shall show, in the case of health protection from radiation exposures—and microwave radiation in particular—data of the second type are scant, and the data that exist have been ineptly evaluated.

Validity of the Present Standards

Each type of environmental protection standards has its own history, and that history has been influential in the development and application of those standards. Microwave radiation as a possible health risk first arose in connection with military applications of radar, so the primary input was from electrical engineers, with scant toxicological data and virtually no epidemiological data, since the exposure was considered to be entirely novel. Although headache and changes in blood counts were noted early, they were not considered relevant to any protective strategy for the military personnel involved (Steneck, Cook, Vander, & Kane, 1980). The dependence on tissue heating as a sole criteria for possible health damage was dominant in standard setting and has continued to be. As I have pointed out, the various committees which have documented their consideration of these standards have not been able to evaluate the epidemiological information available, nor information on nonthermal mechanisms of effects (Goldsmith, 1991).

I am forced to conclude from these findings that a reasonable level of public health protection cannot be assured without incorporation of epidemiological data and analyses in the program of standard setting; it follows that the standards used and cited cannot provide a scientific basis for such protection and thereby are seriously flawed. (Please note that the actual level of the standards, with its various "fudge factors" and safety factors, may or may not be reasonably protective. This discussion speaks only to the adequacy of the scientific input and evaluation.)

Cancer is difficult to study as an endpoint precisely because it is uncommon, but the public and concerned scientists will not accept this as a reason for ignoring its risk. Recall that most cigarette smokers never get lung cancer, but that most of those dying of lung cancer are smokers, and that preventing these deaths is possible by reducing or preventing cigarette smoking. Lung cancer is the most frequent cancer in males and is increasing alarmingly in females. We are just beginning to understand why so relatively few of the individuals heavily exposed to carcinogens get the disease.

Radar exposures are an important occupational risk for aircraft flight traffic controllers. Dr. Goldoni has reported on studies in Zagreb, Croatia (Goldoni, 1990), where changes in blood counts were systematically observed, and chromosomal changes were found for workers exposed accidentally.

I have asked the physician in charge of medical surveillance for U.S. air traffic controllers if comparable studies were done, and the answer was negative, although he writes that there should be data from accidental increases in exposure (D. Watkins, personal communication, January, 1996). I must conclude from these observations that at least the US government has been either indifferent or negatively inclined toward clearly indicated epidemiological studies.

The UK, unlike the US, has a National Cancer Registry. Analyses of cancer experience in the vicinity of broadcast facilities has been reported by Dolk, Elliott, Shaddick, Walls, & Thakrar (1997) and Dolk, Shaddick, et al. (1997). There were significant trend tests for leukemia with distance from the transmitters. I have discussed these findings and some others in a commentary entitled "TV broadcast towers and cancer: The end of innocence for radiofrequency exposures" (Goldsmith, 1997).

A systematic study of data near nuclear facilities in the UK was initiated, but aborted, in part because of a poor choice of statistical criteria for evaluation of expected experience in less exposed areas. Since the data were accessible, I completed the aborted study and reported it (Goldsmith, 1992).

If one adds the distortions produced in what has been published and the absence of data which could have provided better assessment of long term human health risks, it suggests that there seems to have been a policy of obscuring the experiences with radiofrequency exposures of human populations occupationally exposed or exposed as a result of broadcasting. If this supposition has any validity, then it follows that standards for health protection are also likely to be biased due to the lack of such data.

Impressions as to Balance Between Exposures of Phone Users and Exposures in the Vicinity of Broadcast Facilities

The bulk of the material I have seen concerning dose estimation and health risks from microwave communication deals with the handheld phone, recognized to be both a receiver and broadcasting unit. In this case, the person exposed is the one who is directly involved in potential benefit. By contrast, persons living near a broadcasting facility may not be users, and will want to know that their exposures are without appreciable risk. Their exposures are more likely to involve the whole body rather than hands, head, and neck.

Unfortunately, there are no clear interpretations of possible risks associated with broadcasting. Standard forms of broadcasting, usually done in sparsely settled areas, are not associated with any clear exposure limitations for adjacent populations. In my review (Goldsmith, 1995), I mention two reports by a State Health Officer concerning possible, broadcast-related increases in leukemia for children and adults. While these results are of borderline significance, neither was a full-fledged epidemiological study committed to be undertaken.

We must conclude that, even though a smaller number of persons may be exposed to broadcast microwaves than to phone associated microwaves, the levels of exposure are likely to be more varied and some among those will have relatively heavy exposures. Certainly the conclusion must be drawn that collaborative studies of possible health risks from exposure to broadcast microwaves should be undertaken.

Some Interval Suggestions for Broadcast Facilities

Some interval suggestions may be made. A distance criterion from active RF broadcasting sources could be adopted by consensus prior to demonstration of possible risk. Say, for example, that no broadcast facility will emit more than (x, a number to be specified) watts of power closer to a dwelling than 30 meters, or closer to a school or health facility than 60 meters, and that such facilities within twice these distances will be monitored to assure that the exposure levels are sufficiently low. Possibly, for any proposed location, a standardized comparison of exposures and populations will be done for at least two alternative sites. One can also conceive of a minimal exposure configuration, in which the broadcast source is as though from a tethered balloon at, say, 250 meters above the highest point in the broadcast area. This configuration would assure both a high ratio of ground level reception and local protection. Then, any alternate configuration can be evaluated as the minimal exposure above that Level.

Summary

In summary, there is credible evidence of the following types of effects in radar (microwave) exposures under occupational, military, or broadcasting circumstances:

1.   Blood count changes

242

2.   Evidence of somatic mutation
3.   Increased spontaneous abortion (Ouellet-Hellstrom & Stewart, 1993)
4.   Increase in cancer incidence, especially hematopoietic, brain, breast, and testes
5.   Increase in disability of more exposed veterans from major causes after two decades

All but the last effect are found in multiple independent reports. Although exposure levels are not easy to interpret, there is reason to believe that effects can be found at or below average exposures of 100 microwatts/cm^2.

References

Akiyama, M., Umeki, S., Kusunoki, Y., Kyoizumi, S., Nakamura, N., Mori, T., Ishikawa, Y., Yamakido, M., Ohama, K., & Kodama, T. (1995). Somatic cell mutation as a possible predictor of cancer. Health Physics, 68, 643-649.

Bullman, T. A., Watanabe, K. K., & Kang, H. K. (1994). Risk of testicular cancer associated with surrogate measures of Agent Orange exposure among Vietnam veterans on the Agent Orange registry. Annals of Epidemiology, 4, 11-16.

Davis, R. L., & Mostofi, F. K. (1993). Cluster of testicular cancer in police officers exposed to hand-held radar. American Journal of Industrial Medicine, 24(2), 231-233.

DeGuire, L., Theriault, G., Iturra, H., Provencher, S., Cyr, D., & Case, B. W. (1988). Increased incidence of malignant melanoma of the skin in workers in a telecommunications industry. British Journal of Industrial Medicine, 45(12), 824-828.

Dolk, H., Elliott, P., Shaddick, G., Walls, P., & Thakrar, B. (1997). Cancer incidence near radio and television transmitters in Great Britain: II. All high power transmitters. American Journal of Epidemiology, 145(1), 10-17.

Dolk, H., Shaddick, G., Walls, P., Grundy, C., Thakrar, B., Kleinschmidt, I., & Elliott, P. (1997). Cancer incidence near radio and television transmitters in Great Britain: I. Sutton coldfield transmitter. American Journal of Epidemiology, 145(1), 1-9.

Garaj-Vrhovac, V., Fucic, A., & Horvat, D. (1992). The correlation between the frequency of micronuclei and specific chromosome aberrations in human lymphocytes exposed to microwaves. Mutation Research, 281, 181-186.

Garaj-Vrhovac, V., Fucic, A., & Pevelak-Kozlina, B. (1993). The rate of elimination of chromosomal aberrations after accidental exposures to microwaves. Bioelectricity and Bioenergetics, 30, 319-325.

Garaj-Vrhovac, V., Horvat, D., & Koren, Z. (1990). The effect of microwave radiation on the cell genome. Mutation Research, 243(1), 87-93.

Garaj-Vrhovac, V., Horvat, D., & Koren, Z. (1991). The relationship between colony-forming ability, chromosome aberrations and incidence of micronuclei in V79 Chinese hamster cells exposed to microwave radiation. Mutation Research, 263(1), 143-149.

Goldoni, J. (1990). Hematological changes in peripheral blood of workers occupationally exposed to microwave radiation. Health Physics, 58(2), 205-207.

Goldsmith, J. R. (1991). Incorporation of epidemiological findings into radiation protection standards. Public Health Reviews, 19, 19-34.

Goldsmith, J. R. (1992). Nuclear installations and childhood cancer in the UK: Mortality and incidence for 0-9-year-old children, 1971-1980. Science of the Total Environment, 127, 13-35.

Goldsmith, J. R. (1995). Epidemiologic evidence of radiofrequency radiation (microwave) effects on health in military, broadcasting, and occupational studies. International Journal of Occupational and Environmental Health, 1(1), 47-57.

Goldsmith, J. R. (1997). TV broadcast towers and cancer: The end of innocence for radiofrequency exposures. American Journal of Industrial Medicine, 32, 689-692.

Hagmar, L., Brugger, A., Hansteen, I. L., Heims, & Hogstedt, B. (1994). Cancer risk in humans predicted by chromosomal aberrations in lymphocytes. Cancer Research, 54, 2919-2922.

Hayes, R. B., Brown, L. M., Pottern, L. M., Gomez, M., Kardaun, J. W., Hoover, R. N., O'Connell, K. J., Sutzman, R. E., & Javadpour, N. (1990). Occupation and risk for testicular cancer: A case-control study. International Journal of Epidemiology, 19, 825-831.

Leonard, A., Berteaud, A. J., & Bruyere, A. (1983). An evaluation of the mutagenic, carcinogenic and teratogenic potential of microwaves. Mutation Research, 123(1), 31-46.

Lilienfeld, A. M., Tonascia, J., Tonascia, S., Libauer, C. H., Cauthen, G. M., Markowitz, J. A., & Weida, S. (1978). Evaluation of health status of foreign service and other employees from selected Eastern European posts. Baltimore, MD: The Johns Hopkins University and Washington, DC: Department of State, Office of Medical Services. (NTIS No. PB-288-163)

Muhm, J. M. (1992). Mortality investigation of workers in an electromagnetic pulse test program. Journal of Occupational Medicine, 34(3), 287-292.

Ouellet-Hellstrom R., & Stewart W. F. (1993). Miscarriages among female physiotherapists who report using radio- and micro-wave frequency electromagnetic radiation. American Journal of Epidemiology, 138, 775-786.

Robinette, C. D., Silverman, C., & Jablon, S. (1980). Effects upon health of occupational exposure to microwave radiation (radar). American Journal of Epidemiology, 111(1), 39-53.

Silverman, C. (1979). Epidemiologic approach to the study of microwave effects. Bulletin of the New York Academy of Medicine, 55, 1178.

Steneck, N. H., Cook, H. J., Vander, A. J., & Kane, G. L. (1980). The origins of U.S. safety standards for microwave radiation. Science, 208(4449), 1230-1237.

Vagero, D., Ahlbom, A., Olin, R., & Sahlsten, S. (1985). Cancer morbidity among workers in the telecommunications industry. British Journal of Industrial Medicine, 42(3), 191-195.

244

Vecchia, P. (1995, January). Epidemiological studies on long term effects of radiofrequency and microwave electromagnetic fields. In Proceedings of the Commsphere 95 International Symposium on Future Telecommunication and the Electromagnetic Environment, Eilat, Israel, January 22-26, 1995 (pp. 138-145).

Volkers, N. (1992). Speed kills—but what about radar guns? Journal of the National Cancer Institute, 84(17), 1310-1311.

Zhang, Z.-F., Vena, J. E., Zielezny, M., Graham, S., Haughey, B. P., Brasure, J., & Marshall, J. R. (1995). Occupational exposure to extreme temperature and risk of testicular cancer. Archives of Environmental Health, 50(1), 13-18.

Effects on Health of Naval Personnel Exposed to Microwave Radiation (Radar) in 1950-1954, the Korean War

Based on data found in:

Robinette, C. D., Silverman C., & Jablon, S. (1980). Effects upon health of occupational exposure to microwave radiation (radar). <u>American Journal of Epidemiology, 112,</u> 39-53.

The data set reported on here was compiled from official U.S. Governmental sources as described by Robinette et al. in the American Journal of Epidemiology.

The population at risk was derived in large part from the graduates of U.S. Navy Class A School for Technicians 1950-1954 who served on ships. They were divided into two major groups by exposure based on consensus of those who had made measurements according to whether they were maximally exposed, (the maximally exposed groups were mostly repairing radar equipment) or whether they were minimally exposed (mostly using radar equipment). Each of these groups was further divided into three occupational categories. The authors write "Because there were fewer men than estimated in one of the maximally exposed groups (fire control technicians who served on ships), aviation technicians were added to the study group. The vast majority of aviation technicians also graduated from Class A schools during the same period, but served at some time in airborne patrol squadrons."

The following numbers of persons were in these six occupational groups and the numbers of deaths are shown for the period of 1950-1974.

246

Table 1. Persons at risk by occupational categories and deaths, 1950-1974

	"Low Exposure"			"High Exposure"		
	Radiomen	Radarmen	Aviation Electrician's Mate	Electronics Technician	Fire Control Technician	Aviation Electronics Technician
	RM	RD	AE	ET	FT	AT
Number of persons	9,253	10,116	1,412	13,078	3,298	3,733
Deaths	296	308	61	441	144	198
From disease	161	165	22	199	81	77
From malignancy	39	47	8	65	16	27
Of lymphatic and hematopoietic system	6	14	0	18	1	10

Adapted from Robinette et al. (1980, Table 5)

	"Low Exposure"			"High Exposure"		
	Radiomen	Radarmen	Aviation Electrician's Mate	Electronics Technician	Fire Control Technician	Aviation Electronics Technician
	RM	RD	AE	ET	FT	AT
Number of men at risk	9,253	10,116	1,412	13,078	3,298	3,733
Rates, all deaths	32.0	30.4	43.2	33.7	43.7	53.0
All deaths from disease	17.4	16.3	15.6	15.2	24.6*	20.62*
From malignancy	4.21	4.65	5.66	4.97	4.85	7.23*
Of lymphatic and hematopoietic system	0.65	1.38	000	1.38	0.3	2.68*

* Indicates significantly increase (p < 0.05) compared to less exposed groups

Table 2. Crude Death Rates by Occupational Group (per 1000), (Robinette et al., 1980)

| | "Low Exposure" | | | "High Exposure" | | |
| | Radiomen | Radarmen | Aviation Electrician's Mate | Electronics Technician | Fire Control Technician | Aviation Electronics Technician |
	RM	RD	AE	ET	FT	AT
Mean	20.3	20.4	24.7	21.7	21.7	23.4
% over 26	1.9	3.6	31.3	8.0	14.6	18.8
Group mean	20.7			22.0		
% 26 +	4.9			11.3		

From Robinette et al. (1980, Table 4)

Table 3   Mean Age of the Occupational Groups Based on a 5% Sample and Percent Over 26 Years of Age in 1952

We use for statistical tests the comparison between observed and expected numbers, based on Poisson assumptions for expected numbers.

As can be seen from Table 3 , the mean age of the air squadron personnel is older and the % over 26 years of age is also greater in 1952. This may very well have an affect on subsequent mortality from disease.

In fact, the oldest occupational group has the second lowest disease mortality 15.7/1000, whereas the two highest exposed occupational groups have the highest mortality from disease, a significant increase, as well. The occupational category with the presumed highest exposure, the Aviation Electronics Technicians have significantly elevated mortality from malignant disease, most of which is contributed to by hematological and lymphatic malignancies. This can hardly be attributed to age, since the older age group of Aviation Electronics Mate doesn't show such an increase.

Nevertheless it is desirable to compare the data after age-adjustment. However the authors combine, with no reason given, the two groups, Aviation Electronic Technicians and Fire Control Technicians. Each group includes about 3200 men, but the former group had 10 and the latter group 1 death from Lympho-hematopoietic malignancy, this combination leads to a combined age-adjusted ratio which is not significantly elevated, whereas if the Aviation Electronic Technicians data had been separately age-adjusted, it almost certainly would have been statistically significant.

The article presents data for a potential exposure index based on examination of individual work records, only based on the high exposed groups; the data were obtained only for men in these groups who died and for a 5% sample of the living. It is expressed as "Hazard Number", and reflects only the cumulative potential by type of ship and duration of assignments. Table 4 shows the data.

Hazard Number	Electronics Technician	Fire Control Technician	Aviation Electronics Technician
	ET	FT	AT
0	28.0	6.6	13.0
1-2,000	28.4	23.8	16.9
2,001-5,000	19.9	30.9	18.0
5000+	10.8	26.6	48.3
Unknown	12.9	12.1	3.8
MEAN*	1,870	3,317	3,843

* Based on the assumption that the means hazard number by class was 1000, 3500 and 6000, respectively for 1-2,000; 2001-5000; and 5000+.

Table 4. Distribution in percent of the "hazard number" for the three presumably high exxposure groups, based on a sample of naval personnel. The mean values are baed on assumptions given in the above note. (Robinette et al., 1980)

The authors present data for the two most exposed occupational categories combined when they analyze the possible contribution of exposure to likelihood of having disability compensation. Here again, they make the comparisons in an unexpected way, listing both the data for all three "low exposure" job groups and the Electronic Technician group of the "high exposure" set. In Table 5 we conduct the analysis in the most natural way, combining the two most highly exposed occupational groups and comparing them with all the four other groups.

As the Table shows, this most plausible comparison will show that the more exposed men had significantly more disability in the Musculoskeletal, Respiratory, and Cardiovascular groups, and that overall about 100 more men were disabled than would have been expected if the rates for the less exposed men had applied. There were 26.4% men in the two high exposed occupations with disability compensation than would have been expected on the basis of the four lesser exposed groups.

Data are also presented for hospitalizations, which are consistent with men having higher exposure being hospitalized more for hematological problems.

Diagnostic Group	FT + AT Number	FT + AT Rate/1000	All Others Number	All Others Rate/1000	FT + AT Expected Number
Musculoskeletal	119*	16.9	403	11.9	83.7
Special Sense Organs	42	6.0	152	4.49	31.6
Systematic Conditions	5*	0.7	7	0.204	1.45
Respiratory	51*	7.3	171	5.05	35.5
Cardiovascular	47*	6.7	142	4.19	29.5
Digestive	55	7.8	229	6.76	47.6
Genitourinary	19	2.7	99	2.92	20.6
Hemic, Lymphatic	3	0.4	10	0.3	2.08
Skin	58	8.2	227	6.70	47.1

Based on Table 12 of Robinette et al. (1980)

* Significantly increased $p < 0.05$; ** Significantly increased $p < 0.01$

Table 5 (continued on next page). Number of Men Receiving Veterans Administration Compensation in 1976 by Diagnosis Group and for Two High Exposure Groups (FT + AT) Relative to the Remaining (Low Exposure) Groups

Diagnostic Group	FT + AT		All Others		FT + AT Expected Number
	Number	Rate/1000	Number	Rate/1000	
Endocrine	11	1.6	46	1.36	9.55
Neurological	16	2.3	54	1.60	11.2
Nerves	3	0.4	41	1.21	8.5
Epilepsy	00		16	0.47	3.32
Mental conditions	46	6.5	198	5.85	41.1
Other	2	0.3	19	0.56	3.95
TOTAL	477**	67.84		53.61	376.94
POPULATIONS	7,031		33,859		

Based on Table 12 of Robinette et al. (1980)

* Significantly increased p < 0.05; ** Significantly increased p < 0.01

Table 5 (continued from previous page). Number of Men Receiving Veterans Administration Compensation in 1976 by Diagnosis Group and for Two High Exposure Groups (FT + AT) Relative to the Remaining (Low Exposure) Groups

Interpretations

The job category most likely to be heavily exposed, compared to other job categories combined, had significantly more deaths from disease, significantly more deaths from cancer, and significantly more deaths from cancer of the lymphatic and hematopoietic system. The two most heavily exposed job categories had significantly more disability from musculoskeletal, cardiac and respiratory conditions, and highly significantly more disabilities overall.

These epidemiological findings do not <u>prove</u> that radar exposure was responsible for the associations. The findings are suggestive of and consistent with such a set of relationships. To state as the abstract does that "No adverse effects were detected in these indices that could be attributed to potential microwave radiation exposure in 1950-1954" is misleading.

In fact, Dr. Silverman, the second author, gives a much more reasonable interpretation in her report to the New York Academy of Medicine: "While some significant differences among the occupational groups classified by level of potential exposure have been found with respect to all the end-points studies, the difference could not be interpreted as a direct result of microwave exposure." (Bull. N.Y.Acad. Med. <u>55</u>, 1178, 1979) No epidemiologist is likely to affirm that the statistical findings are the <u>direct</u> result of the associated exposures, particularly when the exposures are only potential ones.

Statistical Note

The data in this set (and in a number of other sets), represent the occurrence of relatively rare events among a large population at risk. For example all of the populations are greater than 1000, and risks of cancer less than one in a thousand, even for these long-term follow-ups. These are conditions which are suitable for analysis based on <u>Poisson</u> distributional assumptions.

A convenient feature of using the Poisson assumptions is that the observed mean (or observed value) is numerically equivalent to the variance, or the square of the standard deviation. It follows that for every pair of observed and expected values, say of the frequency of cancer, one can easily evaluate whether the observed value is within 1.96 standard deviations of the expected value. If it is not, then the probability that it could deviate that much or more as a result of random variation is less than 5 %, the usual criterion for statistical significance.

To illustrate from the data in Table 1, we note 10 cases of lympho-hematopoietic cancer among the 3,733 men who were Aviation Electricians' Mates (AE), and 29 such cases among the other 37,157 men. In order to calculate the number expected among AE if the experience of the other men was occurring, we divide 29 by 37,157 and multiply the rate by 3,733 This gives an expected number of 2.91. (The variance of the expected number). The standard deviation is the square root , 1.707, and the 5% cutoff point in its distribution is 1.96 x 1.707 + 2.91, which equals 6.26, much less than 10. In fact the difference between observed and expected is 7.09, more than 4 times the standard deviation, with a probability of being due to random variation of < 0.0001.

When the two most exposed groups are combined, there are 11 cases observed among 7023 men and 28 cases among the remaining 33,859, the number of expected increases to 5.808, 5.192 less than the 11 observed. The standard deviation is 2.41, and the 5% confidence limit is at 10.53, which is a barely significant result at $p = 0.05$. When the result is age adjusted the apparent consequence is to lead to a non-significant difference.

Note on Epidemiological Interpretations

A statistically significant association may or may not indicate a causal relationship In general the epidemiologist with only a single study to report is not able to say that the effect(s) observed are causally related, due to, or a result of, the exposure under study. Other variables, which affect both exposure and effect are the source of the most common reservation.

So for virtually any epidemiological study, regardless of the strength of the association, one could say: "It is not possible on the basis of the research to prove that the exposures led to these results." But such remarks are disingenuous, and may be misleading, if there are strong associations and substantial effort has been made to avoid them being due to other variables. The use of words like "direct" or "Proof" may be a way of qualifying an apparent positive result.

Thus a truly negative outcome of an epidemiological study is likely to be summarized as: "The study showed no evidence of association between the exposure and the health outcome studied."

A suggestive study may be summarized as "The study showed evidence of statistically significant associations, but this does not prove that the exposure was the cause of the health outcomes studied."

An apparently positive study may be summarized "The study shows evidence of a positive association, and the most likely alternative mechanisms having been examined and rejected, the results are consistent with a causative relationship of exposure and the effect studied."

19
THE EPIDEMIOLOGY OF SMALL EFFECTS

Ernst L. Wynder and Joshua Muscat

Abstract

Epidemiology faces significant challenges when dealing with suspected risk factors whose effect is likely to be small. In such cases it is particularly important that epidemiologists carefully consider problems that may be associated with case-control selection, biases, confounders, subgroup analysis, and interactions. As we examine, for instance, the possible effect of cellular telephones on brain cancer general symptomology that may be claimed to be associated with such use, it is vital that all of the problem areas are carefully considered before drawing a conclusion as to causation. However, if these various problematic areas have been carefully considered and to the extent possible, if they have been avoided, then a conclusion as to causation can be made, particularly if they meet the criteria in respect to judgment as well delineated by Bradford Hill. When dealing with weak associations and proper conclusions, the science of epidemiology must be at its optimum.

With the epidemiology of sizable associations such as active smoking and lung cancer, excessive drinking and liver cirrhosis, and severe sunburn and melanoma well-established, what remains generally for the epidemiologist to research involves weak associations with odds ratios of less than two, which, if real, can nevertheless be of public health importance, but often lead to erroneous conclusions as to causality as recently emphasized in an article in *Science* (Taubes, 1995). In fact, the *Science* article quotes some distinguished epidemiologists who say that a relative risk of less than 3 or even 4 might have little etiological significance. We disagree with such conclusions although clearly the lower the relative risk, the more likely errors in study design or conduct could have led to a faulty or misleading outcome. If we examine a report, either as a reviewer or as a reader of a published study, we should consider using a checklist to judge the adequacy of a study and its conclusion (Table 1). Although such a list, at first glance, seems simplistic, it affords an orderly review of some of the most likely missteps an investigator could take that a less organized review may well overlook.

CHECKLIST FOR CRITERIA IN EPIDEMIOLOGIC STUDIES

Author, Title:_____

Year, Vol. No., Page No. _____

	CASES				CONTROLS		
	Yes	**No**	**DK** __N.A.__		**Yes**	**No**	**DK** __N.A.__

1. Case/Control Selection

Type of interview/place

In-person	☐	☐	☐		☐	☐	☐
Telephone	☐	☐	☐		☐	☐	☐
hospital	☐	☐	☐		☐	☐	☐
home	☐	☐	☐		☐	☐	☐

Surrogate

hospital	☐	☐	☐		☐	☐	☐
home	☐	☐	☐		☐	☐	☐

Type of surrogate defined

spouse	☐	☐	☐		☐	☐	☐
sibling	☐	☐	☐		☐	☐	☐
other	☐	☐	☐		☐	☐	☐
Not defined	☐				☐		

% eligible	☐	☐	☐		☐	☐	☐
% enrolled	☐	☐	☐		☐	☐	☐

	Yes	No	Don't Know N.A.
2. Sampling Methodology Defined			
in-person	☐	☐	☐
telephone	☐	☐	☐
mail	☐	☐	☐
3. Confounders adjusted			
Education	☐	☐	☐
Race	☐	☐	☐
Lifestyle habits			
Tobacco	☐	☐	☐
Amount of smoking	☐	☐	☐
Alcohol	☐	☐	☐
Amount of alcohol	☐	☐	☐
Quetelet index	☐	☐	☐
Proxy	☐	☐	☐
4. Causation Criteria Considered			
Strength of the association	☐	☐	☐
Internal consistency (subgroup analysis)	☐	☐	☐
Dose-response	☐	☐	☐
Biological plausibility	☐	☐	☐
Temporality	☐	☐	☐

Table 1. Checklist for criteria in epidemiologic studies

Case-control Selection

Not infrequently we see a mismatch, such as when information on cases is obtained from surrogates while controls are interviewed in person, or when cases may be interviewed in person while a control is interviewed by telephone. Often the nature of the relationship with a surrogate is not given, nor is the percentage of refusals of either cases or controls stated. Does one compare a hospital case against a population control? In terms of cohort studies, how representative are the subjects of the general population? These are just some of the points that we can check against our list. In our own studies we have mostly relied on hospital-based cases and controls because of similar environment and attitudes towards the interviewer.

Confounding

Significant problems may arise if confounding is not properly considered, or if in fact confounding data are not available. Cigarette smoking, for example, is a powerful confounder with respect to many variables (Berger & Wynder, 1994; Figure 1). It is negatively correlated with age and education, which in themselves may have an impact on disease etiology. It is highly correlated with consumption of alcohol and coffee, and negatively associated with fruits and vegetables, while positively related to meat consumption. These interactions are important to consider since diet does have its own impact on several types of cancer and cardiovascular disease. Diet in turn is highly correlated with occupation, so that if we study the impact of diesel exhaust on long-distance truck drivers with lung cancer and we have no reliable study on smoking, no conclusions can be drawn as to an independent effect of diesel exhaust (Boffetta, Harris, & Wynder, 1990). Figures 2 and 3 show excessive cigarette smoking and a high-fat diet among long-distance truck drivers, both variables which, in the case of smoking strongly and in the case of diet moderately, affect lung cancer etiology (Heber et al., 1992). Since smoking especially today is so strongly tied to education and education in turn is related to other variables such as diet, it behooves investigators to correctly adjust for direct and indirect confounders as they contemplate causation. Here we would suggest stratifying each variable one at a time rather than carrying out logistic regression analysis, which is so commonly used now. Such analysis, especially when a study is of limited size and when more than five variables are adjusted for simultaneously, can lead to misleading results.

Bias

A most subtle problem of a weak association is the reporting bias where a respondent may tend to underreport such factors as sexual exposure, fat intake, cigarette and alcohol consumption, and exposure to sunlight. In terms of nutrition, underreporting may occur when using a food frequency questionnaire or even dietary records. Overreporting may occur as we want to put the problem on someone else such as exposure to an environmental factor for which we are not responsible. Bias it should

Partial Correlation Structure of the 1° Variables by Sex

Females

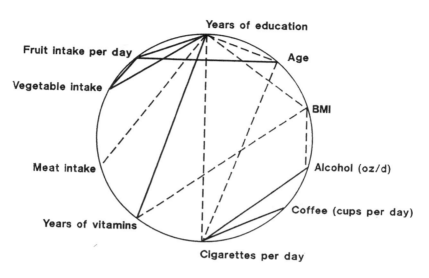

— Positive Correlation   — —· Negative Correlation

— Positive correlation; - - Negative correlation

Figure 1. Partial correlation structure of the 1° variables by sex: Females

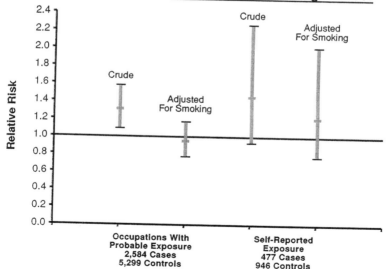

Source: Boffetta, Harris & Wynder, 1990

Figure 2. Diesel exhaust exposure and lung cancer

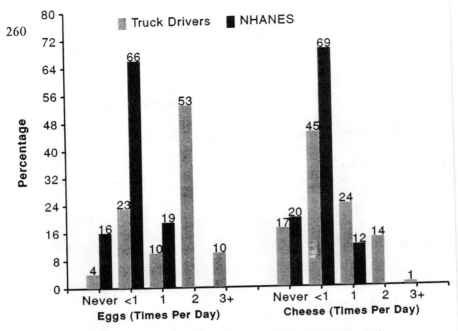

Source: Wynder & Miller, 1988 (Eggs); NCHS, 1979 (Cheese)
Figure 3. Dairy product consumption in long distance truck drivers and NHANES I study

be noted can affect cases and controls to differing degrees. In our ongoing Women's Intervention Nutrition Study, we increasingly observe an underreporting of dietary fat among our cases, no doubt, due to an increased public awareness relative to fat and breast cancer (Buzzard et al., 1996).

A new bias, which has received relatively little attention, is the negative placebo effect. If told by a physician, lawyer, media, or by completing an informed consent form that an exposure to a given factor such as breast implants, cellular telephones, electromagnetic fields, Alar on apples, or dioxin in soil may lead to an unspecific symptomology such as pain, irritability, headaches, insomnia, or joint aches, many of us experience such symptomology by a route from the mind to the body, the nature of which is not fully understood. Medical students will report headaches when told that an electric current has been passed through their brain when, in fact, this did not occur (Schweiger & Parducci, 1981; Figure 4). When told that eye drops will lead to eye irritation when only in fact distilled water is used, a significant percentage of individuals will report eye irritation, a percentage that is twice as high among type A compared with type B personalities (Drici, Raybaud, DeLunardo, Iacono, & Gustovic, 1995; Figure 5). The idea that personality type may relate to the negative placebo is of particular interest. Asthmatics have reported a worsening of symptomology when receiving a benign saline solution when told it would enhance their symptomology, but report an improvement when the same saline solution is given with the suggestion that it would be beneficial (Luparello, Lyons, Bleecker, & McFadden, 1968; Figure 6). Such negative placebo effects will have a particularly wide effect when given broad media publicity such as has been the case with Alar or breast implants and will be

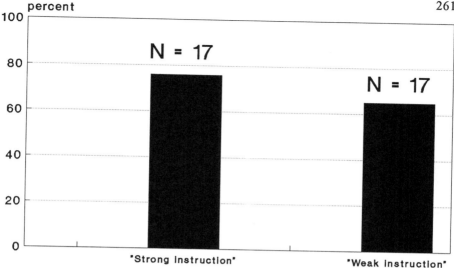

Strong: headache likely; Weak: unlikely
Source: Schweiger & Parducci, 1981
Figure 4. Incidence of reported headaches in subjects receiving nonexistent shock

further enhanced when "secondary gains" may be received in terms of monetary rewards. While in the case of cellular telephones and breast implants this would not apply to brain or breast cancer, there is a likelihood that symptomology such as headaches, dizziness, or joint pains can be a result of the negative placebo.

Subgroup Analysis

To the extent that some investigators search for a positive outcome, they may undertake many subgroup analyses and report only those that fit their theory. Such conduct is bad science both in statistical terms and to the extent that such subgroups may no longer match the initial matching procedure. Particularly troublesome is when the results of a subgroup analysis but not the confidence limits appear in the abstract of the paper.

American Health Foundation Study

A study we are currently conducting on cellular telephones and brain cancer is subject to the concerns discussed in this paper. In our American Health Foundation ongoing study, all cases and controls are interviewed in collaborating hospitals by trained interviewers to assure that the information obtained from cases and controls is obtained under comparable settings. Control subjects are age and sex-matched patients admitted for conditions not related to electromagnetic field exposure. Patients with leukemia

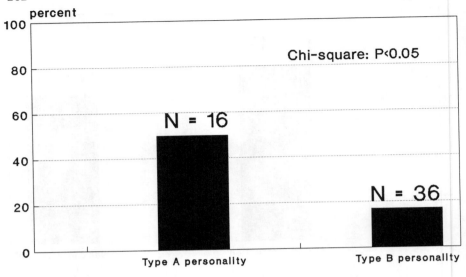

percent

Chi-square: P<0.05

N = 16

N = 36

Type A personality   Type B personality

Phase I study; other eye received drug
Source: Drici et al., 1995
Figure 5. Incidence of reported eye irritation in 52 subjects receiving eyedrop
placebo

and lymphoma are excluded. Tallies are kept of eligible patients who are approached
and interviewed, and if not interviewed, the reasons will be ascertained. Of course, the
type of person who uses a cellular phone may be expected to have a higher
socioeconomic status than the average hospital patient, although there is no data yet to
substantiate this. Detailed information is obtained on possible confounders such as
smoking, alcohol consumption, body weight, and other factors, although so little is
known of brain cancer etiology that it is currently not possible to identify important
cofactors.

The study was designed with the power to detect an odds ratio of two or more,
although with the rapid rate of increase in cellular telephone use since even the
beginning of the study a year ago, there should be greater statistical power. Here, if
there is a causal association, it would be detected by a strong dose-response trend.
Unlike many other lifestyle behaviors or dietary habits where there is often a
homogenous distribution in the population, there is a wide range of cellular phone use.
There are two types of phone users: the occasional user and the daily user. If a causal
association existed, the risk for heavy users would certainly be greater than those for
light users.

As yet, we do not know the magnitude, if any, of the association between cellular
phone use and brain cancer. If case-control studies were completed today, we would
likely find no measurable effect because the data from national cancer registries show
no changes in the incidence of brain cancer after these products were introduced in the
mid-1980s (Ries et al., 1994; Figure 7). Ongoing studies are needed because the
mechanisms by which radiofrequency (RF) fields could cause cancer are unknown.

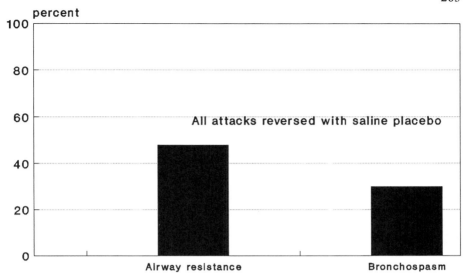

percent

Actual exposure: saline solution
Source: Luparello et al., 1968
Figure 6. Changes in airway reactivity in 40 asthmatics inhaling "allergens"

If RF fields initiate the cancer process in brain cells, the effects wold not be manifested until several decades later. The available in vitro and in vivo studies of RF fields indicate, however, that cellular telephones are not genotoxic although there are several postulated ways in which RF fields may be involved in cancer promotion (Verschaeve, 1995). In terms of epidemiology, it is important to determine the international correlation of cellular phone use and brain cancer rates as well as relative risk in other case-control and cohort studies. If a weak positive association is observed, it needs to be asked whether the observation is consistent for men and women and for all age groups, and if the effect is found in all histologic types. A negative answer does not necessarily rule out an association, but restraint in interpreting results must be taken when conducting subgroup analysis. On the other hand, a necessary condition for causality is a dose-response trend. Unlike other common epidemiologic risk factors that have little heterogeneity in the population, cellular phone usage certainly varies substantially between bankers and salesmen, and housewives and blue-collar occupations.

The biological plausibility of an association between cellular telephones and brain cancer has been addressed (Verschaeve, 1995). There is little evidence that RF fields from cellular phones are genotoxic, or even cause cellular stress from their thermal effects in cell tissues (Verschaeve, 1995). In the classic model of carcinogenesis, the possible effects of cellular phones would be "promotional," where RF fields could, for example, reduce immunocompetence. Epidemiologic studies need to consider whether the site of the tumor is adjacent to the side of the head where the phone is normally held. With respect to temporality, one must reflect on the natural history of tumor growth. Slow growing tumors may not be clinically manifest for months or possibly

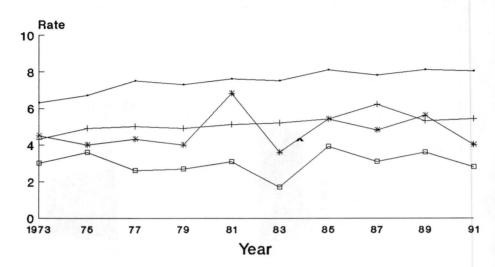

SEER: Age-adjusted, 1970 U.S. population
Figure 7. Incidence of brain cancer in the US per 100,000; 1973-1991

years, and the effects of recent phone usage need to be considered with caution.

Checklist

As mentioned previously, we have recently developed a "checklist" for epidemiologists and journal reviewers for the purpose of determining whether studies conform to generally accepted epidemiologic practices. On the surface, this list appears simplistic in that it cannot account for the individual and unique aspects of a study. However, if one reviews the epidemiologic literature, it can be seen that many reported epidemiologic studies do not conform to good epidemiologic principles. This may occur because researchers and reviewers are lax in their standards, because studies are performed by investigators not formally trained in the discipline, or because an investigator desires to support a preconceived or cherished hypothesis. The checklist provides a simple way of ascertaining that at least the basic features of the study design and the interpretation of results are described in a meaningful way. Although studies that report strong associations between an exposure and a disease outcome (e.g., smoking and lung cancer) may not require close scrutiny, the use of this checklist would be helpful when the magnitude of the effect is weak. The checklist is not to be scored, but as shortcomings are noted, they should caution both the investigator and the reviewer to be cautious while interpreting the data.

Contemplation

In reviewing the evidence as to whether an association is real or artefactual, positive or negative, we need to consider the criteria of judgment first suggested by Bradford Hill, which were properly used in the first Surgeon General Report on Smoking and Health in 1964 when the committee delineated this issue even though the odds ratio was very high, but which are not often considered today when investigators report small effects (Hill, 1965; U.S. Department of Health, Education, and Welfare, 1964). Such omission does injustice to the science of epidemiology, which we must regard as an art as well as a science. As part of these criteria, we must give special attention to biological plausibility. What is the exposure in terms of dose? Does this dose suffice to cause cellular damage and overcome the natural anatomical and physiologic defenses? It is here that laboratory scientists should work in close contact with epidemiologists. It is here that global epidemiology should come into play. Regarding cellular telephones, for example, is there a correlation between brain cancer and the per capita use of such telephones in a country? Causation requires a fit for all of these criteria. With good science and cautious interpretation, we can, in fact, even in the case of small effects, determine whether an association is real or artefactual. With proper experience in the conduct of an epidemiological study, avoiding bias including one's own, and after carefully considering the many pitfalls of our own studies in design and conduct, the science of epidemiology can and will make important contributions to the etiology of disease.

References

Berger, J., & Wynder, E. L. (1994). The correlation of epidemiological variables. Journal of Clinical Epidemiology, 47, 941-952.

Boffetta, P., Harris, R. E., & Wynder, E. L. (1990). Case-control study on occupational exposure to diesel exhaust and lung cancer risk. American Journal of Industrial Medicine, 17, 577-591.

Buzzard, M., Faucett, C. L., Jeffrey, R. W., McBane, L., McGovern, P., & Baxter, J. S. (1996). Monitoring dietary change in a low fat diet intervention study: Advantages of using 24-hour dietary recalls versus food records. Journal of the American Dietetic Association, 96(6), 574-579.

Drici, M.-D., Raybaud, F., DeLunardo, C., Iacono, P., & Gustovic, P. (1995). Influence of the behavior pattern on the nocebo response of healthy volunteers. British Journal of Clinical Pharmacology, 39, 204-206.

Heber, D., Ashley, J. M., McCarthy, W. J., Solares, M. E., Leaf, D. A., & Chang, L. J. (1992). Assessment of adherence to a low-fat diet for breast cancer prevention. Preventative Medicine, 21, 218-227.

Hill, A. B. (1965). The environment and disease: Association or causation? Proceedings of the Royal Society of Medicine, 58, 295-300.

266

Luparello, T., Lyons, H. A., Bleecker, E. R., & McFadden, Jr., E. R. (1968). Influences of suggestion on airway reactivity in asthmatic subjects. Psychosomatic Medicine, 30(6), 819-825.

National Center for Health Statistics. (1979). National Health and Nutrition Survey: Food consumption profiles of white and black persons aged 1-74 years, US 1971-1974 (PHS Publication 79-1685). Washington, DC: U.S. Department of Health, Education, and Welfare.

Ries, L. A. G., Miller, B. A., Hankey, B. F., Kosary, C. L., Harras, A., & Adwards, B. K. (Eds.). (1994). SEER cancer statistics review, 1973-1991: Tables and graphs (NIH Publication No. 94-2789). Bethesda, MD: National Cancer Institute.

Schweiger, A., & Parducci, A. (1981). Nocebo: The psychologic induction of pain. Pavlovian Journal of Biological Science, 16, 140-144.

Taubes, G. (1995). Epidemiology faces its limits. Science, 269, 164-169.

U.S. Department of Health, Education, and Welfare. (1964). Smoking and health: Report of the advisory committee to the Surgeon General of the Public Health Service (PHS Publication 1103). Washington, DC: U.S. Department of Health, Education, and Welfare, Public Health Service.

Verschaeve, L. (1995). Can non-ionizing radiation induce cancer? Cancer Journal, 8, 237-249.

Wynder, E. L., & Miller, S. (1988). Letter. Cancer Research, 48, 1989-1990.

V

NON-BIOLOGICAL HEALTH RISKS FROM RADIO FREQUENCY RADIATION: INTERFERENCE WITH MEDICAL DEVICES

Editor's Note:

Comprehensive surveillance for effects from radio frequency radiation has included the search for impacts that are not directly biological. Interference between wireless phones and hospital equipment is addressed in the comprehensive papers by Drs. Joyner and Segal.

Laboratory studies that have elucidated interference between wireless phones and both implanted cardiac pacemakers and cardiac defibrillators are reviewed in the papers by Dr. Barbaro and colleagues, and Dr. Silny. Drs. Hayes and Carrillo present clinical observations of the same phenomena with public health intervention solutions to those problems.

It is important to note that the collective experience gleaned from the phone-pacemaker interference problem is reassuring for government, industry, and consumers. The surveillance approach to assessing and correcting problems from wireless communication technology being employed worldwide works for the betterment of public health. The interference problem with pacemakers was first suggested in June 1994. In September 1997, following comprehensive in vitro and clinical research conducted throughout the world, recommendations for solving the problem were put forth and implemented in both the wireless industry and the pacemaker industry. This experience argues strongly in favor of propagating the same type of approach for bioeffects surveillance.

G. L. C.

20

STATE OF THE SCIENCE IN WIRELESS INSTRUMENT MEDICAL EQUIPMENT INTERFERENCE

Kenneth H. Joyner

Introduction

With the ever increasing use of the electromagnetic spectrum and the proliferation of electronic devices, including mobile communications devices, it is not surprising that issues of electromagnetic interference (EMI) have gained such prominence. However, EMI is not a new phenomenon associated only with the introduction of mobile communication services. Indeed, Maxwell referred to the phenomenon in 1873 in a discussion about the arrangement of current flows to avoid an "electromagnetic effect."

The effects of EMI on medical electrical equipment are of concern because of the potential to interfere with the safe operation of life-support and other critical care equipment. Numerous incidents involving EMI in medical electrical equipment have been reported to the U.S. Food and Drug Administration (FDA) and these have been summarized and published (Silberberg, 1993). Sources of the interference included communications transmissions, electrosurgical devices, other electrical and electronic equipment, electrical disturbances on the main power distribution systems, and electrostatic discharge. Silberberg reports that many of these incidents had or could have had life threatening consequences. However, mobile communications are seen as an essential adjunct to patient care. The Australian and New Zealand Intensive Care Society supports the continued use of mobile telephones in hospitals especially for doctors treating critically ill patients.

The EMI problem with medical electrical equipment has several aspects. First, much of the equipment in use in hospitals and the home is particularly susceptible to EMI. Secondly, with the explosion in the number of mobile communications devices, there are numerous situations where medical electrical equipment may be exposed to relatively high electromagnetic fields.

Although the introduction of mobile communications services has highlighted the EMI issue, it is certainly not specific to intentional radiators such as wireless or radio communications devices. EMI to medical electrical equipment can be manifested from a number of other sources:

- Unintentional radiators such as computers and other digital electronic equipment which produce spurious electromagnetic emissions. Also included in this category are shortwave and microwave diathermy devices and electrosurgical units. Although these latter devices use electromagnetic energy they may be classed as unintentional radiators because their emissions cannot be fully contained to the treatment area on the patient and subsequently illuminate other medical electrical equipment.

- Any main-powered electrical equipment may generate electrical transients on the 50/60 Hz main power distribution system which may, in turn, cause interference with other medical electrical equipment which is not isolated from that power supply system.

- Electrostatic discharge occurs when equipment and personnel at different potentials come into contact, causing a current to flow and possibly an electrical disturbance in the operation of the medical electrical equipment.

Results of EMI Testing

At the present time, there have been few comprehensive scientific reports on the electromagnetic compatibility of electrical medical equipment and mobile telephones, although a number of preliminary studies have been reported. A number of research efforts have been initiated, including a program at the Center for the Study of Wireless Electromagnetic Compatibility of the University of Oklahoma, and the results of these studies should add greatly to our understanding and strategies for addressing the issues. I shall therefore concentrate on presenting the summary results of the EMI testing performed in Australia on medical electrical equipment. I will also present our results on the EMI testing of hearing aids and a very brief mention of our work on implanted cardiac pacemakers. The following invited paper by Dr. David Hayes concerning the EMI of implanted cardiac pacemakers and defibrillators will address this subject in much more detail.

There are two mobile telephone systems in use in Australia. The Advanced Mobile Phone System (AMPS) is an analogue system employing frequency modulation of the carrier signal. The AMPS mobile telephones transmit between 825 and 845 MHz, with a maximum transmit power of 0.6 W for the hand-held unit, and up to 3 W for the transportable units.

The other mobile telephone system is the Global System for Mobile Communications (GSM) digital system. The GSM mobile telephones transmit between 890 and 915 MHz. The transmission is pulsed with a repetition frequency of approximately 217 Hz and a pulse width of approximately 0.6 ms. There are several other transmission modes from the GSM mobile telephones; a burst of pulses at a rate of approximately 2 Hz, known as the DTX mode, and a single transmission approximately every 8 Hz for internal control purposes. The DTX mode is a discontinuous transmission mode designed primarily to extend battery life by only transmitting during a portion of the available time slots when the GSM user is only listening to the incoming call. The maximum transmit power for the hand-held unit is 2 W peak (0.25 W average) and 8 W peak (1 W average) for the transportable unit.

Comparative typical field strengths for a 0.6 W AMPS, a 2 W GSM, and an 8 W GSM mobile telephone are given in Table 1. Note that these field strengths vary with antenna type and between different manufacturers, and may also be altered by the presence of radiofrequency (RF) wave reflections from nearby objects.

Distance (m)	Field Strengths (V/m)		
	0.6 W AMPS	2 W GSM	8 W GSM
0.1	27.0	42.0	80.0
0.2	13.5	28.0	53.0
0.3	9.2	20.0	40.0
0.4	6.9	15.0	30.0
0.5	5.1	12.0	24.0
1.0	4.2	6.0	12.0
1.5	-	4.0	8.0
2.0	1.4	3.0	6.0
2.5	-	2.4	4.8
3.0	1.0	2.0	4.0
3.5	-	1.7	3.4
4.0	0.89	1.5	3.0
4.5	-	1.3	2.7
5.0	0.62	1.2	2.4

Table 1. Field Strength Measurements—AMPS and GSM Mobile Telephones

Medical Equipment Testing

In the original series of measurements, three types of mobile telephones were placed near various pieces of medical electrical equipment in order to detect any abnormal behavior due to EMI (Clifford et al., 1994). When abnormal behavior was observed, the symptoms were recorded and the telephone moved away until normal operation of the equipment resumed. The three types of mobile telephone equipment were a 0.6 W

AMPS hand-held, a 2 W GSM hand-held, and an 8 W GSM transportable mobile telephone.

Fifteen pieces of medical electrical equipment were selected, including two patient monitors, six drug infusion pumps, a defibrillator/monitor, a cardiac monitor, a pulse oximeter, an oxygen monitor, a blood pressure monitor, a fetal monitor with telemetry, and an ECG telemetry transmitter. The units chosen were not necessarily the latest available models.

The AMPS mobile telephone affected only three pieces of equipment; the ECG trace was distorted on one of the patient monitors and two of the drug infusion pumps initiated false alarms, though one of these pumps gave false alarms only when the antenna of the telephone was within 50 mm of the case of the pump. When the same pieces of equipment were tested with the GSM mobile telephones, seven of them operated normally. The other eight displayed the following symptoms: distortion or loss of ECG traces, false alarms and halting/change of speed of infusion pumps, and the introduction of severe distortion into the telemetry systems, including a 217 Hz audible interference tone on one unit. Use of the higher power GSM mobile telephone did not change the symptoms, except in one case when an alarm was triggered in addition to the other symptoms. Changing from the 2 W to the 8 W unit generally doubled the distance within which interference effects were observed.

Three of the drug infusion pumps were not affected at all and, at distances greater than 200 mm, the other three were free from interference even from the 8 W GSM mobile telephone. Within the critical distances, the three pumps displayed various error messages; two of them then ceased to operate and one continued to operate, but at two-thirds of its selected rate.

The ECG display in the defibrillator/monitor was free of interference, but the three other units with ECG monitors displayed a variety of symptoms, including blanking of one CRT unit and/or horizontal lines, and high levels of noise on the ECG trace which initiated alarms in two of the units. In one of the units, the distortion persisted at distances up to 1 m for the 2 W and 2 m with the 8 W GSM mobile telephone.

The pulse oximeter unit in one of the patient monitors showed a low signal at distances up to 2 m from the 8 W GSM mobile telephone.

Both telemetry systems were affected by the GSM mobile telephones, producing interference and large excursions of the trace. One unit had a 217 Hz interference which was audible. No interference was observed when the telephones were more than 2 m from both the transmitters and receivers of the telemetry systems.

All of the medical electrical equipment tested was immune to EMI at field strengths from the mobile telephones of around 7 V/m. This immunity level was recommended in a 1979 US FDA voluntary electromagnetic compatibility standard. The reader is referred to the section on EMI Standards.

The results of this study and those from another major Australian hospital which showed infant incubators exhibiting adverse effects from EMI at field strengths as low as 1 V/m prompted the Australian Therapeutic Goods Administration (part of the Commonwealth Department of Human Services and Health in Australia) to issue the statement below regarding EMI into medical electrical equipment.

Mobile Telephone Interference with Devices

Various Australian hospitals have or are about to introduce restrictions on the use of mobile telephones and radio transceivers because these devices may cause electrical interference with medical electrical equipment. Although no incidents have yet been confirmed in Australia, tests carried out in at least two hospitals have demonstrated that equipment can be affected.

Most medical electrical equipment has been designed to allow for this kind of interference. However, tests have shown that within a distance of two meters some critical devices like drug infusion pumps, ventilators and settings on infant incubators may be affected. The newer digital (GSM) mobile phones appear to generate more interference than older analogue (AMPS) mobile phones.

Interference to medical equipment is currently being considered by various public and private bodies. The concerns over mobile phones may develop into a broader investigation into the significance of other sources of electromagnetic interference within the medical area.

We strongly recommend that hospitals consider adopting the following policy:

- Patients or visitors entering the hospital environs should turn off their phones. Mobile phones generate interference even when not in use while they are turned on or in standby mode.

- Inform patients and visitors of your institution's policy controlling the use of cellular telephones and other radiofrequency (RF) transmitting devices, explaining that the rationale for formulating such a policy is because of known overseas cases of interference occurring with medical equipment caused by radio transmissions.

- Whilst RF transmitting devices will continue to be a vital component of hospital operations, clinical staff must be alerted that when practical, users should avoid transmissions within two meters of medical devices in such areas as patient rooms, critical care units, emergency rooms, operating theaters, diagnostic and treatment areas, and clinical laboratories.

- Electromagnetic interference must be considered when purchasing or installing medical electrical equipment.

A further joint Australian study is underway between the Therapeutic Goods Administration, Mobile Service Providers such as Telstra, and the Woden Valley Hospital in Canberra to evaluate the electromagnetic compatibility of a range of medical electrical equipment (Dwyer, Englund, Flood, Joyner, & Raiz, 1995). The aim of this study is to evaluate the performance of a number of currently available drug infusion pumps and syringe drivers when subjected to the electromagnetic fields from 2 W GSM and 0.6 W AMPS mobile telephone handsets. Performance is graded into one of four categories:

1.   No interference—normal operation under all conditions.

2.   Permanent failure, but fail-safe, with an appropriate alarm warning. (Fail-safe is defined as the equipment recognizing a problem, giving an alarm, and then shutting down.)

3.   Intermittent interference and reversion to normal operation when the interference source is removed.

4.   Subtle, but permanent interference, where the unit does not fail-safe with an alarm warning and an indication of change of state of operation.

The range of the seventeen devices tested so far has varied from instruments released to the market over ten years ago but which are still in active service to devices registered for use in Australia but not yet released. Eight devices have exhibited a category 2 failure mode. No instruments have entered a failure mode where there was no indication given to the operator and the pump did not fail safe. It is interesting to note that in one instance the infusion pump itself did not exhibit EMI, but when a drip detector was connected to the pump, EMI occurred. EMI testing protocols should address distributed and patient-coupled systems. The testing protocol and preliminary results form part of an ongoing study which will input into standards development and regulations.

Hearing Aids Testing

A joint investigation undertaken between Telstra Research Laboratories (TRL) and the National Acoustics Laboratories (NAL) confirmed that GSM digital mobile telephones caused interference (a "buzzing" sound) in various types of hearing aids (Joyner, Wood, Burwood, Allison, & Le Strange, 1993). A summary of the results are shown in Table 2. It should be noted that these results were obtained with the hearing aids suspended in free space. This arrangement represents the worst possible situation; subsequent subjective testing on hearing impaired persons indicated that the EMI was less severe.

This preliminary study prompted a more extensive joint investigation by NAL, TRL, the Spectrum Management Authority, AUSTEL (the Australian Telecommunications Industry Regulator), other mobile service providers, representatives from the hearing aid industry, and consumer groups, including hearing aid user organizations. The primary aims of this study were to:

1.   assess the degree of interference caused by GSM digital mobiles to a wide range of hearing aids;

2.   assess the effectiveness of various treatments and design modifications to hearing aids to reduce interference;

3.   develop a reliable and practical measurement system;

4.   develop hearing aid standards for immunity to digital mobile interference.

Hearing Aid Type	Field Strength for 10 dB above Noise Floor of Aid (V/m)	Distance from GSM Unit	
		2 W (m)	8 W (m)
Aid 1 (BTE)	0.65	9.2	18.5
Aid 2 (BTE)	1.3	4.5	9.2
Aid 3 (BTE)	2.0	3.0	6.0
Aid 4 (BTE)	2.8	2.1	4.3
Aid 5 (BTE)	3.1	1.9	3.9
Aid 6 (ITE)	9.4	0.64	1.3
Aid 7 (ITE)	9.4	0.64	1.3
Aid 8 (ITE)	32.0	0.17	0.38

BTE = Behind the ear; ITE = In the ear

Table 2. Summary of Results of the Free Space EMI Testing on Various Hearing Aids Using GSM Digital Telephones

A highly effective measurement system — incorporating a terminated waveguide test chamber and a hearing aid manipulator capable of rotation around three perpendicular axes—was designed by TRL and NAL for the GSM frequency bands. TRL has recently designed, manufactured, tested, and installed a further waveguide transition at NAL to expand their measurement capabilities to include the frequency bands from 1.8 GHz to 2.5 GHz.

The results of these studies are summarized in Table 3. The free space immunity test levels for 45 dB Sound Pressure Level (SPL) and 55 dB SPL are shown, as well as the results of subjective testing of hearing aid users.

It should be pointed out that hearing aid 6 is the latest production hearing aid available in Australia. This is a behind-the-ear aid which has a free space immunity in excess of 10 V/m.

Hearing Aid Type & Status	Immunity Level		Class of Use	
	45 dB SPL	55 dB SPL	1 m separation	Use with phone
Aid 1 - ITE experimental	335	596	Usable	Usable
Aid 2 - BTE experimental	150	266	Usable	Usable
Aid 3 - BTE experimental	75	133	Usable	Usable
Aid 4 - BTE experimental	67	119	Usable	Usable
Aid 5 - ITE production	33	60	Usable	Sometimes Usable
Aid 6 - BTE production	17	30	Usable	Unusable

Table 3. Results of Free Space EMI Testing on Modified and the Latest Production Hearing Aids and Subjective Tests Using GSM Mobile Telephones

There have been several recent efforts to evaluate hearing aid interference. All of the Australian research and development work is contained in a detailed report (National Acoustics Laboratories, 1995). Other centers are developing and implementing protocols for the study of wireless phone interaction with hearing aids, including The Center for the Study of Wireless Electromagnetic Compatibility in the School of Industrial Engineering of the University of Oklahoma.

Implanted Cardiac Pacemaker Testing

I will only briefly mention the Australian EMI testing of the implanted cardiac pacemakers because pacemakers are the subject of the following detailed presentation.

The aim of this series of measurements was to investigate the potential for GSM mobile telephones to interfere with the operation of implanted cardiac pacemakers. To simulate the GSM digital signal, a 25 W, 900 MHz carrier was pulsed at a rate of either 2 Hz, 8 Hz, or 217 Hz, with a pulse width of 0.6 ms. This signal was fed into a WG4 coaxial-to-waveguide adaptor which was held 10 cm from the chest of the patient and rotated to check for possible polarization effects of the incident field. Also, the antenna of a 2 W GSM mobile telephone operating at full power was held in contact with the patient and slowly moved over the area above the pacemaker and cardiac leads. Twenty five patients with a range of cardiac pacemakers (DDD, DDDR, VVI, VVIR) were tested with the pacemakers set in bipolar and unipolar modes at maximum sensitivity and at normal settings.

Occasional inhibition of output and oversensing by the atrial channel, manifested as a transient increase in ventricular rate, was observed; it was more common in the unipolar pacing mode. The minute ventilation rate adaptive pacemakers showed no pacing rate changes as a result of changes in measured transthoracic impedance. An expert consulting cardiologist concluded that these disruptions of pacemaker function would cause no consistent, clinically significant effects during pacemaker operation at maximal sensitivities and at normal pacemaker settings.

EMI Standards

Medical Electrical Equipment

The FDA issued a voluntary standard specifying that medical electrical equipment should be immune from EMI in fields up to 7 V/m within the frequency range of 450 to 1000 MHz (Food and Drug Administration, 1979).

The International Electrotechnical Commission (IEC) has published a standard on electromagnetic compatibility for medical electrical equipment which states that an immunity level of 3 V/m shall apply for the frequency range 26 to 1000 MHz (International Electrotechnical Commission, 1993). However, it is stated in this standard that the 3 V/m immunity level may be inappropriate because the physiological signals measured may be substantially below those induced by a field strength of 3 V/m. It is also difficult to understand why, in the face of an explosion in the use of mobile communication devices, the IEC would reduce the immunity level from the previous FDA voluntary level of 7 V/m.

In recognition of the fact that the safety of life-supporting medical electrical equipment requires a higher level of immunity, the IEC issued a draft standard for infusion pumps and controllers which states that an immunity level of 10 V/m shall apply for the frequency range 26 to 1000 MHz (International Electrotechnical Commission, 1994).

Both the 3 V/m and 10 V/m levels referred to above are root mean square (RMS) levels. For the EMI testing, the carrier signal is to be 80 percent amplitude modulated with a 1 kHz sine wave. This effectively means that the peak RMS field strengths are 1.8 times or 5 dB higher.

Immunity levels of 10 V/m are certainly a major step forward, but will not guarantee EMI effects will not occur. However, where mobile communications devices are used inadvertently in the vicinity of medical electrical equipment, a 10 V/m immunity level means that EMI effects will almost certainly be minimized.

Hearing Aids

The Australian/New Zealand standard for hearing aid immunity is designed to ensure that not more than 10 percent of hearing aid users will be annoyed by interference from 2 W GSM mobile telephones operating at a distance of 1 m (Australian/New Zealand Standard Hearing Aids, 1995). This criterion leads to an input related interference level of 45 dB SPL associated with an interrupted 10 V/m RMS carrier field strength, which is the maximum field strength expected from 2 W GSM mobile telephones at the distance of 1 m. The situation where a hearing impaired person wants to use a

GSM digital mobile telephone proximate with a hearing aid is under discussion within the Australian/New Zealand standard committee as a matter of urgency. For the EMI testing of hearing aids, the carrier signal is 80 percent amplitude modulated with a 1 kHz sine wave.

The IEC is in the process of developing an immunity standard for hearing aids and it is understood that an immunity level of 3 V/m is under consideration. Some models of hearing aids currently in production have immunity levels in excess of 10 V/m and the wisdom of the IEC considerations of a 3 V/m immunity level could be viewed as questionable.

Discussion and Recommendations

It must be recognized that EMI to medical electrical equipment is not a recent phenomenon resulting from the introduction of mobile communications devices. In addition, mobile communications are seen as an essential adjunct to patient care. The Australian and New Zealand Intensive Care Society supports the continued use of mobile telephones in hospitals, especially for doctors treating critically ill patients. However, it has to be acknowledged that, with the explosion in the number of mobile communications devices, the EMI problem will only grow if the issues are not dealt with. The following strategies are suggested as a means to manage EMI issues with medical electrical equipment.

Mobile Communications Management Strategy

Mobile communications services used in the medical industry should be configured and controlled to minimize the likelihood of transmission of high electromagnetic fields in the near vicinity of medical electrical equipment.

In Australia, several hospitals have introduced low power (10 mW) mobile communications systems known as CT2. The medical practitioners are extremely happy with the performance of the systems, which have all the functionality of the hospital's internal telephone systems. Extensive EMI testing of the CT2 system in a cardiology ward of one of the hospitals involved in the trial revealed no instances of EMI, even with the CT2 handsets in contact with the medical electrical equipment.

Options for the installation and positioning of antenna systems and radio base stations should take into account field strengths in the vicinity of medical electrical equipment and, if power control for the mobile stations is available, the resultant maximum transmit power of the mobile handsets when attempting to establish a radio link with the base station.

Education Strategy

Personnel in the medical industry and people using medical electrical equipment in the home must be made aware of EMI. Issues include the possible sources, their likely effect on the operation of the medical electrical equipment, and what to do if EMI is suspected.

The educational material produced for health care workers and the general public must be concise and easily understood by ethnic groups and people of wide ranging levels of education.

Prevention Strategy

Biomedical engineers should identify particularly sensitive medical electrical equipment and formulate specific controls for that equipment.

It is recommended that this issue be addressed as a matter of priority, and any equipment identified as particularly sensitive should be notified to a central body such as the Emergency Care Research Institute in the United States for dissemination to all biomedical engineering departments. EMI issues should be considered when designing, purchasing, and installing medical electrical equipment.

EMI Standards Strategy

New medical electrical equipment must have a reasonable degree of immunity to EMI. This issue has to be recognized as a longer term solution but it must be addressed by all standards setting bodies. The regulatory frameworks for medical electrical equipment within Australia and Europe define the following risk categories:

> **High Risk:** Life support devices, key resuscitation devices, and other devices whose failure or misuse is reasonably likely to seriously injure patients or staff.

> **Medium Risk:** Devices whose failure or misuse would have a significant impact on patient care, but would not be likely to cause direct serious injury.

> **Low Risk:** Devices whose failure or misuse is unlikely to result in serious consequences. This category would also encompass an "Annoying" classification.

EMI effects may be similarly categorized, and it is recommended that a minimum level of immunity for the Medium and High Risk categories should be no less than 10 V/m, which is not unduly onerous considering the 7 V/m that applied in the US in 1979. For the Low Risk/Annoying category, the minimum level of immunity should be at least 3 V/m. Consideration must also be given to test protocols which take into account the distributed nature of medical electrical equipment systems and the influence of the dielectric and conducting mass of the patient on the EMI performance of that equipment.

Acknowledgements

The permission of the Director of Telstra Research Laboratories to publish this paper is hereby acknowledged. The author would also like to acknowledge the technical inputs of Steve Iskra (Telstra Research Laboratories), Ian Swinson (Telstra Mobile Communications Services), Mike Flood (Therapeutic Goods Administration), and Grant Symons (AUSTEL).

Update

Kenneth H. Joyner is currently employed with Motorola as Director, EME Strategy & Regulatory Affairs—Asia Pacific.

Since the preparation of this manuscript in mid-1995, several large investigations into the potential of mobile communications devices to cause interference into medical electrical equipment have been published (VIFKA Telecommunicatie, 1995; Electromagnetic Interference Management, 1996; U.K. Department of Health, 1997). The conclusions and recommendations of these studies are in general agreement with the recommendations presented and discussed in this manuscript.

The interference between wireless communications devices and cardiac pacemakers has been very well documented in recent times and interested readers should consult the various studies in PACE 1996;19(10):1405-58 and Hayes et al, N Engl J Med 1997;336(21)1473-9.

The International Electrotechnical Commission is reviewing the EMC requirements and tests for medical electrical equipment (IEC 601-1-2:1993). Currently under consideration are radiated immunity levels of 3 V/m (80 MHz to 2 GHz) for non-life support equipment and 3 V/m (80 to 800 MHz) and 10 V/m (800 MHz to 2 GHz) for life support equipment. The test signals will be 80 percent modulated with either a 2 Hz or 1 kHz, depending on the intended use; 2 Hz will be required for equipment used in the control, monitoring, or measurement of a physiological parameter. This initiative to increase the immunity limits will facilitate the long term management of EMC/EMI issues for mobile communications devices and medical electrical equipment.

References

Australian/New Zealand Standard Hearing Aids. (1995). Part 9: Immunity requirements and methods of measurement for hearing aids exposed to radiofrequency fields in the frequency range 300 MHz to 3 GHz (AS/NZS 1088.9). Standards Australia, 1 The Crescent, Homebush, Sydney, Australia, 2140.

Clifford, K. J., Joyner, K. H., Stroud, D. B., Wood, M., Ward, B., & Fernandez, C. H. (1994). Mobile telephones interfere with medical electrical equipment. Australasian Physical and Engineering Sciences in Medicine, 17, 23-27.

Dwyer, M., Englund, A. M., Flood, M., Joyner, K. H., & Raiz, D. (1995, November). EMI/EMC, mobile phone and medical equipment the continuing story. Paper presented at the Engineering and Physics in Medicine Conference, Queenstown, New Zealand.

Electromagnetic interference management in the hospital environment. Part 1: An introduction. (1996). Norman: University of Oklahoma, Center for the Study of Wireless Electromagnetic Compatibility.

Food and Drug Administration, Bureau of Medical Devices. (1979, October). Electromagnetic compatibility standard for medical devices (BMD Publication No. MDS-201-0004). Rockville, MD: Food and Drug Administration.

International Electrotechnical Commission. (1993). Medical electrical equipment, part 1: General requirements for safety, 2. Collateral standard: electromagnetic compatibility—requirements and tests (IEC 601-1-2). Geneva, Switzerland: International Electrotechnical Commission.

International Electrotechnical Commission. (1994). Draft First Edition 19. Medical Electrical Equipment. Part 2: Particular requirements for safety of infusion pumps and controllers, Draft (IEC 601-2-24). Geneva, Switzerland: International Electrotechnical Commission.

Joyner, K. H., Wood, M., Burwood, E., Allison, D., & Le Strange, J. R. (1993, March). Interference to hearing aids by the new digital mobile telephone system. Global System for Mobile (GSM) Communication Standard, National Acoustics Laboratories, Sydney, Australia.

National Acoustics Laboratories. (1995, May). Interference to hearing aids by the digital mobile telephone system, Global System for Mobile Communications (GSM) (Report No. 131). Sydney, Australia: Le Strange, J. R., Burwood, E., Byrne, D., Joyner, K. H., Wood, M., & Symons, G.

Silberberg, J. (1993). Performance degradation of electronic medical devices due to electromagnetic interference. Compliance Engineering, 10, 25-39.

U.K. Department of Health. (1997). Electromagnetic compatibility of medical devices with mobile communications. London, UK: The Medical Devices Agency.

VIFKA Telecommunicatie. (1995). Recommendations regarding the use of pocket telephones within health care institutions. De Meem, The Netherlands: VIFKA Telecommunicatie.

21

MEDICAL EQUIPMENT INTERFERENCE: RISK AND MINIMIZATION

Bernard Segal

Abstract

To help estimate the risk of medical equipment interference, the hospital electromagnetic environment and the immunity of critical-care medical equipment were characterized. Fields were found to be very low (e.g., 0.1 V/m), except near radiofrequency (RF) sources. Most medical equipment (e.g., 75%) exhibited serious malfunctions beside 5 W transmitters. Malfunctions decreased as other lower power sources or greater separations were employed. Since transmitters are rarely operated near medical equipment, this explains the probable low current risk of such malfunctions. However, minimizing this risk will require cooperative efforts, both short-term (education; management of sources and equipment; ad hoc testing of existing equipment) and long-term (equipment design; standards), all fostered by multi-disciplinary research.

Introduction

This presentation will aim to put the significance of previous work done by others and at McGill into context by reviewing the issues involved in estimating the risk of medical equipment malfunction due to electromagnetic interference (EMI) and in minimizing such risks in the future.

Estimation of Risk of Medical Equipment Interference

Interference Conditions

Medical equipment interference will occur when:

Electromagnetic environment > Equipment immunity.

A very particular condition is required for interference. A source must be radiating energy, the function of the medical equipment must be capable of disruption at the frequencies being radiated, and the source must be close enough so that the electromagnetic fields at the equipment exceed their immunity. There is no single cause of the malfunction, especially when multiple sources are present, when sources radiate at multiple frequencies, or when devices are susceptible at multiple frequencies. The malfunction arises from the *entire combination*. Each side of the above equation will be considered in turn.

The Electromagnetic Environment of Hospitals

As reviewed elsewhere, there are many potential sources of electromagnetic interference which influence the electromagnetic environment of hospitals (Association for the Advancement of Medical Instrumentation, 1997; Health Canada, 1987; Paperman, David, & McKee, 1994; Segal, 1995; Silberberg, 1993). The most common interference sources are: 1) other very nearby medical devices (e.g., monitors,

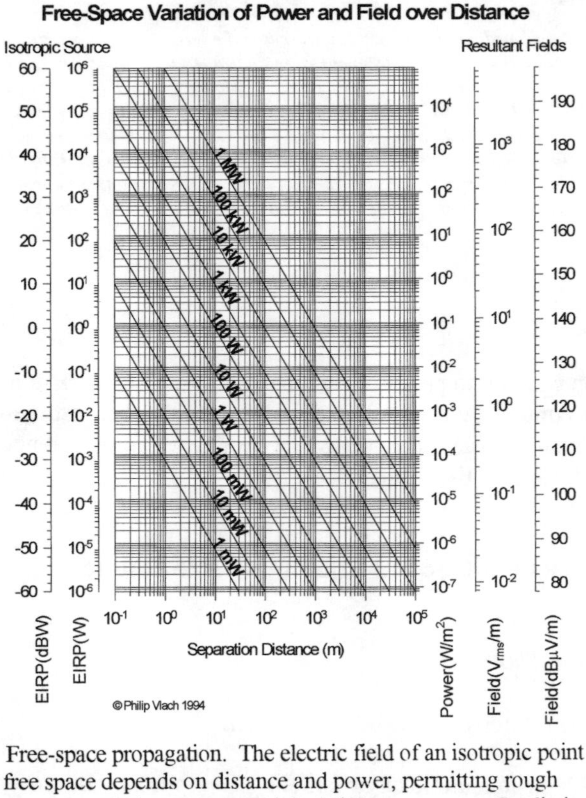

Free-Space Variation of Power and Field over Distance

© Philip Vlach 1994

Figure 1. Free-space propagation. The electric field of an isotropic point source in free space depends on distance and power, permitting rough comparisons of the relative EMI potential of different sources. Predictions are inaccurate in the near-field, with real antennas, and in the presence of absorbers and scatters.

electrosurgical units); 2) fixed sources such as nearby broadcast (AM, FM, or TV) antennas; 3) portable sources (walkie talkies, cell phones, personal communication systems [PCS], wireless computer components); 4) powerline frequency distribution components; 5) electrostatic discharge; or 6) "unknown" sources that, once identified, are often found to be unintentional and unexpected.

Rough estimates of the electric field that might be associated with such sources can be estimated by assuming that a given source can be represented by a point source radiating in free space. Figure 1 shows how this free-space-propagation field changes with distance and power (electric field rises as the square root of the source's power, and falls as the reciprocal of distance). Estimates predict that fields within hospitals should be very small (e.g., less than 0.1 V/m), provided that minimal source-equipment separation distances are maintained.

Measurements within hospitals confirm this prediction. Figure 2 shows electric fields measured in five Montreal hospitals by our McGill Group in collaboration with Industry Canada (Vlach, Liu-Hinz, Segal, Skulic, & Pavlasek, 1995; Vlach, Segal, & Pavlasek, 1995). Typically, eight sites were surveyed at each hospital, both outside and inside (e.g., intensive care units, operating rooms, and patient rooms). The horizontal dashed line shows the 3 V/m level, the current International Electrotechnical Commission immunity level. Fields measured were usually well below this limit. Corresponding results have been obtained by others (e.g., Kole, 1995).

Figure 3 characterizes fields associated with portable sources, showing the probability of observing a given maximal field level in an upper-level hospital room during a 24-hour period. About 32,000 calls were placed in two walkie-talkie bands and in the cellular band, originating both from within the hospital and from nearby surrounding streets. Measured fields were very low-level (e.g., below 0.01 V/m), presumably because no walkie-talkie or cell phone transmissions originated close to this room. However, higher fields were measured when portable sources were operated nearby. Thus, the hospital electromagnetic environment is not that severe if portable sources are appropriately managed so that they operate at sufficient distances from medical equipment.

Medical Equipment Immunity

Estimation of the risk of medical equipment interference also requires consideration of medical equipment immunity. Current knowledge of such immunity generally comes from two sources of information—clinical reports and laboratory reports (Segal, 1995; Silberberg, 1995).

Clinical reports from various sources suggest that, although there have been many equipment malfunctions caused by interference that have had serious implications, the total number of reports is small, typically two to three per year, which represents a very small part of reports due to other causes (Knickerbocker & Barbell, 1995; Segal, 1995; Silberberg, 1993, 1995; Tan & Hindberg, 1995).

Laboratory test results frequently suggest a higher incidence of medical equipment malfunction caused by interference. Tests on apnea monitors and on powered wheelchairs reported large percentages of devices that exhibited serious

286

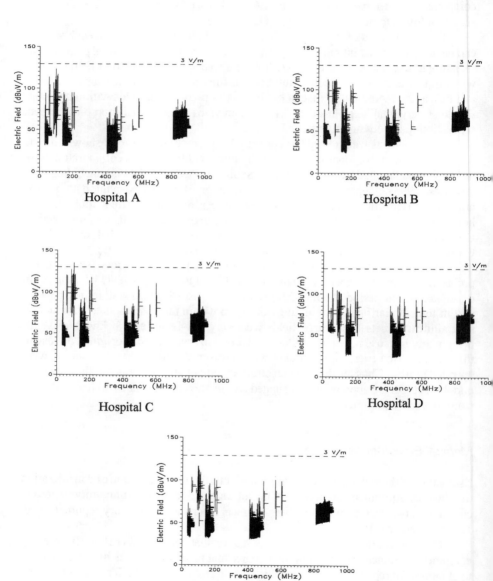

Figure 2. Fields measured inside and outside five hospitals. Horizontal bar shows average of measurements made at 5-13 sites at each hospital, the ends of each bar showing corresponding minimums and maximums.

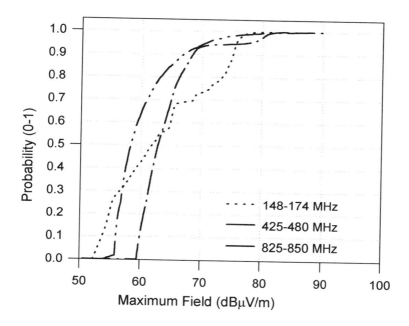

Cumulative distribution function of maximum field per call during a 24 hour period.

Figure 3. Fields of portable sources in hospital room. Measurements were made in a typical, single-patient hospital room with one window, having an upper-level location. The y-axis shows the cumulative probability of observing an electric field level having a magnitude shown on the x-axis. Three bands (business-police: 148-174 MHZ; land-mobile UHF: 425-480 MHZ; cellular: 825-850 MHZ) are shown, representing about 32,000 calls in a 24-hour period.

malfunctions when *full-susceptibility* testing used a wide range of frequencies to assess immunity (Ruggera & O'Bryan, 1991; Witters & Ruggera, 1994). Rice and Smith (1993) reported that a very high percentage of medical devices malfunctioned near cell phones. Significantly, this study was one of the first to describe results based on ad hoc testing. In such tests, common sources are brought close to medical devices and any resulting malfunction is noted. Such testing can be viewed as a *"partial-frequency" susceptibility* test, rather than a full-frequency susceptibility test. Others have reported similarly high percentages of malfunctioning results (Joyner, 1995; Kisilevich & Tan, 1995). Such results have caused concern, to the point that some hospitals are banning certain products.

McGill Ad Hoc Testing

Interpretation of this situation is clarified by tests performed at McGill (Segal et al., 1995). Using our ad hoc test procedure, we took six common RF sources and operated them near typical critical-care medical devices found in the hospital. Only common realistic configurations (e.g., relative positions, device operation modes) were examined. Only serious malfunctions were considered (e.g., device shut downs requiring operator intervention; device operation out of specification without alarm; repair or factory reprogramming required; etc.). Figure 4 summarizes our results. The y-axis represents the percentage of medical equipment that malfunctioned, going from zero to 100%. The x-axis represents the distance between the source and the medical device at which a serious malfunction first occurred. As would be expected, walkie talkies, being the most powerful sources used, caused the most malfunctions. Bringing walkie talkies very close—perhaps unreasonably close—to these medical devices caused most medical devices (about 55-75%) to exhibit serious malfunctions. As the walkie talkies were moved farther away, the percentage of devices that malfunctioned decreased. Only two devices continued to malfunction as the separation was increased beyond three meters—both older, unusually susceptible devices, which continued to malfunction at a distance of eight meters. When testing was done using cellular phones, many fewer devices malfunctioned. When the separation was about an inch, the percentage was around 20%. At a separation of about one meter, only one of the unusually susceptible devices continued to malfunction. Similar results were obtained using both analog and digital phones. When testing was done using a very low power source (10 mW), no malfunctions were observed.

These results perhaps explain the different perspectives that emerge from consideration of clinical reports and laboratory reports. Laboratory tests were performed using very high field levels or included testing at very small separation distances, whereas in most clinical situations RF sources are rarely brought so close to medical devices.

Estimation of Current Risk of Medical Equipment Interference

Clinical reports probably *underestimate* the potential EMI risk. For example, it is unlikely that every EMI malfunction is identified as such and subsequently reported. Also, although the function of some devices may be disrupted by interference, some malfunctions may not be identified by medical staff (Segal, Retfalvi, & Pavlasek, 1995).

Laboratory tests probably *overestimate* the potential EMI risk. Although there have been a large number of malfunctions that have been reported based on ad hoc testing, it is unclear whether such sources will ever be operated so close to medical equipment. Also, even if this occurs and the equipment malfunctions, the clinical impact of the malfunction is uncertain. If medical staff react appropriately to the malfunction (e.g., quickly restore normal function to the device), there will be no clinical impact. Finally, the risk of EMI malfunction has to be compared to other iatrogenic risks.

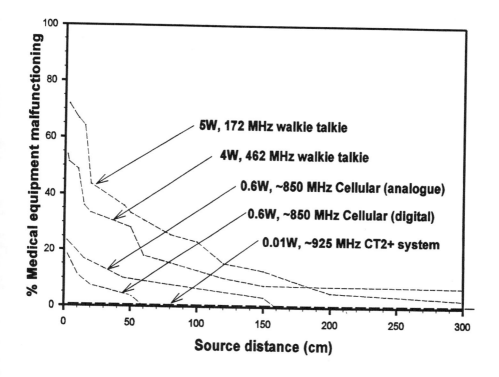

Figure 4. Percent of medical equipment affected by EMI. Sources transmitting at different power levels were operated at progressively smaller separations from critical-care medical devices until a serious malfunction was observed. The percent of devices that malfunctioned at given separations is shown. Thirty-nine, 33, 27, 15, and 15 devices were tested with a 5-watt walkie talkie, 4-watt walkie talkie, 0.6 watt analogue cell phone, 0.6-watt digital cell phone, 0.01-watt CT2+ portable unit, and its corresponding base station, respectively.

Thus, the current EMI risk can only be estimated roughly, since the actual incidence of EMI malfunction is currently unknown. Knowledge of the electromagnetic environment in hospitals and equipment immunity is available in isolated cases, but much more data is required to increase the sample size. Discussion with those within hospitals indicates that there have been millions and millions of hours of safe operation of medical devices, indicating that current EMI malfunctions are probably rare. However, it is incumbent upon us to try to minimize any future occurrences of EMI malfunction as much as possible. Predictions of future EMI risks are confounded by the fact that we now are aware of, and know how to minimize, the EMI risk; our success in doing so will influence any predictions of the future.

Minimizing the Risk of EMI Malfunctions

There are two main categories of activities that will minimize the future EMI risk: those that will be effective within the next five to ten years and those that will be optimally effective only afterwards (Segal, 1995).

EMI Risk Minimization: The Next Five to Ten Years

We are currently in a transition period during which the existing medical equipment inventory, whose EMI immunity is largely unknown, is gradually being replaced with new equipment having improved EMI immunity, and the RF sources now being used in hospitals are gradually being replaced by lower-power sources. However, until this transition period is over, three groups of parallel activities are required to minimize the risk of EMI malfunction.

The first involves education. All concerned parties must be educated to aid EMI prevention. For example, *medical personnel* must be educated to aid identification of EMI malfunctions. If no one notices that a device is malfunctioning, this malfunction cannot be prevented or analyzed so that other similar ones can also be prevented. *Manufacturers* must consider electromagnetic compatibility at all stages of product development and distribution. *Biomedical engineers* must know how to manage electromagnetic compatibility in hospitals (see below). The *public* must understand why cell phones, or walkie talkies, must only be used in designated areas of the hospital.

The second activity that will minimize the risk of EMI malfunctions involves management of the heath care environment, where possible. Minimal separations between more powerful sources and medical devices have to be established and enforced. If it is found that a device is unusually susceptible, the manufacturer of the device should be asked whether its immunity can be increased. If this is not possible, the use of such devices may have to be restricted. The power of sources should be minimized wherever possible.

The data in Figure 4 show that most medical devices malfunctioned when operated very close to higher-powered sources (e.g., 5 W walkie talkies)—fewer malfunctioned as the power of the source fell, and still fewer malfunctioned as the separation distance increased. These data suggest that a separation distance can be specified for each source that should insure that medical devices of a given immunity will not be affected by EMI. For minimal separation distances of about three meters for a walkie talkie, and of about one meter for a cellular phone operating at 600 mW, the likelihood of a malfunction was small. Larger separation distances would be required when unusually susceptible devices are involved, when devices are in rooms having large reflective surfaces, or when multiple sources are simultaneously active (Liu-Hinz, Segal, Skulic, & Pavlasek, 1995). But how large should the separation distance be? Table 1 shows several examples. Using minimal distances, roughly five percent of devices malfunctioned in our own study. More effective separation distances might be based on trying to ensure that devices are not exposed to fields which exceed the proposed "3 V/m" level (Table 1, center column), or even more conservative values might be appropriate in other situations (e.g., equipment immunity is unknown, or equipment is located in reflective environments). The appropriate separation distance is likely to vary from hospital to hospital.

Source	Minimal	3 V/m	Conservative
5 W walkie talkie	3	6	12
0.6 W cell phone	1	2	4
0.01 W PCS	0.15	0.3	0.6

Table 1. Source-device separation distances (m)

The third activity is especially challenging. The immunity of the existing medical equipment inventory must be estimated since this is largely unknown. However, it is not cost effective to test every piece of medical equipment in every hospital using full susceptibility testing. Instead, a national program is required to estimate the immunity of critical-care medical equipment using ad hoc test procedures such as those described above or elsewhere (American National Standards Institute, 1997). Although care must be taken in interpreting results from such a test program, this program would be the minimal and the most cost-effective means of identifying those unusually susceptible devices that probably exist. This must be done before all wireless communication can be safely used throughout the health care system.

These three activities form the basis of a set of draft recommendations for electrocompatibility in health care (Segal, Retfalvi, Townsend, & Pavlasek, 1996) which are currently being considered by a Canada-USA Task Force (Tan, Segal, Townsend, & Stedman, 1995). After suitable review, it is anticipated that recommendations very similar to these will be endorsed by Health Canada, the Canadian government agency that is analogous to the U.S. Food and Drug Administration.

EMI Risk Minimization: The Next 10 to 20 Years

A second category of activities must be initiated today, but will not have optimal impact until the next decade, when all of the present medical equipment inventory is replaced by EMI- resistant counterparts. Those familiar with the design of EMI-resistant medical equipment believe that such EMI-resistant equipment will eventually become available without substantial cost increases. Achieving this goal remains a great engineering-design challenge, because most medical devices have patient-applied parts which, when connected to the patient, present such devices with poorly defined EMI antennas consisting of the patient and the patient connection lines (either conductive wire or fluid).

It is only once the above engineering-design problems have been resolved that it will be possible to define appropriate standards for medical equipment. Such standards will also have to address issues such as specifying appropriate immunity levels, specifying realistic clinical pass/fail criteria, and so on.

Ongoing research is needed to foster all of the above activities. However, the above activities cannot be implemented without solving another key problem—the human one. In order to optimize health care delivery, there must be ready communication of information within the hospital, whether that be between patients communicating with medical systems, or between medical staff communicating with each other. The success with which this can be done depends on the cooperation of six groups. Medical device users are at the front line. If the nurses and doctors do not recognize when EMI is causing a device to malfunction, then no one else can analyze the malfunction and find out how to prevent it. Medical device manufacturers and RF source manufacturers and providers have to cooperate with each other to help prevent EMI malfunctions. Next, regulators and standards agencies, as well as government bodies, have to work with all other groups to overcome many legal and practical hurdles so that emerging solutions can be implemented (Townsend, 1995). And, of course, researchers building a new field—electromagnetic compatibility health care research—must help to provide the theoretical and practical solutions that are required to resolve the above problems. By working together, this challenge can be met.

Combining Health Care and Health Research

Understanding an EMI malfunction of a medical device within the body (e.g., a pacemaker), or effectively within it (e.g., a hearing aid), first requires the solution of a classical health research problem: How electromagnetic fields are distributed in part of the body, here the region adjacent to a within-body device. Such understanding also requires the solution of a classical electromagnetic compatibility health care research problem: How EMI affects a medical device, here the within-body one. Clearly, optimal understanding of such malfunctions requires input from both health and health care research. It is also interesting to note that both areas of research should benefit from the usage of identical research tools. For example, understanding of fields within the body, or within a hospital room, both require solution of electromagnetic equations in complex environments. Thus, Okoneiwski, Stuchly, and Stuchly have recently used the FD-TD technique both to compute fields in the head of the user of a cellular phone, and to compute fields within a hospital room. Both health care and health research will benefit from such cross disciplinary efforts.

Acknowledgments

The following individuals made significant contributions to this presentation: P Vlach, C Liu-Hinz, S Retfalvi, T Pavlasek, B Skulic, and other members of The McGill Biomedical Engineering Group on Electromagnetic Compatibility. The collaboration of Industry Canada is greatly appreciated. The support of various sponsors over the past six years is gratefully acknowledged.

References

American National Standards Institute. (1997). Recommended practice for an on-site, ad hoc test method for estimating radiated electromagnetic immunity of medical devices to specific RF transmitters (Standard C63.18). Piscataway, NJ: Institute of Electrical and Electronics Engineers.

Association for the Advancement of Medical Instrumentation. (1997). Guidance on electromagnetic compatibility of medical devices for clinical/biomedical engineers — Part 1: Radiated radiofrequency electromagnetic energy in health care facilities (Tech. Information Rep. No. 18-1997). Arlington, VA: Association for the Advancement of Medical Instrumentation.

Health & Welfare Canada. (1987). Proceedings of the workshop on electromagnetic interference and electromagnetic compatibility in health care facilities. Edmonton, Canada: Health Canada, Electronics Test Center.

Joyner, K. H. (1998). State of the science in wireless instrument medical equipment interference. In G. L. Carlo (Ed.), Wireless phones and health: Scientific progress (pp. 269-281). Norwell, MA: Kluwer Academic Publishers.

Kisilevich, D., & Tan, K. S. (1995). Effects of EMI on medical devices - Inside the hospital. In K. S. Tan, B. Segal, D. Townsend, & J. Stedman (Eds.), Proceedings of a round-table discussion on electromagnetic compatibility in health care (pp. 25-27). Spruce Grove, Canada: Care Technology.

Knickerbocker, G. G., & Barbell, A. S. (1995). Medical device malfunction caused by electromagnetic interference: The ECRI perspective. In B. Segal (Ed.), Proceedings of a workshop on electromagnetics health care and health (pp. 24-28). Piscataway, NJ: Institute of Electrical and Electronics Engineers. Also in: Proceedings of 1995 IEEE Engineering in Medicine & Biology Society Annual Meeting and the 21st Canadian Medical & Biological Society Conference [CD-ROM web edition], (pp. 1775-1779). Piscataway, NJ: Institute of Electrical and Electronics Engineers.

Kole, B. (1995). Preliminary broadband survey of electric fields in hospitals. In K. S. Tan, B. Segal, D. Townsend, & J. Stedman (Eds.), Proceedings of a round-table discussion on electromagnetic compatibility in health care (pp. 39-41). Spruce Grove, Canada: Care Technology.

Liu-Hinz, C., Segal, B., Skulic, B., & Pavlasek, T. (1995). Electromagnetic fields near portable radiofrequency sources: Estimates using image theory and measurements. Proceedings of the 1995 IEEE Engineering in Medicine & Biology Society Annual Meeting and the 21st Canadian Medical & Biological Society Conference (pp. 1589-1590). Piscataway, NJ: Institute of Electrical and Electronics Engineers.

Paperman, W. D., David, Y., & McKee, K. A. (1994). Electromagnetic interference: Causes and concerns in the health care environment (Healthcare Facilities No. 055110). Chicago, IL: American Society for Hospital Engineering, American Hospital Association.

Rice, M. L., & Smith, J. M. (1993). Study of electromagnetic interference between portable cellular phones and medical equipment. Proceedings of the Canadian medical & biological engineering conference, 17, 330-331.

294

Ruggera, P., & O'Bryan E. R. (1991). Studies of apnea monitor radio frequency electromagnetic interference. Proceedings of 1991 IEEE Engineering in Medicine & Biology Society, 1641-1643.

Segal, B. (1995). Sources and victims: The potential magnitude of the electromagnetic interference problem. In S. Sykes (Ed.), Proceedings of electromagnetic compatibility for medical devices: Issues and solutions (pp.24-39). Arlington, VA: Association for the Advancement of Medical Instrumentation.

Segal, B., Retfalvi, S., & Pavlasek, T. (1995). "Silent" malfunction of a critical-care device caused by EMI. Biomedical Instrumentation Technology, 29, 350-354.

Segal, B., Retfalvi, S., Townsend, D., & Pavlasek, T. (1996). Recommendation for electromagnetic compatibility in health care. Proceeding of the Canadian Medical and Biological Engineering Conference, 22, 22-23.

Segal, B., Skulic, B., Liu-Hinz, C., Retfalvi, S., Orange, M., & Pavlasek, T. J. F. (1995). Preliminary study of critical-care medical-device susceptibility to portable radiofrequency sources [abstract]. Proceedings of 30th Annual Meeting of the Association for the Advancement of Medical Instrumentation, 83.

Silberberg, J. (1993). Performance degradation of electronic medical devices due to electromagnetic interference. Compliance Engineering, 10, 25-39.

Silberberg, J. (1995). What can/should we learn from reports of medical devices EMI. In B. Segal (Ed.), Proceedings of a workshop on electromagnetics health care and health (pp. 10-19). Piscataway, NJ: Institute of Electrical and Electronics Engineers. Also in: Proceedings of 1995 IEEE Engineering in Medicine & Biology Society Annual Meeting and the 21st Canadian Medical & Biological Society Conference [CD-ROM web edition], (pp. 1763-1772). Piscataway, NJ: Institute of Electrical and Electronics Engineers.

Tan, K. S., & Hindberg, I. (1995). Investigation of EMI in Canadian hospitals. In B. Segal (Ed.), Proceedings of a workshop on electromagnetics health care and health (pp. 20-28). Piscataway, NJ: Institute of Electrical and Electronics Engineers. Also in: Proceedings of 1995 IEEE Engineering in Medicine & Biology Society Annual Meeting and the 21st Canadian Medical & Biological Society Conference [CD-ROM web edition], (p. 1773). Piscataway, NJ: Institute of Electrical and Electronics Engineers.

Tan, K. S., Segal, B., Townsend, D., & Stedman, J. (1995). Executive summary. In Proceedings of a round-table on electromagnetic compatibility in health care (p. 5). Spruce Grove, Canada: Care Technology.

Townsend, D. (1995). The challenges of implementing engineering solutions into national laws: Looking ahead at electromagnetic compatibility standards for medical devices. In B. Segal (Ed.), Proceedings of a workshop on electromagnetics health care and health (pp. 110-111). Piscataway, NJ: Institute of Electrical and Electronics Engineers. Also in: Proceedings of 1995 IEEE Engineering in Medicine & Biology Society Annual Meeting and the 21st Canadian Medical & Biological Society Conference [CD-ROM web edition], (p. 1757). Piscataway, NJ: Institute of Electrical and Electronics Engineers.

Vlach, P., Liu-Hinz, C., Segal, B., Skulic, B., & Pavlasek, T. (1995). The electromagnetic environment due to portable sources in a typical hospital room. Proceedings of the 1995 IEEE

Engineering in Medicine & Biology Society Annual Meeting and the 21st Canadian Medical & Biological Society Conference (pp. 683-684). Piscataway, NJ: Institute of Electrical and Electronics Engineers.

Vlach, P., Segal, B., & Pavlasek, T. (1995). The measured and predicted electromagnetic environment at urban hospitals. Proceedings of the 1995 International Symposium on Electromagnetic Compatibility, Atlanta, GA (pp. 4-7). Piscataway, NJ: Institute of Electrical and Electronics Engineers.

Witters, D., & Ruggera, P. (1994). Electromagnetic compatibility (EMC) of powered wheelchairs and scooters. Proceedings of 1994 IEEE Engineering in Medicine & Biology Society (pp. 894-895). Piscataway, NJ: Institute of Electrical and Electronics Engineers.

22

IN VITRO AND IN VIVO OBSERVATION OF DIGITAL AND ANALOG CELLULAR PHONE INTERFERENCE WITH CARDIAC PACEMAKERS

Vincenzo Barbaro, Pietro Bartolini, Andrea Donato, and Carmelo Militello

Introduction

At the annual Bioelectromagnetic Society scientific conference held in Copenhagen in June 1994, the capacity of Groupe Systemes Mobiles (GSM) cellular phones to interfere with pacemakers was dramatically brought to light by three research groups (Barbaro, Bartolini, Donato, & Militello, 1994a; Eicher et al., 1994; Joyner, Anderson, & Wood, 1994). Recently, the effect of cellular-phone-induced electromagnetic interference (EMI) on pacemakers has been further investigated in the USA (Carrillo et al., 1995; Hayes, Von Feldt, Neubauer, Christiansen, & Rasmussen, 1995a, 1995b) and Europe (Barbaro, Bartolini, Donato, Militello, Altamura, et al., 1995; Moberg & Strandberg, 1995; Wilke, Grimm, Hoffman, Funck, Maisch, 1994).

By the end of 1993, the Italian Minister of Health assigned the Istituto Superiore di Sanità the task of verifying whether the interference of cellular telephones with pacemakers might pose a public health risk. To this purpose, a series of in vitro trials was carried out at the Laboratory of Biomedical Engineering of the Istituto Superiore di Sanità, adopting an experimental model designed and constructed by the authors to simulate an implanted pacemaker (Barbaro, Bartolini, Donato, & Militello, 1994b). First, we tested digital phones working with the GSM European standard, and then those working with the analog Total Access Communication System (TACS) standard. Since no permanent malfunctioning was recorded in the pacemakers tested, we felt encouraged to perform a few ad hoc trials in vivo in order to verify the suitability of our experimental model. In vivo tests were carried out at the Cardiology Department of the San Camillo Hospital.

In order to verify the EMI effects induced by GSM phones, we conducted a series of trials at the Cardiology Department of the San Filippo Neri Hospital on a wide population of informed pacemaker patients (Barbaro, Bartolini, Donato, Militello, Altamura, et al., 1995). On that occasion we also carried out some preliminary in vivo observations with TACS apparatuses (Barbaro, Bartolini, Donato, Militello, & Santini,

1995).

It was not within the scope of the present study to rank the performance of pacemakers subject to telephone-induced EMI, so the results do not appear directly correlated with brands.

Experience with GSM Cellular Phones

Materials and Methods for GSM In Vitro Trials

Twenty seven pacemakers of widespread use on the international market were chosen as representative of the most common operating modes. Tests were carried out in a Plexiglas parallel piped (30x20x15 cm) filled with 0.9 percent saline solution (NaCl), which contained the pacemaker and its lead(s). A depression of 9x7 cm was made on the lid of the box (1 cm thick); in this area thickness was reduced to 2 mm. Two external PVC screws, perpendicular to the lid, allowed us to regulate the level of immersion of a Plexiglas plane on which the pacemaker lay. The proximity to the source of interference could thus range from 2 mm to a few centimeters. The lead(s) were fixed to the inner surface of the lid, 1 cm from the outside environment, in a configuration which simulated the actual implant as closely as possible. For the sake of repeatability, a reference grid was traced on the external surface of the lid. In order to monitor the pacemaker function, two pairs of stainless steel plaques were positioned on two opposite sides of the simulator. Each plaque was accessible from the outside through a BNC connector. The pacemaker signal was detected, with no galvanic contact, by one pair of plaques, and sent to the input of a differential amplifier (CMRR = 130 dB, input impedance > 100 MΩ). The differential output was sent to an oscilloscope (PHILIPS PM3394). Pacemaker inhibition was effected by using a signal generator simulating the electrocardiac activity (square waves 500 μs of duration) and connected to a third plaque. The fourth plaque was connected to a ground common to all instruments.

The GSM telephones used for the tests were Dynatac™ and Micro TAC™. The former has a removable dipole antenna, 14 cm long. The latter has a dual antenna system. When the primary antenna, a half wave dipole 12 cm long, is collapsed above the telephone case, there is a 1.75 cm long helical wire which forms the radiofrequency radiator with the metal in the radio case. Both systems have a maximum radiated power of 2 W. It is worth noting that the telephones using the GSM standard (a sinusoidal signal in the 900 MHz range, pulse modulated at 217 Hz) feature automatic power regulation (from a few tens mW to maximum available power), according to the distance from the base station (Déchaux & Scheller, 1993).

Each pacemaker was programmed at its minimum sensing threshold, placed inside the trunk simulator, and connected to proper lead(s) according to its stimulation and sensing configuration. Initially, the pacemaker was placed at 2 mm from the external surface and, with a robot arm positioning the telephone antenna (mid point for Dynatac, helical radiator for Micro TAC) on each area of the grid, the effect of the following operative phases was observed:

i.   switch on and connection between telephone and base station;
ii.   ringing; and
iii.   switch off and end of connection.

For each position of the antenna, two trials were made:

a.   in the presence of an inhibition signal to verify whether the interference made the pacemaker switch into asynchronous mode; and

b.   in the absence of the inhibition signal to monitor pacemaker inhibition by, or synchronization with, the interfering signal.

When EMI effects were detected, trials were repeated in order to find maximum sensing threshold, maximum pacemaker depth, and maximum distance between antenna and pacemaker at which interference persisted.

For the purpose of characterizing the GSM signal timing, the radio signal from the telephone was acquired with an oscilloscope (Tektronix mod. TDS- 684A, 1 GHz digital real time) during the three phases of the cycle.

In order to assess the validity of the experimental model, an ad hoc series of in vivo trials was conducted on seven informed, nondependent patients implanted with pacemaker models that were among those that had already been tested in vitro, with and without effect. The selection criteria we adopted accounted for different geometrical characteristics and different pacing and sensing configurations.

GSM In Vitro Results

Upon "switch-on," the telephone emits a burst (access burst) of about 321 ms duration and a sequence of three 4-burst packets. Each burst lasts approximately 546 ms, and has a repetition frequency of about 217 Hz. The distance between the first and the second packets is either 70 ms or 130 ms, and between the second and the third packets either 130 or 70 ms, respectively. The repetition frequency of this three-packet sequence is 2.2 Hz. During this handover phase, the telephone scans radio channels in search of a free one; when found, the telephone goes into standby. In the "switch-off" phase, the signal looks as in the switch-on phase but lacks the access burst.

It is worth underlining that handover duration is not rigorously constant but depends on a number of factors such as signal propagation, traffic volume, atmospheric conditions, etc. The amplitude of the signal is also variable. Under our in vitro experimental conditions, telephone power was calculated to be about 0.5 W (25% of the maximum available telephone power) on the basis of the measured signal amplitude.

When the antenna was in close proximity to the pacemakers, some sort of interference occurred in 15 of the 27 devices tested. More specifically, pulse inhibition in 3 of 27 cases, asynchronous pacing in 4 of 27 cases, and ventricular triggering in 4 of 27 pacemakers. Pulse inhibition was also observed combined with asynchronous pacing and ventricular triggering in 4 of 27 cases. Interference was observed

300

regardless of telephone model tested or sensing configuration. EMI effects were detected at a maximum distance of 13 cm. Electromagnetic interference effects occurred at maximum ventricular and atrial sensing thresholds of 4 mV and 5.6 mV, respectively and at maximum depth of about 5.5 cm with the antenna in direct contact to simulator lid and the pacemaker programmed at its minimum sensing threshold. No permanent malfunctioning or changes in the programmed parameters were detected.

It is interesting to note what happens when the connection has not succeeded. Even if there is no ringing, the GSM telephone emits a series of bursts that can last for over 20 seconds and inhibit the pacemaker during this phase.

As far as the validation of the experimental model is concerned, the results obtained under the above described experimental conditions showed good repeatability. Although the trunk simulator does not account for the nonhomogeneity of tissue, it has yielded impedance values between the pacemaker electrodes quite close to the values measured on implanted pacemakers (500 Ohm). Inhibition, synchronization, and asynchronous pacing phenomena were detected in vivo as well and were in good agreement with in vitro results.

Materials and Methods for GSM In Vivo Trials

In vivo trials were conducted to verify the GSM-induced effect on a wider population. One hundred and one informed pacemaker-implanted patients volunteered for trials. All the pacemakers were positioned in the right subpectoral site and connected to endocardial leads. Forty-three pacemaker models from 11 manufacturers were tested in all (Barbaro, Bartolini, Donato, Militello, Altamura, et al., 1995). With a robot arm keeping the telephone antenna (mid point for Dynatac, helical radiator for Micro TAC) in contact with the skin over the pacemaker and its leads, we observed the effects of the ringing phases while the heart function of the patients was continuously monitored with an electrocardiograph.

Tests were conducted following two protocols:

a.   to detect inhibition and synchronization phenomena, basic rate was programmed at 20 ppm faster than patient's spontaneous rhythm; and

b.   to detect whether the device switched to its EMI asynchronous mode, basic rate was 20 ppm slower than patient's rhythm.

GSM In Vivo Results

Inhibition, synchronization, and asynchronous pacing phenomena were detected in vivo as well. When the PMK's sensing threshold was set at a minimum and the antenna was in direct contact with the patient's chest, interference was detected in 26 out 101 patients. Pulse inhibition was observed in 10 of 101 cases, ventricular triggering with the interfering signal in 9 of 101 patients, and 4 of 101 devices turned into asynchronous pacing. Pulse inhibition occurred in combination with asynchronous pacing in 1 of 101 cases and with ventricular triggering in 2 of 101 cases.

Minimum effect length was approximately three seconds, but in six cases effects continued as long as the interfering GSM signal was on. The maximum distance at which EMI occurred was 10 cm.

Experience with TACS Cellular Phones

Materials and Methods for TACS In Vitro Trials

We used two analog cellular telephones (Hitachi mod. Butterfly, and Bosch model Cartel SX\1) of 0.6 W maximum power, working with the TACS standard. Both telephones have a dual antenna system. The TACS standard is a 900 MHz sinusoidal continuous wave, which has only a few bursts during the handover phase. TACS telephones are power regulated, just as GSM systems.

Observations were carried out on 32 pacemakers from nine manufacturers well known on the international market on the experimental model previously described. Pacemaker inhibition was induced by using a test signal waveform simulating the electrocardiac activity in compliance with the EN 50061 standard. The device was placed inside the trunk simulator at 0.5 cm (typical depth of an actual implanted pacemaker) and connected to proper lead(s) according to its stimulation and sensing configuration.

With a robot arm positioning the helical radiator (tests with collapsed antenna) or the mid point (tests with fully extracted antenna) in contact with each area of the reference grid, we observed the effects of the incoming call and of the actual ringing of the telephone. Tests were repeated varying the orientation of the antenna inside each grid area, and following two protocols:

a. in the absence of the test signal, to monitor pacemaker inhibition or synchronization with the interfering signal; and

b. in the presence of the test signal, to verify whether the interfering signal—being a continuous wave—sensitized or desensitized the pacemaker, or made it switch into its asynchronous mode (Barbaro, Bartolini, Donato, & Militello, 1996).

TACS In Vitro Results

EMI effects were recorded in 15 pacemakers out of the 32 tested; maximum distance at which effect persisted was 13 cm.

Protocol a). During the ringing phase, the worst case of pulse inhibition consisted of the skipping of three nonconsecutive beats. When the connection failed, pacemakers skipped a maximum of three beats and then resumed their normal pacing.

Protocol b). We observed three instances of desensitizing and one of sensitizing. These phenomena did not show a linear behavior, and in one case we observed a combined effect. The effects were triggered approximately seven seconds before the telephone actually started ringing.

No pacemaker switched into its EMI asynchronous mode, and in no case was there permanent malfunctioning or reprogramming. Again, effects were independent of telephone model and sensing configuration of the pacemaker.

Preliminary TACS In Vivo Trials

Preliminary TACS observations were carried out on 15 patients with 15 pacemaker models from seven manufacturers. TACS-induced EMI effects were observed in 3 of the 15 implanted patients.

Discussion and Conclusions

Since interference was always found to occur when the telephone antenna was in line with the pacemaker head, the electromagnetic field radiated by the cellular telephone can be reasonably supposed to couple with the unscreened connectors.

The effects observed are attributable to a nonlinear behavior of the pacemaker input stages. If the signal coupling with connectors reached the pacemaker input stages at an amplitude high enough to saturate them, the stages would work nonlinearly and detect the envelope of the GSM or TACS signal. The low-frequency components of the GSM envelope would then be able to induce pacemaker asynchronous pacing, ventricular triggering, and/or pulse inhibition effects; the initial bursts of the TACS signal would result in pulse inhibition, and the 900 MHz envelope would induce sensitizing and desensitizing phenomena.

The absence of effect could be the result of the following: 1) the EM field emitted does not couple with connectors; or 2) the induced voltages are attenuated, for instance by an anti-EMI capacitor. The interfering signal would therefore reach the pacemaker input stages with too low an amplitude to saturate them.

The pulse inhibition effects induced by TACS telephones are less dangerous than those observed with GSM. This is because of the TACS signal timing; the signal presents only a few bursts during the initial part of the ringing phase which can cause, at most, the skipping of three nonconsecutive beats.

Interference was observed regardless of telephone model tested or sensing configuration, (i.e., the effect was independent of the fact that leads were unipolar or bipolar); therefore, bipolar leads, currently believed to reject EMI better than unipolar leads, would not warrant immunity against the GSM and TACS signals.

Our results are strongly dependent on TACS and GSM telephone power regulation, and have been obtained at approximately 70% and 25% of the available power, respectively. In view of the fact that pacemakers were inhibited during handover and when the connection did not succeed, and considering that these occurrences are wholly unpredictable, we believe this phenomenon deserves to be thoroughly studied. With TACS, the pacemakers missed only a few nonconsecutive beats, but they were seriously inhibited by GSM (20 seconds). We also believe in the usefulness of in vitro trials because they allow us to conduct the tests in a controlled and repeatable manner, and vary programmable parameters without interfering with the patient.

References

Barbaro, V., Bartolini, P., Donato, A., Militello, C. (1994a, June). GSM cellular interference with implantable pacemakers: In vitro and in vivo observations. Paper presented at the 1994 Bioelectromagnetics Society Conference, Copenhagen, Denmark.

Barbaro, V., Bartolini, P., Donato, A., & Militello, C. (1994b, September). GSM cellular phones interference with implantable pacemakers: In vitro observations. Proceedings of the International Symposium on Biomedical Engineering, Santiago de Compostela, Spain, 275-276.

Barbaro, V., Bartolini, P., Donato, A., & Militello, C. (1996). Electromagnetic interference of analog cellular telephones with pacemakers. Pacing and Clinical Electrophysiology, 19, 1410-1418.

Barbaro, V., Bartolini, P., Donato, A., Militello, C., Altamura, G., Ammirati, F., & Santini, M. (1995). Do European GSM mobile cellular phones pose a potential risk to pacemaker patients? [Abstract] Pacing and Clinical Electrophysiology, 18, 1218-1224.

Barbaro, V., Bartolini, P., Donato, A., Militello, C., & Santini, M. (1995). GSM and TACS cellular phones can alter pacemaker function. Abstract book of the Bioelectromagnetics Society, 24-26.

Carrillo, R., Saunkeah, B., Pickets, M., Traad, E., Wyatt, C., & Williams, D. (1995). Preliminary observation on cellular telephones and pacemakers [Abstract]. Pacing and Clinical Electrophysiology, 18, 863.

Déchaux, C., & Scheller, R. (1993). Che cosa sono il GSM e il DCS? [What are the GSM and DCS systems?] ALCATEL: Prospettive di Telecomunicazioni, Rome, Italy, 1118-1127.

Eicher, B., Ryser, H., Knafl, U., Burkart, F., Naegeli, B., et al. (1994). Effects of TDMA-modulated hand-held telephones on pacemakers. Abstract book of the Bioelectromagnetics Society, 67.

Hayes, D. L., Von Feldt, L., Neubauer, S., Christiansen, J., & Rasmussen, M. J. (1995a). Does cellular phone technology cause pacemaker or defibrillator interference. Pacing and Clinical Electrophysiology, 18, 842.

304

Hayes, D. L., Von Feldt, L., Neubauer, S., Christiansen, J., & Rasmussen, M. J. (1995b). Effect of digital cellular phones on permanent pacemakers [Abstract]. Pacing and Clinical Electrophysiology, 18, 863.

Joyner, K. H., Anderson, V., & Wood, M. P. (1994). Interference and energy deposition rates from digital mobile phones. Abstract book of the Bioelectromagnetics Society, 67.

Moberg, B. L., & Strandberg, H. G. (1995). Effects of interference on pacemakers. Pacing and Clinical Electrophysiology, 5, 146-157.

Wilke, A., Grimm, W., Hoffmann, J., Funck, R., & Maisch, B. (1994). Influence of handy telephones on pacemaker function: A prospective study in 30 patients with permanent pacemakers. Cardiostimolazione, 12, 236-237.

23
INTERFERENCE OF CARDIAC PACEMAKERS IN THE NEAR FIELDS OF PORTABLE DIGITAL TRANSMITTERS
Jiri Silny

Introduction

As is generally known, implanted cardiac pacemakers are sensitive to electromagnetic fields. In most cases, unipolar pacing systems seem to be more endangered by electromagnetic interference than bipolar simulators (Hauser, Edwards, & Stafford, 1985). The electronic circuits of cardiac pacemakers are resistant to electromagnetic fields only up to a low level of radiation. In the case of stronger continuous electromagnetic interference, the pacemaker reacts by switching to the fixed rate mode. Strong, amplitude-modulated, low or high frequency electromagnetic fields can even cause a fast asynchronous pacing as well as an inhibition of the stimulation function of the pacemaker. The latter two perturbation situations must be avoided at any rate as they could be highly dangerous for the pacemaker patient.

Numerous investigations have been conducted to develop a basic understanding of the possible effects of electric, magnetic, and electromagnetic fields produced by different technical sources on implanted cardiac pacemakers (Barbaro et al., 1995; Carillo et al., 1995; Smith & Toler, 1981). All studies have focused on particular electromagnetic emissions and therefore have only limited validity for other situations.

Since the introduction of wireless hand-held phones, the user carries not only a receiver but also a transmitter close to his body. This transmitter emits relatively strong electromagnetic fields into the direct neighboring parts of the body. The emitted electromagnetic waves, with their analog, digital, or both kinds of modulation, penetrate the body where they can possibly influence existing electronic implants.

Already today cellular phones are very popular because they have enormously improved the possibility to communicate wirelessly with others, almost from every place in the world. It is probable that this technology will play an important role in the future not only in business, but also in social connections, for healthy people and even more so for the sick. Therefore this technology must be safe also for patients, especially those with a cardiac pacemaker or other electronic implants.

Recently, the interference behavior of implanted cardiac pacemakers in the proximity of cellular telephones has been investigated by several research groups in the United States, Europe, and Australia. But one cannot simply compare the results as there are a number of differences in the kind of implanted pacing system, the way of implantation in the body, and in the currently used communication technologies.

This presentation focuses on the conditions found in Europe. In Europe, cardiologists prefer to implant unipolar aggregates. In Europe, the digital GSM standard (Global System for Mobile Communication) has been established according to the Time Division Multiple Access (TDMA) procedure for the communication of hand-held wireless phones. Most cellular telephones in Europe today use the D-net in a frequency range between 890 and 960 MHz. These hand-held portables transmit the voice as well as the coding information by sending bursts of electromagnetic waves at frequencies between 890 and 915 MHz, with a maximum power of up to 2 W.

Research Activity in Germany

Possible influences of the cellular D-net phones on cardiac pacemakers have been treated recently in several German studies with different experimental approaches. Most investigations have been initialized and supported by the "Forschungsgemeinschaft Funk" (German Radio Research Association).

Hansen (1995) developed an analytical and a numerical model for calculations of impedance and voltage at the input of implanted pacemakers in a high frequency electromagnetic near field of a dipole. The aim was to find an equivalent electrical circuit which adequately simulates the transmission loss between the dipole and the pacemaker input. Irnich, Batz, Müller, and Tobisch (1995) measured the interference of cellular C-, D-, and E-net phones with 231 different cardiac pacemakers. The pacing systems, with a defined geometry, were arranged in a horizontal plain and immersed 2 cm deep into a saline solution. About 35% of the tested aggregates were disturbed by a 2 W cellular D-net phone at a distance of 10 mm from the water surface, whereas the E-net phone with a power up to 1 W did not produce any disturbances.

Meckelburg, Jahre, and Matkey (1995) investigated the disturbance threshold of 95 selected cardiac pacemakers via a calculated network of electromagnetic waves in the frequency range between 30 kHz and 2.5 GHz at the sensing input. The tests were carried out at different modulation patterns of the applied signal.

Silny (1994) is investigating the interference of cardiac pacemakers in bench tests as well as in complementary studies in vitro and in vivo. The first steps and the results are treated in the following paragraphs.

Design of the Study

In order to develop a basic understanding of the effects of microwaves from cellular D-net phones on implanted cardiac pacemakers, comparative and complementary investigations were projected (Figure 1). The first fundamental question was how the electronic circuits of the sensing input inside the pacemaker react to the application of strong high frequency signals. In the next step, the signals which are transmitted from the cellular telephone in different modes were analyzed in time and frequency range. In further bench investigations, corresponding test signals were injected into the inputs of 13 selected pacemakers to obtain the individual thresholds for oversensing in pacemakers, resulting in false inhibition or false synchronization, as well as in switching to the fixed rate mode. The transmission of the electromagnetic fields from different portables to the pacemaker input was checked in a thorax phantom. Currently, all results are being verified in patients with cardiac pacemakers which have shown a high liability to interference by wireless phones in in vitro tests.

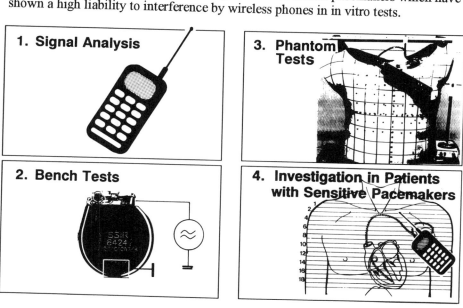

Figure 1. Design of the study

The ultimate objective of this project is to develop a reliable procedure for testing the electromagnetic compatibility of implanted cardiac pacing systems in in vitro investigations.

Behavior of the Electronic Circuit of the Pacemakers at a High Frequency Signal

The sensing part of each pacemaker requires an amplifier and a band-pass filter at its input (Figure 2). The characteristics of these circuits are adapted to the amplitude and the frequency spectrum of the intracardial electrocardiogram (IECG). As Figure 3 shows, the essential frequency components of the IECG range between 10 and 120 Hz. Therefore, the band-pass filters in the sensing channel of all pacemakers are generally adapted to this bandwidth. The electronic circuits of the cardiac pacemakers are

308

principally designed for the processing of low frequency signals. In the case of a strong high frequency signal, the semiconductor circuits behave nonlinearly. The consequence is a demodulation of the microwave signals in the input circuits of the pacemaker. In this way, during the operation of the cellular phone, a low frequency response to the emitted bursts arises within the input circuits of the pacemaker. In the sensing channel these new signal components are filtered, amplified, and processed in the same manner as the IECG, and can ultimately oversense the pacemaker.

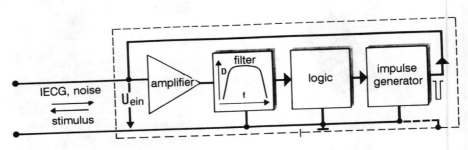

Figure 2. Equivalent circuit design of a pacemaker

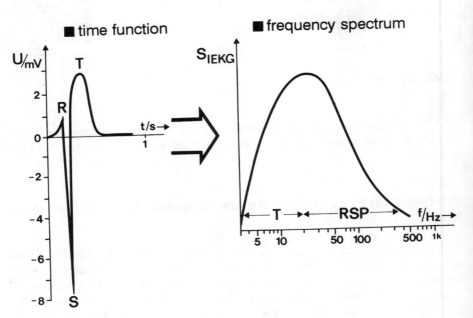

Figure 3. Intracardial ECG and its frequency spectrum

309

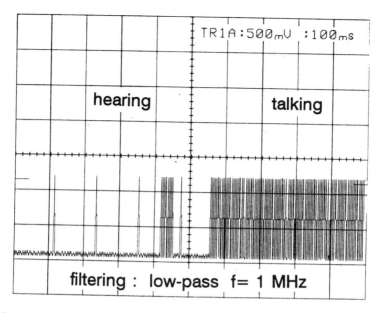

Figure 4. Burst trails emitted from a D-net cellular phone during the listening and talking phases

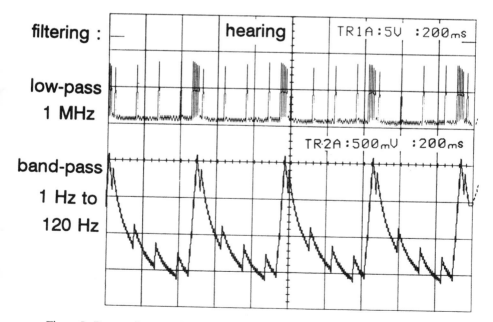

Figure 5. Burst trails transmitted from a D-net cellular phone during the listening phase and its response in the sensing channel of the pacemaker

310

Burst Sequences Transmitted from D-Net Portables

The burst sequences transmitted by the cellular telephones have a very complicated timing depending on the operating mode. After demodulation and low pass filtering at a cut frequency of 1 MHz, the tracings show dominant patterns of different frequencies during the dialing, listening, and talking phases (Figure 4). The demodulation and the band-pass filtering in the first electronic stages of the pacemaker form saw-tooth signals with a strong amplitude of a 2 Hz and a weak 8 Hz component during the dialing and listening phases (Figure 5).

Figure 6 depicts the typical burst trails during the talking phase. Here, burst frames with a frequency of 217 Hz and 8 Hz are predominant.

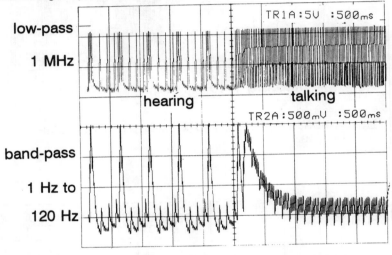

Figure 6. Burst trails emitted from a D-net cellular phone during the listening and talking phases and its responses in the sensing channel of the pacemaker

Bench Tests with Pacemakers

The purpose of these investigations was to characterize the interference performance of selected cardiac pacemakers. In this study, high frequency signals, which simulate the fields of the D-net cellular phones at different operating modes, were directly injected into the pacemaker sensing input. Table 1 shows that the oversensing thresholds vary in a wide range between 90 mV and 15,000 mV (peak to peak) in the selected pacemakers.

Older aggregates seem to be more sensitive to disturbances than recent models. As Figure 7 depicts, the lowest interference threshold results in the case of the application of a D-net signal, which is emitted during the listening or dialing phases, when a 2 Hz saw-tooth signal is predominant. The injection of a 217 Hz saw-tooth signal as it appears during the talking phase of the portable phone results in a higher oversensing threshold for the pacemaker to switch to the fixed rate mode.

Unipolar Pacemaker		Threshold of Inhibition	
Model	Manufactured	Input	Input Voltage Uss/mV
Paragon 2010	1991	A	12.500
		V	14.800
Minix 8341	1994	V	6.500
Legend 8417	1991	V	7.000
Finesse 2273 SCHA	1992	V	1.200
Astra 6	1988	V	700
Implatronic μp 61	1988	V	96

Table 1. Threshold of the inhibition of different pacemakers in the bench test

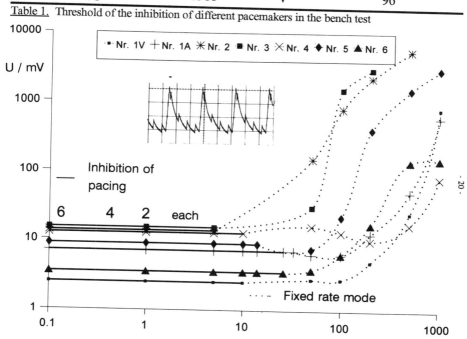

Figure 7. Oversensing of the pacemakers induced by a D-net test signal of different burst frequencies which are injected at the sensing input of the pacemaker

Phantom Tests

The interference threshold of the selected pacemaker systems was investigated in a tank model of a thorax considering:

- the unfavorable position of the cellular phone on the thorax;

- the interference threshold in comparison to the bench tests;

- the guiding of the leads; and

- the material of the leads.

The thorax phantom is made of thin plastic and modeled after the thorax of an adult male with a chest circumference of 120 cm. For the simulation of the electric and dielectric properties of the body at the frequency of 900 MHz, the phantom was filled with a specific saline solution (Hartsgrove, Kraszewski, & Surowiec, 1987). Each pacemaker and the lead were placed in the model in correspondence with the actual position of a pacemaker-lead system in the left pectoral position of a patient. Additionally, in a separate test, the guiding and the material of the lead were varied in adaptation to possible realistic situations.

Figure 8 visualizes that the maximal transmission of the electromagnetic field from the antenna of the phone to the input of the pacemaker occurs when the portable phone lays directly on the case of the pacemaker, and its antenna is oriented in the lead-direction (positions 1 and 2). For the coupling of the electromagnetic field from the phone to the pacemaker input, the guiding of the first 20 cm of the lead, beginning in the pacemaker case, is responsible.The transmission loss factor between the near electric field strength of the antenna and the voltage at the input of the pacemaker varies between 15 and 35. The factor remains constant in all investigated pacemakers for the same lead guiding, as documented in Table 2. The insulation material of the lead does not influence the transmission factor essentially.

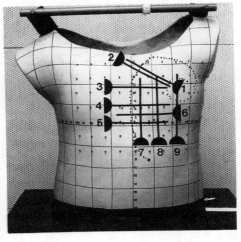

Postion	M-3200	T-D1-324
	Input voltage Upp / mV	
1	610	800
2	600	780
3	480	670
4	240	320
5	150	210
6	180	270
7	110	140
8	240	350
9	200	330

Figure 8. Voltage at the pacemaker input in dependance on the position of the cellular phone

Unipolar Pacemaker		Threshold of Inhibition	
Model	Manufactured	Input	Power W
Paragon 2010	1991	A	1.952*
		V	2.737*
Minix 8341	1994	V	528*
Legend 8417	1991	V	612*
Finesse 2273 SCHA	1992	V	18
Astra 6	1988	V	6, 12
Implatronic µp 61	1988	V	0, 12

* calculated data

Table 2. Minimal emitted power of the cellular phone situated in an unfavorable position on the thorax for the oversensing threshold of pacemakers

Investigation in Patients with Sensitive Pacemakers

The first comparative investigations in voluntary patients bearing implanted pacemakers of the same types tested in vitro have been started. The attention focuses on those pacemakers which have shown high sensitivity to interference by digital mobile transmitters. Preliminary results indicate that the oversensing thresholds of the pacemakers, as they were derived from simple models, seem to be estimated too low.

Conclusion

The interference of digital D-net cellular phones with implanted cardiac pacemakers was investigated in in vitro and in vivo studies. All tests confirmed that the pacemakers can be principally oversensed in different manners by signals emitted from portable transmitters. Bench tests showed that primarily the 2 Hz impulse component of the phone signal is responsible for the oversensing of cardiac pacemakers. These signal components are not predominant in the talking, but in the listening and dialing phases, of the phone operation. Results from investigations with a phantom confirm that the pulse modulated electromagnetic fields which are emitted by 2 W digital cellular telephones can alter the normal operation of certain unipolar cardiac pacemakers. This situation is given when the cellular phone is placed in the range of 2 to 20 cm from the highly sensitive pacemaker. The thresholds of interference depend strongly on many different factors such as the lead configuration, the location of the pacemaker system in the body, the characteristics of the individual pacemaker, and the position of the phone on the body of the patient.

It is concluded that complementary studies in pacemaker patients and in adequate models must be carried out in the future to gain the information that is necessary to rule out safety hazards in implanted pacemakers caused by electromagnetic disturbances. The majority of these tests can be conducted in in vitro investigations.

Update

Dr. Silny's most recent work has been concentrated in interference of cardiac pacemakers in the vicinity of GSM system base stations. The interference of cardiac pacemakers with the electronic fields of GSM system base stations was investigated under consideration of different realistic urban situations. The results show that the implanted cardiac pacemakers could be disturbed only within the near field of the transmitter (i.e., immediately surrounding the antenna). Therefore, it should not be allowed that patients with cardiac pacemakers enter these special areas. In the normal, everyday environment, however, there is no danger for this group of patients, either in the long distance or in the close range around the base station.

References

Barbaro, V., Bartolini, P., Donato, A., Militello, C., Altamura, G., Ammirati, F., & Santini, M. (1995). Do European GSM mobile cellular phones pose a potential risk to pacemaker patients? Pacing and Clinical Electrophysiology, 18(6), 1218-1224.

Carillo, R., Saunkeah, B., Pickels, M., Traad, E., Wyatt, C., & Williams, D. (1995). Preliminary observations on cellular telephones and pacemakers [abstract]. Pacing and Clinical Electrophysiology, 18(4), 863.

Hansen, V. (1995). Entwicklung eines Verfahrens zur Berechnung der Eingangsimpedanz von Herzschrittmachern und der durch einen externen Dipol am Herzschrittmacher-eingang erzeugten Störspannung Studie im Auftrag der Forschungsgemeinschaft Funk e.V. [Computation of the input impedance of parameters]. Bonn, Germany: Forschungsgemeinschaft Funk, 1-26.

Hartsgrove, G., Kraszewski, A., & Surowiec, A. (1987). Simulated biological materials for electromagnetic radiation absorption studies. Bioelectromagnetics, 8, 29-36.

Hauser, R. G., Edwards, L. M., & Stafford, J. L. (1985). Bipolar and unipolar sensing: Basic concepts and clinical applications. In S. S. Barold & M. D. Mount Kisco (Eds.), Modern Cardiac Pacing (pp.137-160). New York: Futura Publishing Company.

Irnich, W., Batz L., Müller, T. A. R., & Tobisch, R. (1995). Störbeeinflussung von Herzschrittmachern durch Mobilfunkgeräte [Interference of pacemakers by mobile phones]. Bonn, Germany: Forschungsgemeinschaft Funk, 1-29.

Meckelburg, H. J., Jahre, K., & Matkey, K. (1995). Störfestigkeit von Herzschrittmachern im Frequenzbereich 30 kHz bis 2,5 GHz [Electromagentic immunity of the cardiac pacemakers in the frequency range 30 kHz to 2.5 GHz]. Bonn, Germany: Forschungsgemeinschaft Funk, 1-69.

Silny, J. (1994). Störbeeinflussung von Herzschrittmachern durch die Mobilfunkanlagen im D-Netz [Interference of cardiac pacemakers by cellular phones (GSM) in D-net]. Bonn, Germany:

DeTeMobil, 1-48.

Smith, G. S., & Toler, J. C. (1981). Analysis of the coupling of electromagnetic interference to unipolar cardiac pacemakers. Medical and Biological Engineering and Computing, 9(1), 97-109.

24

STATE OF THE SCIENCE IN WIRELESS INSTRUMENT PACEMAKER AND DEFIBRILLATOR INTERFERENCE

David L. Hayes

Introduction

Electromagnetic interference (EMI) is a phenomenon that may occur when an electronic device is exposed to an electromagnetic field. Any device that has electronic circuitry can be susceptible to interference. Radiated emissions are a common source of EMI. When an electronic device is exposed to radiofrequency (RF) signals, RF energy is absorbed by the electronic circuitry and other components and the device's function may be altered. The counterpart to EMI is electromagnetic compatibility (EMC). EMC is a science of its own in which specific areas of interference are identified, circuits are redesigned, or shielding is put in place to avoid any interference potential. EMI can be inconsequential from a public health perspective (e.g., a radio causing interference on a computer screen). However, interference can sometimes result in a life threatening situation when critical care medical instruments are involved. The U.S. Food and Drug Administration (FDA) recently published a report that cites 101 instances of alleged interference that had come to the attention of the FDA between 1979 and 1993 (Silberberg, 1993). Pacemakers pose a unique problem. Not only do they often act as life-sustaining devices, they are implanted in ambulatory patients who are not confined to a hospital or other controlled environment. These people encounter electromagnetic fields in their homes, work, and other everyday environments.

EMC issues between wireless hand-held phones and pacemakers were highlighted in June 1994 when three separate papers were presented at the annual Bioelectromagnetics Society scientific conference. The studies presented consisted of both in vitro and human experimental studies in which phones were manipulated around pacemakers in an attempt to produce effects. The results indicated that interference could be produced when the phone was held very close to the pacemaker. The phones used in these studies employed a European technology that is not currently available in the United States. Nevertheless, the reports of interference generated valid questions about the technologies employed in the United States and indicated the need for further investigation.

Phone technologies that have not been investigated for this type of interaction are currently available in the United States and many more will be introduced in the near future. Wireless telephones conform to strict standards adopted by the Federal Communications Commission (FCC), setting limits on power levels and frequencies used. These factors have an important impact on the potential for interference with implantable pacemakers. In addition, medical devices such as pacemakers have voluntary standards to guide shielding specifications. There is a deficiency, however, of empirical studies investigating interactions between RF sources and pacemakers. Therefore, it is important that a scientific database be developed that identifies how implanted pacemakers react while a patient is exposed to RF fields from wireless telephones in real life situations.

Cellular Telephone Technology

All devices that transmit radio signals—such as radio broadcast towers and cellular telephones—emit RF radiation. RF radiation is electromagnetic energy emitted in the form of waves (electric and magnetic fields that vary periodically in time and space). Cellular telephones transmit voice messages by sending signals from an antenna using radio waves at frequencies between 824 and 894 megahertz (MHz). With the system currently in widespread use in the United States, digital cellular hand-held phones use up to a maximum of 0.6 W of power to transmit messages to a cellular transmitter tower. The power level used by the phone fluctuates throughout a call. At a great distance from the tower, the instrument may use the full 0.6 W. If the caller is closer to the tower, the telephone may only need 0.05 W to transmit the signal. The number of phones being used on a system at any one time also affects the power.

Cellular telephones transmit either analog or digital voice messages, depending on the type of instrument and the service available. In analog radio systems, messages are transmitted by modulating, or varying, either the wave's amplitude (height), or the frequency (number of wave crests per second). In digital systems, messages are transmitted in a series of rapid bursts, or pulses. An advantage of digital transmission is that it increases channel capacity by allowing several users to transmit messages at the same frequency at the same time. Analog signals are continuous waves; digital systems are pulsed. Because digital technology is more efficient in its use of channels, the industry is focusing on it for future use.

There are two types of digital technology relevant to the question of pacemaker/phone interaction in the United States: Code Division Multiple Access (CDMA) and Time Division Multiple Access (TDMA). In CDMA, messages are transmitted as various sequences of ones and zeroes with a special code attached so that only the intended receiver is able to decode the message. Under TDMA, data are transmitted in bursts by turning the signal on and off 50 times per second, causing it to appear to pulse. This signal is sometimes described as "pulse-modulated" RF radiation.

Global Standard for Mobile Communications (GSM) technology uses the TDMA technology and operates in a frequency range between 890 and 960 MHz. The GSM uses a 217 Hz pulse rate. The power generated by a GSM portable ranges from 0.020 W to 2 W. Generally, the power generated from European instruments is higher because of the greater distance they have to transmit to base stations; the density of base stations is lower in Europe than in the United States.

Another technology in evolution is that of 1.8 to 2.2 GHz personal communication systems (PCS). In this system, pocket-sized communication devices that use digital technology will deliver voice, data, and images. They will operate using less power than the current generation of cellular phones.

Cardiac Pacemaker Technology

In order to understand the potential effect that EMI created by cellular telephones may have on implantable devices, it is necessary to have some basic understanding of the operation of the implantable devices. Permanent pacemakers may be single-chamber, i.e. pacing only the atrium or only the ventricle, or they may be dual-chamber, i.e. pacing in both atrium and ventricle. They may also be unipolar or bipolar configuration. In a unipolar system, the insulated wire stimulating the heart utilizes a single electrode (the cathode) and the surface of the implanted pacemaker serves as the anode. In a bipolar device, bipolar leads have two electrodes in close proximity at the tip of the lead, placed within the heart chamber that is being sensed or paced. The pacemaker's sensitivity to spurious signals increases with the distance between the electrodes (the greater the distance, the more susceptible the device to EMI; see Sager, 1987). In a bipolar system, the interelectrode distance is small compared to that of a unipolar pacing system, which makes bipolar pacemakers less sensitive to EMI.

Pacemaker nomenclature is designated by the NBG code (Bernstein et al., 1987; see Table 1). In this code, Position I indicates where pacing takes place; Position II indicates where the pacemaker senses spontaneous depolarizations; Position III indicates what the pacemaker does in response to sensing. If sensing capability is absent, it does nothing (O). If sensing occurs in either chamber alone, it may inhibit (I) pacing, or trigger (T) a pacing stimulus immediately. If sensing occurs in both chambers, the response depends on the pacemaker channel and the portion of the pacemaker's timing cycle in which it takes place: in some circumstances it may inhibit pacing in one or both chambers, while in others ventricular pacing may be triggered after a suitable delay in response to atrial sensing (dual response, D); Position IV serves a dual purpose, describing two distinctly different device characteristics: the degree of programmability and the presence or absence of rate modulation (R); Position V indicates the presence of one or more active antitachyarrhythmia functions (i.e., excluding normal-rate competition or fixed-rate pacing to suppress a tachyarrhythmia), and is rarely used.

As may be seen from the definition of the NBG Code, a VVI pacemaker is one that paces the ventricle alone (V), senses only in the ventricle (V) and inhibits (Hayes, Von Feldt, Neubauer, Christiansen, & Rasmussen, 1995a) a ventricular stimulus in response to ventricular sensing. Table 2 gives specific examples of the applied NBG code.

Position:	I	II	III	IV	V
Category:	Chamber(s) paced	Chamber(s) sensed	Response to sensing	Programmability, rate modulation	Antitachyarrhythmia function(s)
	O = None A = Atrium V = Ventricle D = Dual (A+V)	O = None A = Atrium V = Ventricle D = Dual (A+V)	O = None T = Triggered I = Inhibited D = Dual (T+I)	O = None P = Simple programmable M = Multi-programmable C = Communicating R = Rate modulation	O = None P = Pacing (antitachyarrhythmia) S = Shock D = Dual (P+S)
Manufacturer's designation only:	S = Single (A or V)	S = Single (A or V)			

Note: Positions I through III are used exclusively for antibradyarrhythmia function

Adapted with permission from Bernstein et al., 1987

The NASPE/BPEG generic pacemaker code for antibradyarrhythmic and adaptive-rate pacing and antitachyarrhythmia devices.

Table 1. NBG code

Code	Meaning
VOO	Asynchronous ventricular pacemaker; no adaptive rate control or antitachyarrhythmia functions
VVI	Ventricular "demand" pacemaker with electrogram-waveform telemetry; no adaptive rate control or antitachyarrhythmia functions
DVI	Multiprogrammable AV-sequential pacemaker; no adaptive rate control
DDD	Multiprogrammable "physiologic" dual-chamber pacemaker; no adaptive rate control or antitachyarrhythmia functions
DDI	Multiprogrammable DDI pacemaker (with dual-chamber pacing and sensing but without atrial-synchronous ventricular pacing); no adaptive rate control or antitachycardia functions
VVIR	Adaptive-rate VVI pacemaker with escape interval controlled adaptively by one or more unspecified variables
DDDR	Programmable DDD pacemaker with escape interval controlled adaptively by one or more unspecified variables

AV = atrioventricular
Adapted with permission from A. D. Bernstein, EngScD
Table 2. Examples of NBG code.

Electromagnetic Interference (EMI)

For pacemakers, EMI can be defined as any interference or disturbance from electromagnetic activity which compromises normal pacemaker operation (Hayes, Maue-Dickson, & Stanton, 1993). EMI can come from a conducted or a radiated source. Conducted interference occurs when the body comes into direct contact with an electrical source (usually accidentally). This type of contact can cause permanent pacemaker damage. Radiated interference results from indirect exposure to an electromagnetic field (Sager, 1987). An electromagnetic field surrounds a moving electrical charge in a wire or an electric device, or around a device that transmits various forms of electromagnetic waves such as radio waves (Sager, 1987). Pacemaker interference may also be caused by the body itself which can cause interference through electrical signals called myopotentials, which originate in the muscle tissue. Bipolar pacemakers are less susceptible than unipolar devices because of their relatively small antenna area afforded by the electrodes located within the heart. In the overwhelming majority of cases, EMI is temporary—lasting only as long as the pacemaker is within range of the source; however, it is possible for radiated interference to cause permanent damage to a pacemaker device under certain conditions, especially within the medical environment (Warnowicz-Papp, 1983).

The development of sensing and demand pacing introduced the problem of interference from external sources such as electric and electromagnetic fields. Demand pacemakers are capable of detecting spontaneous cardiac depolarizations, and therefore, are inherently susceptible to interference that mimics the characteristics of the heart's natural activity (Denny & Jenkins, 1993). The development of dual-chamber pacing compounded the problem because when the two leads are placed perpendicularly within the two chambers, they can serve as antennas (Sager, 1987).

The factors that contribute to the effects of EMI on a pacemaker include the power of the electromagnetic field, the spectrum of the signal, the distance and positioning of the pacemaker relative to the source, the electrode configuration (unipolar or bipolar), the programmed sensing threshold, and the pacing mode (Sager, 1987). Response to EMI is described in a multitude of ways in the literature. The most frequent responses are inappropriate inhibition or triggering of pacemaker stimuli and reversion to asynchronous (noise-mode) pacing. Less frequent responses include reprogramming of pacing parameter settings and permanent damage to the circuitry or the electrode/tissue interface.

Since most responses are temporary, occurring only when the pacemaker is in proximity to the source of interference, it has been difficult for researchers and clinicians to define what kind of response is clinically significant. Also, what is clinically significant in a patient that is dependent on their pacemaker (i.e. without the pacemaker they would be symptomatic), may not be significant in a non-dependent patient who relies on a pacemaker only to improve quality of life. Moreover, there is no consensus on the actual definition of pacemaker dependency within the clinical community.

Evaluating EMI's effects on pacemaker-dependent patients differs from evaluating the majority of patients who are not pacemaker-dependent. A delay in the pacemaker's return to normal function could be serious for a dependent patient; however, many nondependent patients may not even be aware of a change in their pacemaker's function. This fact contributes to the difficulty in establishing how prevalent EMI is in pacemakers. It is often hard to determine the difference between an effect which might have been caused by EMI or which was actually a mechanical or electrical malfunction in the pulse generator or lead.

In response to an increasing number of reports of EMI in pacing, the FDA established guidelines for the design and manufacture of pacemaker devices which restricted their susceptibility to EMI through shielding. Pacemakers manufactured and sold in foreign countries follow these guidelines also (Sager, 1987). Though studies and reports of EMI before these guidelines were established offer a picture of the problems that were being encountered, it is necessary to realize that pacemakers made after FDA guidelines offer more protection from EMI.

Modern devices guard against EMI through metallic shielding, low-pass filtering, and algorithms that identify noncardiac sources of EMI. Along with shielding and noise analysis, most modern pacemakers are designed to revert to fixed-rate or asynchronous pacing if noise gets through. This reversion will occur in the presence of continuous interference signals above 10 to 15 Hz (Denny & Jenkins, 1993). Reversion causes the pacemaker's output to compete undesirably with the patient's natural cardiac rhythm. Since the pacemaker's design requires continuous interference for a certain period of time before it will revert to the fixed-rate mode, a noncontinuous or pulsed signal may cause the pacemaker's output to pause, or become inhibited, instead of reverting to the fixed-rate mode (D'Cunha, Nicoud, Pemberton, Rosenbaum, & Botticelli, 1973). There are still some interference sources such as ionizing radiation, magnetic-resonance devices, and electrocautery that bypass noise protection and can be a concern, particularly for pacemaker-dependent patients.

A 1978 report (Irnich, de Bakker, & Bisping) describes VVI and AAI pacemaker models which were popular at the time as being sensitive to amplitude modulated or pulsed fields which had frequencies in the physiological range (1 Hz to > 1 kHz). This type of interference was found near welding equipment, in electric steel plants, and in certain medical therapies such as diathermy. The authors reported that shielding and/or filtering were effective protection against other sources of high frequencies.

The Georgia Tech Research Institute in Atlanta began testing pacemakers' reactions to high power EMI in 1971. Researchers there exposed demand pacemakers (in vitro) to pulsed 450 MHz and continuous 2450 MHz (microwave) signals at varying power levels. They report that since 1977 (coinciding with the FDA's design guidelines for pacemakers in 1976), almost all pacemakers tested have been immune to interference from 450 MHz fields with field strengths as high as 220 to 260 V/m (Denny & Jenkins, 1993). Similar results were obtained in the microwave susceptibility tests. They add that some prototype pacemakers sent to their laboratory for testing were susceptible at power levels less than 200 V/m, at which time the manufacturers were notified and the designs were corrected.

There have been some studies and case reports of pacemaker interference from electromagnetic sources in recent years. The observed effects have varied—both positive and negative—and some studies that investigated devices in vitro and then in vivo found effects in the former case, but not in the latter. The accounts have been primarily about medical and diagnostic devices— electrocautery, diathermy, nuclear magnetic resonance, and nuclear magnetic resonance imaging—however, there have been a few investigations of nonmedical sources like antitheft devices and point-of-sale terminals.

Clinical Significance of Electromagnetic Interference

In an effort to categorize EMI that occurs as a result of any source, it is desirable to have some framework in which to classify the events. In an attempt to establish such a framework, a group of pacemaker experts were convened to develop a classification scheme of the clinical significance of EMI. The recommendations of this group are provided in Appendix 1.

In Vitro Assessment of Cellular Phones and Pacemaker Interference

A limited number of preliminary in vitro studies on cellular phone interference with pacemakers have been conducted to date.

Multiple in vitro studies have been performed at Siemens-ElemaAB in Sweden. In a 1992 study, they assessed three NMT phones (Strandberg, 1992)—a 450 MHz system with 15 W as a car station with movable roof antenna, a 450 MHz system with 15 W as a suitcase station with integrated antenna, and a 900 MHz system with 1 W hand-held unit with integrated antenna. A VVI pacemaker was tested in a saline tank and in the tank without solution (air only). The pacemaker was programmed to the most sensitive programmable setting. The activated phones were placed in positions near the pacemaker and various portions of the pacing lead. No interference was seen when the pacemakers were tested in the saline tank. In the air-only environment, EMI was seen with all 3 phones. The conclusion was that EMI would not be seen with the pacemaker implanted but only externally or with other electronics that were not well grounded.

In a later 1992 study from the same testing center, Vock, Strandberg, and Pillekamp assessed a unipolar VVI pacemaker under similar circumstances but with a Gigaset 952 (Siemens-Elema) TDMA mobile telephone. Again, no interference was seen when tested in a saline bath. The only EMI seen was in the air-only environment.

In 1993, another GSM phone was tested by this group (Strandberg, 1993). Three pacemakers were tested programmed to unipolar AAI, unipolar VVI, and a rate-adaptive pacemaker programmed to single-chamber mode (SSI) with the sensor in the "passive" model. Testing was again performed in saline baths—two types—and one pacemaker was tested in the air-only environment. No interference was seen in the saline baths, but the single pacemaker tested without saline was affected by EMI.

In a more recent publication, Moberg and Strandberg (1995) report on the testing of a 7.6 W Siemens type S24859-2000 GSM car telephone with an integrated antenna. Three pacemakers programmed to the most sensitive programmable setting were tested in a saline tank. Once again, no EMI occurred with the pacemakers exposed to the GSM phone during immersion in the saline bath but EMI was seen in an air-only environment. This study also included assessment of the telemetry transfer of the pacing system, and interference was seen at distances shorter than 0.4 m between the telemetry head and the telephone antenna.

In a similar Italian study (European Telecommunications Standards Institute, 1991), an unspecified number of unipolar and bipolar pacemakers were tested in a phantom model (saline bath) and then compared to those tested in the air. No inhibition was seen with the pacemakers in the phantom model. An electric field was increased to a level of 200 V/m, corresponding to 208 W transmit peak power at 0.5 m distance, and no interference was seen. During the air testing, an electric field of at least 40 V/m, corresponding to 8 W transmit peak power of a GSM phone at 0.5 m distance, was required to cause inhibition of a unipolar pacemaker. For bipolar pacemakers, it required an electrical field > 75 V/m— transmit peak power of 28 W at 0.5 m—to cause pacemaker inhibition.

Irnich and colleagues assessed 231 pacemaker models from 20 manufacturers (Irnich, Batz, Müller, & Tobisch, 1995). A pacemaker with lead was placed in a saline tank and the antenna of the mobile phone was positioned as close as possible to the pacemaker. If EMI was noted, the antenna was elevated until EMI was no longer seen. Of the 231 pacemakers tested, some form of interference occurred with 106 pacemakers (45.9%). The interference was seen with either C-net or D-net mobile phones. The authors went on to state that it would be pessimistic to think that such a high incidence of EMI would be seen in vivo, because no patient would simultaneously use C- and D-net phones. When separated into C- or D-net phones, the incidence of EMI was 30.7% and 34.2%, respectively, of all models tested. No interference was seen with the E-net phones. With respect to D-net phones, all pacemakers of six manufacturers proved to be unaffected. Of pacemakers from the eleven other manufacturers, some pacemaker models were affected and others were not. They concluded that although 27% of patients may experience interference with D-net phones, general use of cellular phones by pacemaker patients should not be questioned. They advised that a distance of 25 cm is sufficient to guarantee integrity of the pacemaker with respect to hand-held mobile phones. In addition they advised that larger transportable phones should have a distance of approximately 0.5 meter from the pacemaker.

An Italian study (Barbaro, Bartolini, Donato, & Militello, 1994) tested GSM cellular phone interference with implantable pacemakers in vitro and in vivo. Results from the same group's in vivo studies are described in the following section (Barbaro et al., 1995). Approximately thirty pacemakers were tested in vitro. The outcome parameters were listed as asynchronous, synchronization, and inhibition. The effects occurred when the phones were in close proximity to the pacemaker. No information was supplied on the power generated by the instrument. In vitro testing revealed no interference in 48.1%, asynchronous pacing in 18.5%, synchronization in 11.1%, and some combination of inhibition, asynchronous, and synchronization in 22.2%.

A large-scale in vitro study is currently underway at the Center for the Study of Wireless Electromagnetic Compatibility at the University of Oklahoma and there are no published outcomes to date (H. Grant, personal communication). While the results from this in vitro study should help to determine whether the presence of a public health risk exists and the extent of that risk, the study was also designed to identify the possible mitigation approaches, and what implementation measures could be taken to mitigate the risk. The objectives of the in vitro study are to determine if there are interactions between cellular phones and pacemakers, as well as to investigate the conditions which might promote these interactions and increase our understanding of the mechanism for the interaction.

In Vivo Assessment of Cellular Phones and Pacemaker Interference

In vivo data about pacemaker response to cellular telephones are also limited at this time.

Carillo and colleagues (Carillo et al., 1995) were among the first to perform in vivo investigations in the United States. They reported testing 59 nondependent patients with digital cellular phones that transmitted in the 800 to 900 MHz range. Pacemakers were programmed to a more sensitive level prior to testing. A total of 170 tests were performed, with a mean of 2.8 tests per patient. Each patient was tested by placing the phone in the talking position and then moving the telephone over the pacemaker while constantly monitoring the patient electrocardiographically. No interference was detected with the phone in the talking position. Interference was seen in 21 patients (35.6%), 39 tests (22.9%), and 19 pacemakers models (54%) when the phone was held over the pacemaker. The type of interference observed was inhibition in 21 tests, asynchronous pacing in 14 tests, atrial channel tracking of interference in 12, and ventricular safety pacing in five. Of the 39 positive tests, eight were in the unipolar configuration and 31 were in the in bipolar configuration.

Hayes and colleagues also reported pilot studies with analog (Hayes, Von Feldt, Neubauer, Christiansen, & Rasmussen, 1995a) and digital (Hayes, Von Feldt, Neubauer, Christiansen, & Rasmussen, 1995b) cellular phones. In the first study, 30 patients were tested with analog phones: two hand-held phones operating to a maximum of 0.6 W and one transportable phone operating to maximum of 3 W. All three phones operated in the 824 to 846 MHz range. Of the 30 nondependent patients tested, 24 patients had pacemakers, eight had implantable cardioverter defibrillators (ICD), and 2 patients had both. There were 19 pacemaker models from four manufacturers and two varieties of ICDs. Testing consisted of placing the mouthpiece and earpiece of the activated phone over the pacemaker as well as performing standard trans-telephonic transmission via the cellular telephone. All testing was performed during continuous electrocardiographic monitoring. The pacemaker was interrogated at the end of testing to document that there had not been any reprogramming of the pacemaker. No interference or reprogramming was seen with any device during any of the maneuvers.

In the study performed with digital phones (Hayes et al., 1995b), 30 nondependent patients were tested with four time division multiple access (TDMA) cellular phones. Three of the phones were hand-held with pulsed power of 0.6 W and one was transportable with power output of 3 W. Pacemaker testing was conducted during continuous electrocardiographic monitoring and after the pacemaker had been programmed to the most sensitive programmable value and a pacing rate that would assure pacing. Pacemakers that were polarity programmable were tested in both unipolar and bipolar configurations. The phones were tested in a normal talking position and with the mouthpiece, earpiece, and base of the antenna over the pacemaker at approximately 1 to 2 centimeters from the chest wall. Pacemakers tested were from five different manufacturers. There were nine single-chamber and 21 dual-chamber pacemakers tested, of which 8 were tested bipolar only, three unipolar only, and 19 tested in both. Of the 30 pacemakers tested, no interference was seen with seven dual-chamber and seven single-chamber pacemakers tested. With the other 16 pacemakers, interference was seen and categorized as tracking interference on the atrial lead in 55 tests, oversensing in seven, undersensing in five, reversion to magnet mode in eight, and ventricular safety pacing in three tests. Tracking interference on the atrial lead was the most common type of interference seen; interference was most likely to occur when the pacemaker was tested with the base of the antenna over the pacemaker and interference was more likely to occur with the 3 W transportable phone. A total of 32 positive tests were seen during unipolar configuration and 45 positive tests were during bipolar configuration.

Naegeli and colleagues (Naegeli, Deola, Eicher, & Osswald, 1995) performed 672 provocation tests in 39 patients with four different phones: three hand-held phones with power output of 2 W and one portable model with output of 8 W. Six pacemaker models from four manufacturers were tested. Tests were performed during dialing and during talking. Pacemakers were set to different sensitivity levels in the unipolar and bipolar mode and the mobile phones were placed directly over the pacemaker or the lead tip. In seven patients (18%), 20 (3%) reproducible episodes of interference were seen. In 22 dual-chamber pacemakers, atrial oversensing was observed in six and ventricular oversensing with pacemaker inhibition in three. In 17 patients with VVI pacemakers, inhibition was induced in 11 tests. Interference occurred with phones < 10 cm from the pacemaker. Interference was more frequent with the high output 8 W phone than the hand-held models. In the bipolar mode, ventricular inhibition never occurred. In the unipolar mode, pacemaker inhibition was induced in 14 tests, nine with maximum sensitivity and five defined as having "adjusted" sensitivity. No dysfunction of sensors of rate-responsive pacing systems was noted. They summarized by stating that, of the mobile phones tested, inappropriate tracking occurred in 1.4 percent of otherwise normally functioning pacemakers and potentially dangerous pacemaker inhibition occurred in 2.1%. However, permanent pacemaker dysfunction or changes in the programmed parameters were not observed.

In another recently reported study, Grimm, Wilke, Hoffmann, Funck, and Maisch (1995) tested 30 patients with D-net, 2.5 W hand-held phones. Thirteen patients had single-chamber pacemakers and 17 dual-chamber pacemakers; 17 were unipolar and 13 were bipolar. Each patient was asked to make several calls with the hand-held phone during electrocardiographic monitoring. Calls were repeated after pacemaker programming to minimum ventricular rate of 90 bpm and previous sensitivity and then to minimum rate of 90 bpm and maximum sensitivity without T-wave oversensing. No reprogramming or reversion to VOO mode was seen. Two of 30 patients (3%) reproducibly showed intermittent pacemaker inhibition, both being unipolar configuration. Both were asymptomatic and neither were pacemaker-dependent.

Interference with rate-responsive pacemakers at peak field strengths of approximately 80 V/m was reported by Joyner, Anderson, and Wood (1994). In abstract format, they also state that no interference effects were seen in vivo when a simulated peak digital signal of 25 W was generated 20 cm from the patient's chest.

Eicher and colleagues at Swiss Telecom PTT (Eicher et al., 1994) investigated the effects of TDMA-modulated, hand-held telephones. Thirty-nine pacemaker patients with unipolar and bipolar electrode configurations were exposed to hand-held phones and their pacemakers were tested for speeding up and inhibition. There was some discrepancy in the reports about whether or not the pacemakers were all implanted in the patients. The effects they reported occurred when the phones were placed directly over the pulse generators.

Barbaro and colleagues assessed 101 patients with 43 pacemaker models from 11 manufacturers with two European GSM phones of 2 W power (Barbaro et al., 1995). When programmed to the most sensitive setting and with the antenna of the phone in direct contact with the patient's chest, interference was seen with 26 implanted pacemakers. Types of interference included inhibition of the pacemaker in 10, ventricular triggering from interference sensed on the atrial sensing circuit in 9 of 46 pacemakers in the DDD or VDD pacing mode, and asynchronous pacing in 4 of 52 cases. Pacemaker inhibition and asynchronous pacing was seen in one patient and inhibition and ventricular triggering in two cases. The duration of the interference was described as having a minimum effect for approximately three seconds but in six patients it lasted for the duration of the interfering GSM signal. No pacemaker reprogramming was seen. Interference was detected at a maximum distance of 10 cm with the pacemaker programmed to the most sensitive setting available. When the antenna of the phone was in direct contact with the patient's skin over the implant site, interference occurred at maximum ventricular and atrial sensitivities of 4 mV and 2.5 mV, respectively.

The difficulty in evaluating these data is that most are not published in manuscript form and there are some discrepancies in the data reported. In addition, study methods vary considerably. Although there is some indication of interference which deserves further investigation, these studies are far from comprehensive. There is insufficient information to allow definitive safety guidelines to be issued. Furthermore, it is essential to point out the differences between a GSM digital system which is prevalent in Europe, Asia, and Australia (and under which the studies presented at the Bioelectromagnetic Society meeting were conducted), and the frequency modulated systems used in the United States. Aside from the DTX mode used exclusively in the GSM, the systems operate with different pulse rates and maximum power levels.

Defining and Solving the Issues of Implantable Devices and Cellular Phone Technology

Investigations of potential interference from cellular phones and implantable mechanical devices are underway in multiple clinical centers in the United States and Europe. Members of the cellular phone industry and pacemaker industry are also conducting independent in vitro studies or collaborating with clinical centers on in vitro and/or in vivo studies. An independent research group, Wireless Technology Research (WTR), LLC in Washington, DC, has a major interest in research activities involving wireless technology and defining whether any potential health risks exist (Scientific Advisory Group on Cellular Telephone Research, 1994).

WTR has applied a three phased approach to investigate the implanted device and wireless technology interference issue. The first phase is to conduct clinical studies to assess if and how implanted devices and phones interact in vivo and assess other relevant information.

The second phase is to assess the clinical and public health significance of EMI in pacemakers and defibrillators through a panel of experts (Appendix 1).

The third phase includes risk management research and making recommendations for corrective interventions if necessary. This will include devising possible intervention strategies, coordinating clinical and in vitro testing regarding intervention, and making recommendations as needed.

The program for this multi-center clinical study has been divided into three tiers. The first is the development of the protocol for the clinical study. A multi-disciplinary committee, coordinated by the WTR, has held numerous meetings, conducted pilot tests, and edited protocol drafts in an effort to gather information and complete the collaborative development of the protocol. The second tier is the implementation of the clinical study and the analysis and reporting of the results. The third tier includes the interpretation of the results of the clinical study. An expert panel of cardiologists will be convened to advise on the clinical significance and the public health impact of specific types of pacemaker interference.

The goal of this study is to provide comprehensive, clinically relevant information on patients with pacemakers using hand-held wireless telephones that will serve as a foundation for future investigations. This study will also assist those responsible for making decisions on regulatory considerations, pacemaker and cellular telephone user guidance, and manufacturing recommendations. The study will assess the prevalence of interference in patients with implanted pacemakers set at their clinically appropriate settings while using hand-held, wireless telephones. Testing will be conducted under conditions that simulate daily life telephone usage.

The study population will be selected from patients of all ages presenting at the pacemaker testing center for routine pacemaker checkups. The study is seeking to enroll approximately 1200 patients. All patients with implantable pacemakers who present at the pacemaker testing centers will be considered for inclusion. All patients including pacemaker-dependent and nondependent patients will be allowed to participate in the study. The patient's condition will be classified and noted on a standardized data collection form. Pacemaker dependency will be defined for the purpose of this study as a patient with an implanted pacemaker who does not exhibit an intrinsic ventricular rhythm within 30 seconds following the pacemaker being set at the lowest programmable rate in the VVI mode.

Patients with implanted defibrillators will be excluded from this study but other pilot studies investigating ICDs and potential interference from cellular phones are planned or underway (see below).

The patients will be tested with a series of wireless technologies, both those available currently (analog and TDMA) and those soon to be available in the United States (PCS and CDMA). The patient will be tested with the phones held in normal use position and in a series of movements over the pacemaker. The phones will be operated in the test mode programmed to highest power and in actual transmission during dialing and ringing. The patients will be monitored electrocardiographically throughout the testing procedure to determine primary responses of the pacemaker to any EMI, as well as the patient's clinical responses.

Pilot Studies With Implantable Cardioverter Defibrillators

ICDs are devices that detect abnormal rapid rhythm disturbances of the lower chamber of the heart, the ventricle, and electrically treat by means of cardioversion or defibrillation. The specific rhythm disturbances treated by ICDs are ventricular tachycardia and ventricular fibrillation—both are potentially life-threatening rhythm disturbances. There is a theoretic risk that electromagnetic interference could interfere with detection of the abnormal rhythm and fail to electrically terminate the abnormal rhythm disturbance. Alternatively, the electromagnetic interference could be interpreted by the device as an abnormal rhythm disturbance resulting in inappropriate electrical discharge, cardioversion or defibrillation, in an asymptomatic patient with a normal rhythm.

These potential clinical scenarios are as much or more of a potential health risk as interference with permanent pacemakers.

To date there is really no clinical information published in abstract or manuscript form regarding interference with ICDs from cellular telephones. Hayes et al. reported on a small number of patients tested with analog cellular telephones and no interference was seen. The real concern is, once again, digital cellular phones. Studies are underway at multiple clinical centers.

Public Safety Significance

The clinical study currently underway under the auspices of WTR, and in coordination with the in vitro study at the Center for the Study of Wireless Electromagnetic Compatibility at the University of Oklahoma, should provide much needed information regarding the potential public safety significance of cellular phone influence on permanent pacemakers. The studies noted previously (Barbaro et al., 1995; Carillo et al., 1995; Eicher et al., 1994; Grimm et al., 1995; Hayes et al., 1995a; Hayes et al., 1995b; Joyner et al., 1994; Naegeli et al., 1995) raise the issue of public safety as well as more recent case reports that are just beginning to emerge in the medical literature (Yeşil, Bayata, Postaci, & Aydin, 1995). The multi-center clinical study along with the in vitro study will hopefully provide definitive answers to the following questions:

1.   Is there a public health risk posed by the interaction between pacemakers and wireless instruments?

2.   If yes, what is the extent of the risk?

3.   What are the appropriate interventions to mitigate that public health risk?

4.   What is the appropriate implementation strategy for those interventions?

Simultaneously, clinical engineering groups are attempting to develop standards to minimize interference with medical devices (Bostrom, 1991). As early as 1991, a working group was established to develop standards by considering the potential problems of electromagnetic interference with medical devices (Bostrom, 1991). It is believed that there will never be a universal technical solution for all safety problems, but that standards and type-testing will reduce the incidence of medical device malfunction due to electromagnetic interference.

Summary

No definitive information exists at this time regarding the potential public health risk posed by the interaction between pacemakers and/or implantable cardioverter defibrillators and wireless instruments. Studies to date have clearly demonstrated interference in selected patients with permanent pacemakers, but the data to date are inconclusive and fraught with discrepancies.

At this time, patients are being told that the risk of interference from digital cellular technology has not yet been determined and no definitive clinical answer can be given to questions regarding interference. As a general rule, it is wise for the patient to avoid carrying their activated phone in a breast pocket overlying the pacemaker. In addition, pacemaker-dependent patients, (i.e., patients that are theoretically at the most risk from interference), should take special caution until more definitive information is available.

It is hoped that clinical information from both the multi-center clinical study being performed via WTR and the in vitro study at the University of Oklahoma should be available by Spring 1996.

Update

David L. Hayes is still the Director of the Pacing Laboratory and a cardiologist at the Mayo Clinic in Rochester, MN, United States.

Since the presentation of this manuscript, Dr. Hayes, in cooperation with two other clinical sites and Wireless Technology Research, LLC, completed the multi-center clinical study of interference with cardiac pacemakers by cellular telephones. The results of this study were published in *The New England Journal of Medicine* (Hayes, D. L, Wang, P. J., Reynolds, D. W., et al, N Engl J Med 1997;336(21)1473-9).

The three sites involved in the testing procedures were: Mayo Clinic, Rochester, MN; New England Medical Center, Boston, MA; and University of Oklahoma Health Sciences Center, Oklahoma City, OK. Using Good Clinical Practices, Good Epidemiology Practices, and Good Laboratory Practices, 980 patients were electrocardiographically monitored for interference while exposed to five wireless phone technologies: analog, NADC, TDMA-11 Hz, PCS-1900, and CDMA. The phones were positioned at the patient's ipsilateral ear and maneuvered through a series of positions 1-2 cm over the pacemaker. Throughout testing, all phones operated in test mode and at their maximum power. The NADC phone was also tested using actual transmission.

Data were collected from three sources: electrocardiogram output, pacemaker's programmed settings, and clinical symptoms reported by patients. Interference was further evaluated by the definitions of clinical significance previously defined. Of 5533 phone exposures, the incidence of any interference was 20.0% and the incidence of symptoms was 7.2%. No pacemaker reprogramming was detected. The incidence of clinically significant interference was 6.6%, and there was no clinically significant interference at the ear position.

The results indicate that although clinically significant interference can occur between wireless phones and cardiac pacemakers, this interference does not occur during normal use as represented by the ear position.

References

Barbaro, V., Bartolini, P., Donato, A., & Militello, C. (1994). GSM cellular phones interference with implantable pacemakers: In vitro and in vivo observations. Paper presented at the annual meeting of the Bioelectromagnetics Society, Copenhagen, Denmark.

332

Barbaro, V., Bartolini, P., Donato, A., Militello, C., Altamura, G., & Ammirati, F. (1995). Do European GSM mobile cellular phones pose a potential risk to pacemaker patients? PACE, 18, 1218-1224.

Bernstein, A. D., Camm, A. J., Fletcher, R. D., Gold, R. D., Rickards, A. F., Smyth, N. P. (1987). The NASPE/BPEG generic pacemaker code for antibradyarrhythmic and adaptive-rate pacing and antitachyarrhythmia devices. PACE,10(4, Part 1), 794-799.

Bostrom, U. (1991). Interference from mobile telephone - A challenge for clinical engineers! Clinical Engineering Update, 10, 1-2.

Carillo, R., Saunkeah, B., Pickets, M., Traad, E., Wyatt, C., & Williams, D. (1995). Preliminary observations on cellular telephones and pacemakers [Abstract]. PACE, 18, 863.

D'Cunha, G. F., Nicoud, T., Pemberton, A. H., Rosenbaum, F. F., & Botticelli, J. T. (1973). Syncopal attacks arising from erratic demand pacemaker function in the vicinity of a television transmitter. American Journal of Cardiology, 31, 789-791.

Denny, H. W., & Jenkins, B. M. (1993, April). EMC history of cardiac pacemakers. EMC Test & Design, 33-36.

European Telecommunications Standards Institute. (1991). Potential GSM hazards on cardiac pacemakers (Technical Report 61/91:1-6). Sophia Antipolis, France: Author.

Grimm, W., Wilke, A., Hoffmann, J., Funck, R., & Maisch, B. (1995). Interactions between handy phones and pacemaker function in patients with permanent pacemakers [Abstract]. Journal of the American College of Cardiology, 66A.

Hayes, D. L., Maue-Dickson, W., & Stanton, M.S. (1993). Dictionary of cardiac pacing electrophysiology and arrhythmias. Miami Lakes, FL: Peritus Corporation.

Hayes, D. L., Von Feldt, L., Neubauer, S., Christiansen, J., & Rasmussen, M. J. (1995a). Does cellular phone technology cause pacemaker or defibrillator interference [Abstract]? PACE, 18, 842.

Hayes, D. L., Von Feldt, L., Neubauer, S., Christiansen, J., & Rasmussen, M. J. (1995b). Effect of digital cellular phones on permanent pacemakers [Abstract]. PACE, 18, 863.

Irnich, W., Batz, L., Müller, R., & Tobisch, R. (1995). Störbeeinflussung von Herzschrittmachern durch Mobilfunkgeräte [Interference of pacemaker parameters (function) by mobile phone/transmitters]. Herz-schrittmacher, 15, 5-20.

Irnich, W., de Bakker, J. M. T., & Bisping, H. J. (1978). Electromagnetic interference in implantable pacemakers. PACE, 1(1), 52-61.

Joyner, K. H., Anderson, V., & Wood, M. P. (1994, June). Interference and energy deposition rates from digital mobile phones. Bioelectromagnetics Society Abstract Book, 67.

Moberg, B. L., & Strandberg, H. G. (1995). Effects of interference on pacemakers. European Journal of Cardiac Pacing and Electrophysiology, 5, 146-157.

Naegeli, B., Deola, M., Eicher, B., & Osswald, S. (1995). Pacemaker dysfunction caused by interference with Natel-D mobile phones [Abstract]. PACE, 18, 842.

Sager, D. P. (1987). Current facts on pacemaker electromagnetic interference and their application to clinical care. Heart Lung, 16(2), 211-221.

Siemens Elema A. B. (1992, January). Investigation of pacemakers relative to mobile phones Sweden: Strandberg, H.

Siemens Elema A. B. (1992, September). Investigation: EMC of pacemakers to cordless telephones DECT. Sweden: Vock, J., Strandberg, H., & Pillekamp, H.

Siemens Elema A. B. (1993, April). Investigation of pacemakers relative to GSM mobile phones. Sweden: Strandberg, H.

Scientific Advisory Group on Cellular Telephone Research. (1994). Potential public health risks from wireless technology: Research agenda for the development of data for science-based decision making. (Available from Wireless Technology Research, L.L.C., 1711 N St., NW, Washington, DC 20036).

Silberberg, J. (1993). Performance degradation of electronic medical devices due to electromagnetic interference. Compliance Engineering, 10, 25-39.

Warnowicz-Papp, M. A. (1983). The pacemaker patient and the electromagnetic environment. Clinical Progress in Pacing and Electrophysiology, 1(2), 166-76.

Yeşíl, M., Bayata, S., Postaci, N., & Aydin, Ç. (1995). Pacemaker inhibition and asystole in a pacemaker-dependent patient [Abstract]. PACE, 18, 1963.

Appendix

Clinical Significance of Electromagnetic Interference

On June 7, 1995, a panel of experts in the field of cardiac pacing were convened to discuss the clinical significance of various forms of electromagnetic interference (EMI). Panelists included: David L. Hayes, MD, Mayo Clinic, Rochester, MN, Michael J. Osborn, MD, Mayo Clinic, Rochester, MN, Jay Gross MD, Montefiore Medical Center, Bronx, NY, Paul Wang, MD, New England Medical Center, Boston, MA, Alan D. Bernstein, Newark Beth-Israel Hospital, Newark, NJ, Marleen Irwin, RCPT, Grey Nuns Hospital, Edmonton, Alberta, Canada.

Clinical significance was considered in a three-tiered scheme:
Class I: clinical responses that are definitely be clinically significant;
Class II: clinical responses that are probably clinically significant;
Class III: clinical responses that would not be clinically significant.

Inhibition
I. Definitely Clinically Significant
    A   Symptomatic bradycardia (any symptoms should be considered, i.e. syncope, pre-syncope, dyspnea, chest pain, etc.)
    B.   ≥ 3.0 second pause
    C.   Ventricular tachycardia
    D.   Asymptomatic ventricular tachycardia
II. Probably Clinically Significant
    A.   < 3.0 second pause - asymptomatic
    B.   Asymptomatic bradycardia
    C.   One beat inhibition*
    D.   Rhythms slower than the programmed lower rate limit
III. Probably not Clinically Significant
    A.   Random ventricular safety pacing

*It is realized that the length of a pause that results from one beat inhibition will depend on the patient's paced rate. For one beat inhibition to result in a 3 second [3000 ms] pause, (I-B), the patient would have to be programmed to a lower rate of 40 ppm [1500 ms x 2]. However, it is possible that 'one beat inhibition' could result in an event that may be clinically significant or one that is not clinically significant depending on the paced rate and the degree of the patient's pacemaker dependence. For example, if the patient were totally pacemaker-dependent, i.e. had no intrinsic escape rhythm, and was paced at a rate of 40 ppm, one-beat inhibition would result in a 3 second pause.

Noise reversion
I. Definitely Clinically Significant
    A.   Induction of ventricular tachycardia, symptomatic or asymptomatic,

secondary to competitive pacing
    B.   Symptomatic bradycardia
II.   Probably Clinically Significant
    A.   Symptomatic asynchronous behavior
III.   Probably not Clinically Significant
    A.   Asymptomatic asynchronous behavior
    B.   Asymptomatic bradycardia

Undersensing

I.   Definitely Clinically Significant
    A.   Induction of symptomatic arrhythmias
    B.   Induction of ventricular tachycardia, symptomatic or asymptomatic
    C.   Induction of supraventricular tachycardia and/or reentrant tachycardia requiring intervention
II.   Probably Clinically Significant
    A.   Induction of supraventricular tachycardia and/or reentrant tachycardia NOT requiring intervention
III.   Probably not Clinically Significant
    A.   Isolated premature ventricular contractions
    B.   Isolated competitively paced beats
    C.   Asymptomatic functional non-capture, i.e. pacing in the physiological refractory period

Triggering*

I.   Definitely Clinically Significant
    A.   Symptomatic bradycardia (any symptoms should be considered, i.e. syncope, pre-syncope, dyspnea, chest pain, etc.)
    B.   Symptomatic tachycardia (any symptoms should be considered, i.e. syncope, pre-syncope, dyspnea, chest pain, etc.)
    C.   Asymptomatic ventricular tachycardia
    D.   Induction of supraventricular tachycardia and/or reentrant tachycardia requiring intervention
    E.   Symptomatic tachycardia due to abnormal adaptive-rate behavior when the abnormal behavior is secondary to EMI
II.   Probably Clinically Significant
    A.   Induction of supraventricular tachycardia and/or reentrant tachycardia NOT requiring intervention
    B.   Palpitations
III.   Probably not Clinically Significant
    A.   Isolated premature ventricular contractions
    B.   Isolated competitively paced beats

(* Triggering was used to encompass both 'triggering' and 'tracking'. This would therefore include abnormalities induced by EMI in pacemakers programmed to the VVT or AAT modes. Triggering is also expanded for the purposes of this classification to include triggering or pacing by a sensor-driven device, i.e. activation of the sensor in a rate-adaptive pacemaker by EMI resulting in an inappropriate pacing rate for the patient's level of activity.)

Permanent reprogramming
I.   Definitely Clinically Significant
      A.   Any change in programmed parameters

Runaway pacemaker
I.   Definitely Clinically Significant
      A.   This event would always be considered a Class I event

Device damage
I.   Definitely Clinically Significant
      A.   Any permanent damage to the pacemaker would be considered a Class I event

Tissue damage
I.   Definitely Clinically Significant
      A.   Permanent or temporary increase in pacing and/or sensing thresholds

25

UNLOCKING THE SECRETS OF HEART STOPPING PHONE CALLS

Roger G. Carrillo

Introduction

Wireless technology is a rapidly growing science. Industry sources report 50 million cellular telephone subscribers in 1995, a number which is expected to double by the

transmitters has brought about a new
ctromagnetic field of the antenna to
of EMI (electromagnetic interference)
4 to the present day. In summary, the
tions cellular telephones may produce
wth in wireless communications with
to analyze this interaction. Through
re have been able to identify certain
ication of this knowledge will enable
r future technology to interact with
edical electronics could be improved.
it by predicting which patients are at
unctions may occur.
nts a cooperative labor of physicians
Ir. Q. Balzano and Mr. Oscar Garay.

We have conducted two types of studies: clinical and laboratory. In the clinical study, the methodology involved the use of 65 volunteer patients who are not pacemaker-dependent. They were asked to perform a test with a cellular telephone. Depending upon their time, they were subjected to one or more tests, up to a number of nine, for a mean of 2.8 tests per patient. We have done 211 tests. Ten cellular telephones were used, including analog and digital cellular telephone technologies. The digital technology tested was Time Domain Multiple Access (TDMA), e.g., Global System Mobile Communications (GSM), Motorola Integrated Radio System (MIRS), and the North American Digital System (NADC). The cellular telephones transmitted in a range of 800 to 900 MHZ. The maximum power varied from 0.6 to 3.0 W. Both hand-held and transportable units were evaluated. The procedure involved a pre-test analysis by interrogating the pacemaker to verify proper function. Then it was reprogrammed to the most clinically sensitive settings in both atrial and ventricular channels. During ECG monitoring, two positions were tested: 1) with the telephone held toward the ear; and 2) with the antenna of the telephone held in close proximity to the pulse generator. If a dysfunction was observed, the test was repeated and was only called interference if it was reproduced two or more times. Then, threshold distances were obtained and orientation of the antenna was recorded. The interference was categorized in four areas. Inhibition of pacemaker function was noted in 25 tests. P-wave tracking of electromagnetic noise was seen in 17 cases. Asynchronous pacing was seen in 15 tests and activation of a ventricular safety pacing was seen in five tests. The most significant clinical interaction was inhibition of pacemaker function, followed by P-tracking of electromagnetic noise. These interactions have the potential to cause symptoms varying from syncope to discomfort. Both asynchrony and activation of ventricular safety pacing have less clinical significance.

The second group of studies were conducted in the laboratory. They involved the use of pacemakers with leads submerged in a saline tank. Constant electrocardiographic monitoring was performed. Cellular telephones were approached to the pacemaker. Antennas of cellular telephones were rotated on the horizontal plane at 15° intervals and in the vertical plane at 1 cm intervals. Pacemaker dysfunction end points were defined as inhibition of pacemaker or P-wave tracking of electromagnetic noise. A label of interference was assigned only if the event was reproducible.

Discussion

We will discuss in detail some preliminary observations obtained in our studies.

Power of Cellular Telephone

When comparing interference patterns and cellular telephones of different powers, we observed a direct correlation between frequency of interference and transmitting power. As we see in Figure 1, comparing the North American Digital System of .6 W (hand-held unit) to the same digital system of 3 W, the frequency of interference was significantly different.

Cellular Telephone Peak Output

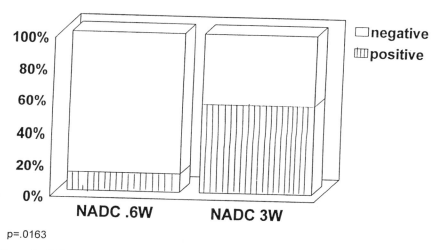

p=.0163

Figure 1. Cellular telephone peak output

Modulation or the Transmission Pattern

The cellular telephones transmit signals in two different patterns: analog or digital. Current digital transmitting patterns are TDMA or CDMA. We tested analog and TDMA cellular telephones. No interaction was seen with the analog system, but production of interaction was seen with the TDMA system. All TDMA telephones—GSM, MIRS, and NADC—were able to produce interference. Due to the small sample size, we could not make statistical conclusions on their frequency of interference. The difference between the analog and the TDMA system is that the latter have a burst transmission. In other words, the pattern of transmission is based on pulses or a train of pulses. For the digital systems that we tested (TDMA), GSM cellular telephones have pulses in the range of 217 Hz. There is another group of pulses in the GSM system, called DTX, designed to save battery power, that are 4 Hz. In the MIRS system, the pulses have a frequency of 11 Hz, and in the NADC, the pulses have a frequency of 50 to 60 Hz.

It should be noted that we did not test the ringing or dialing mode—this adds another train of pulses to both analog and digital systems. Since the duration of both dialing and ringing is not prolonged enough to cause a sustained electrocardiographic pause, we decided to concentrate on the transmitting mode of the telephone.

Antenna

The antenna of cellular telephones is the most significant source of electromagnetic energy. Studies of near-field antennas reveal the presence of electric and magnetic fields (E-Field and H-field). They are related; where the highest magnetic field is found, the electric field has the lowest value. Measurements of the fields revealed different morphology and intensity for different models. We have measured the E-field and the H-field on tested cellular telephones. Furthermore, we have proven that the H-field is responsible for producing more interaction when compared with the E-field.

Orientation of Antenna

Positioning of the H-field over the sensitive part of the pacemaker is a critical factor for production of interference. Clinical studies reveal that both unipolar and bipolar pacemakers have the same rate of susceptibility to cellular telephone interference. Laboratory studies have confirmed that the epoxy header of the pacemaker is more sensitive to interference than the leads or metal case. The metal case is highly shielded, with an attenuation factor of 200 decibels, and is the most resistant part of the pacemaker system to EMI. The connectors and the feed-through in the epoxy header will carry the energy inside the sensing circuitry. Therefore, positioning the vector of the magnetic field in the proper angle of incidence will translate to a higher grade of interference or a worst case scenario.

We have measured the electromagnetic fields at the point of inhibition inside saline solution. They are attenuated when compared with the ones measured in free space. The attenuation range is between 30% and 50%.

Distance

The maximum distance at which the interaction disappeared was called threshold distance. Laboratory studies have shown a range of threshold distances from 0.8 to 12.9 cm. This gives a mean distance of 3.9 cm with standard deviation of 3.3 cm. Clinical studies have shown an even closer distance, with a range of 1.0 to 5.0 cm and a mean of 1.4 cm and standard deviation of 0.6 cm.

Depth of Implanted Pacemaker

The deeper the pacemaker is implanted, the less likely it is to be affected by the electromagnetic fields of the antenna of the cellular telephone. The magnetic field penetrates the skin and subcutaneous tissue. Once it reaches the electrolytic solution like the saline tank or the body fluids, the magnetic field transforms into an electrical field. These fields are conducted to the epoxy header of the pacemaker into the feed-through wires and gain access into the sensing circuitry. Once inside, the oscillation or pulsation of energy is interpreted as heart signals by the band-pass filter of the pacemaker.

Sensitivity of the Pacemaker

The higher the sensitivity of the pacemaker, the more likely it is to be affected by the electromagnetic field.

When the penetrating pulse energy is minimal, we first see P-wave tracking of the electromagnetic noise. This outcome is the result of a lower sensitivity setting in the atrial channel of dual chamber pacemakers. As the amount of energy increases, we then see inhibition of the pacemaker function caused by inhibition of the ventricular channel. Due to the different angles and location of feed-through wires, coupling could vary in atrial or ventricular channels. All these outcomes—P-wave tracking of electromagnetic noise, inhibition of pacemaker function, asynchronous pacing, and activation of ventricular safety pacing—are variations of a single phenomenon. The different outcomes are determined by the amount of penetrating pulse energy to which the sensing circuitry is exposed.

Sensing Electronics

Most of the clinical data reveal that there were some manufacturing companies that have models that were susceptible to this interference and had models that were resistant to it. In one manufacturing company, all the models tested were resistant to the digital cellular telephone interference. In analyzing all the models from that particular company, it was clear that a feed-through electromagnetic filter was present. Further experimentation was performed with standard, off-the-shelf units from the above-mentioned manufacturer and custom-made units without the feed-through filter. Our results demonstrate that the units with the filters were resistant to interference, while units without filters were susceptible. Therefore, the presence of a feed-through electromagnetic filter is a reliable and an efficient way of protecting the pacemaker from the digital cellular telephones.

Conclusions

There are some pacemakers that are sensitive to digital cellular telephone interaction when the antenna is held in close proximity to the pulse generator.

Patients that are pacer-dependent should not use their digital cellular telephones in close proximity to the pulse generator, for example, storage of an active cellular telephone in the breast pocket of their jackets.

Once the source of interference was removed, no permanent malfunction was seen in the pacemakers or in any of their programmable features.

Further testing should be done in order to clarify the importance of the variables that determine this phenomenon. This knowledge will be helpful in predicting how future cellular telephone technologies will affect implantable medical devices. In

342

addition, it will be helpful for the medical professional in determining the extent of the risk to which a given patient may be subjected when using a digital cellular telephone.

APPENDIX A

STATE OF THE SCIENCE COLLOQUIUM AGENDA

sponsored by
Wireless Technology Research, LLC in conjunction with the International Committee on Wireless Communication Health Research (ICWCHR)

UNIVERSITY "LA SAPIENZA" OF ROME
Faculty of Engineering
Via Eudossiana 18
00184 Rome, Italy

13-15 NOVEMBER 1995

Monday, 13 November 1995

2:00-2:30 PM	Introduction to Colloquium	Professor Guglielmo D'Inzeo University "La Sapienza" of Rome
		George L. Carlo, Ph.D., M.S., J.D. Wireless Technology Research, LLC

Session I
Dosimetry/Measurements/Certification

Session Chair: Arthur W. Guy, Ph.D.
Wireless Technology Research, LLC

Session Rapporteurs: Martha Embrey, M.P.H.
Marta Cavagnaro, M.S.

2:30-3:15 PM	Invited Paper: *State of the Science Regarding RF Dosimetry, Measurements, and Certification*	Om Gandhi, Sc.D. University of Utah
3:15-4:00 PM	Invited Panel Responses	Niels Kuster, Ph.D. Swiss Federal Institute of Technology
4:00-4:15 PM	Break	
4:15-4:45 PM	Floor Statements and General Discussion	

Monday, 13 November 1995
Session I, continued
Dosimetry/Measurements/Certification

4:45-5:30 PM	Invited Paper: *State of the Science Regarding In Vitro and In Vivo Exposure Systems for RF Studies*	C.K. Chou, Ph.D. City of Hope National Medical Center
5:30-6:15 PM	Invited Panel Responses	Camelia Gabriel, Ph.D. Microwave Consultants Limited Luc Martens, Ph.D. University of Gent
6:15-6:30 PM	Break	
6:30-7:00 PM	Floor Statements and General Discussion	
7:00-7:15 PM	Remarks	Arthur W. Guy, Ph.D. Wireless Technology Research, LLC
7:15-7:30 PM	Closing	Professor Guglielmo D'Inzeo University "La Sapienza" of Rome George L. Carlo, Ph.D., M.S., J.D. Wireless Technology Research, LLC

Tuesday, 14 November 1995

Session I
Epidemiology

Session Chair: Dr. Paolo Vecchia
Istituto Superiore di Sanità

Session Rapporteurs: Rebecca Steffens, M.P.H.
Mirka Zago, M.S.

9:00-10:00 AM	Invited Paper: *State of the Science in RF Epidemiology*	Kenneth Rothman, Dr.P.H. Epidemiology Resources Incorporated
10:00-11:00 AM	Invited Panel Responses	Robert W. Morgan, M.D., S.M.Hyg. Environmental Health Strategies, Inc. John Goldsmith, M.D., M.P.H. Ben Gurion University of the Negev

Tuesday, 14 November 1995
Session I, continued
Epidemiology

10:00-11:00 AM (continued)	Invited Panel Responses (continued)	Ernst L. Wynder, M.D. American Health Foundation
11:00-11:15 AM	Break	
11:15-12:15 PM	Floor Statements and General Discussion	
12:15-12:30 PM	Remarks	Dr. Paolo Vecchia Istituto Superiore di Sanità

Session II
Interference with Medical Devices

Session Chair: Gerd Friedrich
Forschungsgemeinschaft Funk e.V.

Session Rapporteurs: Gretchen K. Findlay
Andrea Donato, M.S.

2:00-2:30 PM	Invited Paper: *State of the Science in Wireless Instrument Medical Equipment Interference*	Kenneth H. Joyner, Ph.D. Telstra
2:30-2:45 PM	Invited Panel Responses	Bernard Segal, Ph.D. McGill University SMBD-Jewish General Hospital
2:45-3:00 PM	Break	
3:00-3:30 PM	Floor Statements and General Discussion	
3:30-4:00 PM	Invited Paper: *State of the Science in Wireless Instrument Pacemaker and Defibrillator Interference*	David L. Hayes, M.D. The Mayo Clinic
4:00-4:45 PM	Invited Panel Responses	Vincenzo Barbaro, Ph.D. Istituto Superiore di Sanità Jiri Silny, Ph.D. Aachen University of Technology Roger Carillo, M.D. Mount Sinai Hospital
4:45-5:00 PM	Break	
5:00-5:30 PM	Floor Statements and General Discussion	

Tuesday, 14 November 1995
Session II, continued
Interference with Medical Devices

5:30-5:45 PM	Remarks	Gerd Friedrich Forschungsgemeinschaft Funk e.V.
5:45-6:00 PM	Closing	Professor Guglielmo D'Inzeo University "La Sapienza" of Rome
		George L. Carlo, Ph.D., M.S., J.D. Wireless Technology Research, LLC
6:30-8:30 PM	Industry Forum	Charles L. Eger, Esq. Motorola, Inc.

Panel I: The Wireless Technology Explosion
Panel II: Technology and Public Health: Achieving the Balance

Wednesday, 15 November 1995

Session I
Biological Responses

Session Chair: Gary M. Williams, M.D.
American Health Foundation

Session Rapporteurs: Graham Hook, Ph.D.
Micaela Liberti, M.S.

9:00-10:00 AM	Invited Paper: *State of the Science in Determining* *the Potential for Genetic Effects of RF*	David Brusick, Ph.D., F.A.T.S. Corning Hazleton
10:00-11:00 AM	Invited Panel Responses	Luc Verschaeve, Ph.D. VITO
		Martin Meltz, Ph.D. University of Texas, San Antonio
		Joseph Roti Roti, Ph.D. Washington University Medical Center
		Sheldon Wolff, Ph.D. University of California
11:00-11:15 AM	Break	

Session I, continued
Biological Responses

| 11:15-12:15 PM | Floor Statements and General Discussion | |
| 12:15-12:30 PM | Remarks | Gary M. Williams, M.D.
American Health Foundation |

Session II
Biological Responses

Session Chair: Professor Guglielmo D'Inzeo
University "La Sapienza" of Rome

Session Rapporteurs: Kelly G. Sund, M.S.
Francesca Apollonio, M.S.

2:00-3:00 PM	<u>Invited Paper:</u> *State of the Science in Recent Advances in Mechanisms Potentially Related to RF*	Alessandro Chiabrera, Ph.D. University of Genoa
3:00-4:00 PM	Invited Panel Responses	Asher Sheppard, Ph.D. Asher Sheppard Consulting
		Bernard Veyret, Ph.D. Université Bordeaux I
		Thomas S. Tenforde, Ph.D. Battelle Pacific Northwest Laboratories
		Andrew Sivak, Ph.D., F.A.T.S. Environmental Health Sciences Consultant
4:00-4:15 PM	Break	
4:15-5:15 PM	Floor Statements and General Discussion	
5:15-5:30 PM	Remarks	Professor Guglielmo D'Inzeo University "La Sapienza" of Rome
5:30-6:00 PM	Colloquium Summation	George L. Carlo, Ph.D., M.S., J.D. Wireless Technology Research, LLC

APPENDIX B

COLLOQUIUM PARTICIPANTS

Dr. George L. Carlo
Chairman
Wireless Technology Research, LLC
1711 N Street, NW
Suite 400
Washington, DC 20036
United States

Dr. Guglielmo D'Inzeo (Biological Responses, Session II Chair)
University of Rome "La Sapienza"
Department of Electronic Engineering
Via Eudossiana 18
Rome 00184
Italy

Dosimetry/Measurements/Certification

Dr. C. K. Chou
Motorola, Inc.
Corporate Research Laboratory
8000 West Sunrise Boulevard
Fort Lauderdale, FL 33322
United States

Dr. Camelia Gabriel
Managing Director
Microwave Consultants Limited
Josilu, 17B Woodford Road
London E18 2EL
United Kingdom

Dr. Om P. Gandhi
Professor and Chairman
University of Utah
Department of Electrical Engineering
3280 Merrill Engineering Building
Salt Lake City, UT 84112
United States

Dr. Arthur W. Guy (Session Chair)
Bioelectromagnetics Consulting
18122 Sixtieth Place, NE
Seattle, WA 98155
United States

Dr. Niels Kuster
Professor
ETH Zurich
Laboratory for EMF and Microwave Electronics
CH-8092 Zurich
Switzerland

Dr. Luc Martens
Professor
University of Gent
Department of Information Technology
Sint-Pietersnieuwstraat 41
Gent B-9000
Belgium

Epidemiology

Dr. John R. Goldsmith
Professor
Ben Gurion University of the Negev
Department of Epidemiology and Health Services Evaluation
Faculty of Health Sciences
P.O. Box 653
Beer Sheva 84 120
Israel

Dr. Robert W. Morgan
President
Environmental Health Strategies, Inc.
149 Commonwealth Drive
Menlo Park, CA 94025
United States

Dr. Kenneth J. Rothman
Senior Epidemiologist
Epidemiology Resources Inc.
One Newton Executive Park
Newton Lower Falls, MA 02162-1450
United States

Dr. Paolo Vecchia (Session Chair)
Head, Nonionizing Radiation
National Instiute of Health
Physics Laboratory
Nonionizing Radiation Section
Viale Regina Elena 299
Rome 00161
Italy

Dr. Ernst L. Wynder
President and Medical Director
American Health Foundation
320 East Forty-third Street
New York, NY 10017
United States

Interference with Medical Devices

Dr. Vincenzo Barbaro
Istituto Superiore di Sanità
Department of Bioengineering
Via Regina Elena 299
Rome 00161
Italy

Dr. Roger G. Carrillo
Cardiovascular Surgeon
Mount Sinai Medical Center
Department of Thoracic and Cardiovascular Surgery
4300 Alton Road
Suite 211
Miami Beach, FL 33140
United States

Dr. Gerd E. Friedrich (Session Chair)
Forschungsgemeinschaft Funk e.V.
Rathausgasse 11a
Bonn D-53111
Germany

Dr. David L. Hayes
Director of the Pacing Laboratory
The Mayo Clinic
Department of Cardiology
200 First Street, SW, East 16
Rochester, MN 55905
United States

Dr. Kenneth H. Joyner
Director, EME Strategy and Regulatory Affairs, Asia-Pacific
Motorola Australia Pty. Ltd.
6 Carribbean Drive Scoresby
Melbourne, Victoria 3179
Australia

Dr. Bernard Segal
Associate Professor, Otolaryngology
McGill University, SMBD-Jewish General Hospital
Department of Otolaryngology
Room E-266 3755 Cote Ste-Catherine Road
Montreal, Quebec H3T 1E2
Canada

Dr. Jiri Silny
Professor
Research Center for the Environmental Compatibility of Electromagnetic Fields
Aachen University of Technology
Pauwelsstraße 20
D-52074 Aachen
Germany

Industry Forum

Mr. Luca Caroli
Telecom Italia Mobil SpA
Via Luigi Rizzo 22
Rome 00136
Italy

352

Dr. John Harry Causebrook
(formerly)
Technical Manager
Vodafone Limited
Radio Engineering
The Courtyard 2-4 London Road
Newbury, Berkshire RG13 1JL
United Kingdom

Mr. Chuck Eger (Session Chair)
Director, Regulatory Affairs
Motorola, Inc.
Cellular Subscriber Group
1350 I Street, NW
Suite 400
Washington, DC 20005
United States

Mr. Fred Harrison
Cellnet
260 Bath Road
Slough, Berkshire SL1 4DX
United Kingdom

Mr. Matthias Meier
Program Manager of Governmental Relations
Motorola
Corporate Development
Im Gretenhof 4
D-53424 Remagen
Germany

Mr. Norman D. Sandler
Director, Global Strategic Issues
Motorola, Inc.
Corporate Issues Management
1303 East Algonquin Road
Seventh Floor
Schaumburg, IL 60196
United States

Dr. Veli Santomaa
Principal Scientist
Nokia Research Center
Department of Radio Communications
P.O. Box 45
Helsinki
FIN-00211
Finland

Mr. Richard M. Smith
(formerly)
Chief
Federal Communications Commission
Office of Engineering and Technology
2000 M Street, NW Suite 480
Washington, DC 20554
United States

Mr. Christer Tornevik
Expert, Electromagnetic Fields
Ericsson Radio Systems
Research and Development, T/U
Torshamnsgatan 23
SE-16480 Stockholm
Sweden

Biological Responses

Dr. David Brusick
Scientific Director
Corning Hazelton, Inc.
9200 Leesburg Pike
Vienna, VA 22182
United States

Dr. Alessandro E. Chiabrera
University of Genoa
Department of Biophysical and Electronic Engineering
DIBE
ICEMB Interuniversity Center
Via Opera Pia 11A
Genoa 16145
Italy

Dr. Martin L. Meltz
Director
The University of Texas Health Science Center at San Antonio
Center for Environmental Radiation Toxicology
7703 Floyd Curl Drive
San Antonio, TX 78284-7800
United States

Dr. Joseph L. Roti Roti
Chief, Section of Cancer Biology
Washington University School of Medicine
Mallinckrodt Institute of Radiology
Radiation Oncology Center
4511 Forest Park Boulevard
Suite 411
St. Louis, MO 63108
United States

Dr. Asher R. Sheppard
Asher Sheppard Consulting
108 Orange Street, Suite 8
Redlands, CA 92373-4719
U.S.A.

Dr. Andrew Sivak
Consultant
Environmental Health Sciences
P.O. Box 2128
Saint Augustine, FL 32085-2128
United States

Dr. Thomas S. Tenforde
Chief Scientist, Environmental Technology Division
Pacific Northwest National Laboratory
Mailstop P7-52; P.O. Box 999
902 Battelle Boulevard
Richland, WA 99352
United States

Dr. Luc Verschaeve
Project Leader
Vlaamse Instelling voor Technologisch Onderzoek
Environmental Toxicology
Boeretang 200
Mol B-2400
Belgium

Dr. Bernard Veyret
CNRS Senior Scientist
Universite Bordeaux 1
Ecole Nationale Superieure de Chimie et de Physicque de Bordeaux
Laboratoire de Physique des Interactions Ondes-Matiere
URA 1506 CNRS
Avenue Pey Berland, BP 108
Talence
33 405 Cedex
France

Dr. Gary M. Williams (Session I Chair)
Director, Naylor Dana Institute
American Health Foundation
One Dana Road
Valhalla, NY 10595-1599
United States

Dr. Sheldon Wolff
Vice Chairman and Chief of Research
Radiation Effects Research Foundation
5-2 Hijiyama Park
Minami-ky
Hiroshima
Japan

APPENDIX C

COLLOQUIUM INTRODUCTION AND CHARGE TO PARTICIPANTS

George L. Carlo

Thank you, Professor D'Inzeo, for your hospitality, your hard work, and the hard work of your staff in making this colloquium possible. I would also like to thank the WTR staff who have tirelessly looked after the many details required to bring us together for this important meeting.

On behalf of both the WTR and the International Committee on Wireless Communication Health Research, I would like to thank you for your participation and your willingness to assist us in moving forward and advancing the science addressing the public health impact of wireless technology.

The theme bringing us together for the next three days is at once simple and complex. I believe we all share a common interest in identifying public health problems associated with wireless communication technology, and in prescribing and implementing workable solutions to those problems. This straightforward common interest, however, is complicated by the difficult and complex nature of the science upon which our decisions about risk and risk management must be made.

- How should the abundant existing scientific information generally applicable to radio frequency radiation be applied to this new question of low-power, head-concentrated emissions from cellular telephones?

- What safety standards should apply to new generations of wireless technology and how can compliance be measured?

- Do we have the scientific tools necessary to study near-field, low-power exposures at all with a reasonable degree of scientific certainty?

- How do we address indirect biological effects such as those that might follow from interference between digital signals and cardiac pacemakers or defibrillators?

Identifying and solving these problems requires an integration of scientific and medical knowledge from multiple and diverse disciplines. No one discipline, be it epidemiology, toxicology or physics, no one study, and no one scientist can provide definitive answers. On the other hand, every discipline, every study, and every scientist here today can make a positive contribution. Thus, we have the reason for our colloquium and the basis for my belief that this represents an important step forward.

Over the next three days, we will hear of and learn more of this complex scientific field. However, appropriate public policy decisions about wireless technology will require wisdom, and in this case, I believe wisdom is defined not so much by how we use the knowledge we have in hand, but by how we identify and pursue the knowledge we do not yet have, but need in order to make informed judgements. It is my hope that this colloquium will prove to be an asset as we collectively pursue this necessary knowledge and strive to achieve the wisdom we need to make the right public health choices, decisions, and recommendations about wireless communication technology.

I am elated that we have been able to bring together some of the finest scientific minds in the world to assist us in our learning through the course of this colloquium. In planning this colloquium, we have challenged each of the invited speakers to bring to us new and innovative scientific thinking and insight regarding wireless communication public health risks and solutions. We have challenged them to go beyond the status quo, to scratch beneath the surface, and to think practically about how their science can be applied to the betterment of public health in this area.

I am challenging you, the participants, as well. I urge you to actively participate, to roll up your sleeves, and to bring to this forum your knowledge and your most creative insights. Whether you work within a government agency, the news media, a university laboratory, or an industrial manufacturer, I also challenge you to suspend your parochial thinking and interests, and to put forth your best "science-first" thinking and ideas. Please consider the "science first" theme to be central to this colloquium as you move through the next three days. If we all rise to these challenges, this colloquium will be a success.

I ask you now to take up your colloquium binder, and to take careful note of the colloquium format. Invited papers will be followed immediately by invited panel responses. When invited panel responses are completed, there will be a fifteen-minute break during which those participants in the audience who wish to be recognized during the floor statements and general discussion session should complete a question card and place it in one of the baskets. Participants will be recognized by name and asked to come to the podium to make their statements, ask a question of the panel, or present data. We will do our best to recognize all who wish to be recognized; however, we are committed to stay within the time schedule published in the agenda binder.

Of special interest to you will be the Industry Forum being held tomorrow evening from 6:30 until 8:30. This special session, being chaired by Charles Eger of Motorola, will include a panel addressing the wireless technology explosion and another addressing how industry is working to achieve balance between technological development and public health protection. I urge you to make time for this session as well.

APPENDIX D-1

DOSIMETRY/MEASUREMENTS/CERTIFICATION

Martha Embrey and Marta Cavagnaro

Summary

A key feature to conducting bioeffects research using radiofrequency radiation is how the biological material is exposed—either in vitro or in vivo. In an in vitro system, controlling temperature and characterizing the uniformity of the exposure through experimental or analytical measurement methods are crucial factors. Traditionally, in vivo studies have been performed by exposing animals' whole bodies to the radiofrequency radiation source. A challenge in designing systems to test the effects of wireless communication instruments is to recreate the head-focused exposure that mimics cellular phone use in humans. Characterizing the exposures in vitro or in vivo is reliant on many factors, including the dielectric properties and the geometric configuration of the tissues under test and the location of the radiation antenna as a power source.

In his presentation, Dr. Chou covered a wide range of issues related to exposure systems. He first discussed the difficulties inherent in measuring exposure in animals and extrapolating those measurements to humans. Specific absorption rate (SAR) is used to quantify power absorbed in tissue, which can be calculated from the measurements using an electric field (E-field) or a rise in temperature. However, when using the same incident power density to expose animals and humans, the resulting SAR variation is large.

Dr. Chou summarized the different methods for in vitro exposure including waveguides, coaxial lines, horn antennas, and transverse electromagnetic (TEM) cells. An important aspect of in vitro exposure systems is temperature control. Dr. Chou described several systems and their methods to control temperature from many laboratories around the world. He then described WTR-sponsored efforts to characterize exposure in a TEM cell using the finite-difference time-domain (FD-TD) mathematical modeling method. Examining different types of flasks, different locations and orientations within the cell, and different amounts of medium in the flasks, a computer can model the SAR distribution.

Dr. Chou reviewed the variety of in vivo exposure systems developed internationally, using both whole- and partial-body exposures. Different systems in use include a cavity exposure, waveguide, TEM cell, and strip line. He described exposing a variety of species: mice, rats, rabbits, and monkeys. He pointed out that the orientation and the geometry of the animal within the system can drastically alter the SAR pattern; for example, if the E- field is parallel to the long axis during exposure, peak SAR measurements will occur in a rat's tail.

Dr. Chou described several head-only exposure systems that investigated cataract production, microwave hearing, and blood-brain barrier effects. No exposure system exists that duplicates exposure from wireless communication instruments. WTR has contracted with Dr. Chou's laboratory at the City of Hope to develop such a system for use in rodents. They began their design by characterizing the exposure of an ellipsoid rat phantom filled with brain-like material. The City of Hope researchers discovered that a loop antenna produces a more representative SAR pattern in the phantom than a dipole antenna. The next step is to model the loop antennas using a computed tomography scan of an actual rat.

Another important issue is that of animal restraint during exposure. Some animal behaviorists believe that restraint causes stress in the animals, which can confound results. City of Hope is waiting for project biologists to determine whether the system will use restrained or unrestrained animals.

Dr. Chou concluded by stating the importance of using the same frequencies and SAR patterns produced by wireless technology in both in vitro and in vivo systems to gather appropriate exposure data. He stressed the need for collaboration between biologists and physical scientists to reach that goal.

Dr. Gabriel presented information relating to the role of dielectric spectroscopy in in vitro and in vivo dosimetry and about the theories of microscopic dosimetry. She showed data generated in her laboratory on the dielectric properties of various tissues using three different pieces of equipment. The equipment allowed an evaluation of the dielectric spectrum ranging from 10 Hz to 20 GHz. Dr. Gabriel compared the data from her laboratory to measurements reported in the literature over the past 45 years. The data were presented graphically for each tissue type. Generally, Dr. Gabriel reported values falling within the expected range. She pointed out that within the literature, there is not one value per tissue, but a range, suggesting that the values vary according to the composition of the tissue. Composition can deviate from one part of the tissue to another, from one animal to another, and from one species to another; however, she commented that there was no way to relate differences between species in the same tissue types. For example, there is no consistency between rat tissues and human tissues. She therefore concluded that we need a representative value at each frequency rather than searching for one true value.

Dr. Gabriel presented the results of modeling based on four dispersions known to exist in the spectrum of biological material. Her laboratory's calculations have shown good agreement with values reported in the literature and with their own measurements. In the presentation, Dr. Gabriel showed several graphs representing these various values in different tissues and at different frequencies. Her laboratory has studied and modeled more than 40 different tissues.

In the second half of her presentation, Dr. Gabriel discussed dosimetry at the molecular level—microscopic dosimetry. She suggested carrying out an analysis of the dielectric properties of a simple system made up of a single organic molecule in water. This analysis allows us to study the dielectric properties of water dispersion in greater detail. We can apply these observations to more complex systems, such as tissues. Using this model, she found that tissues with high water content (e.g., aqueous humor) hardly differ from values of water. As the water content decreases, the dielectric value decreases, and the relaxation time increases. For example, the relaxation time for bone is more than twice that of pure water. Using this information, Dr. Gabriel showed an example of uneven energy distribution at the molecular level. She concluded that exposing identical solutions, which differ only in concentration, may be giving different doses to the organic macromolecule.

Dr. Gabriel finished her presentation with a recommendation to do thermal modeling in concert with SAR modeling in in vivo experiments. She felt it important to establish the thermal distribution within organs and that thermal analysis would help in the difficult job of extrapolating animal results to humans.

Dr. Luc Martens' presentation began with a discussion of the different specifications that must be considered when designing an in vitro or in vivo exposure system. One major consideration is what Dr. Martens termed the biological structure under test (BSUT), which consists of the animal or cell culture being exposed in a system. The BSUT will completely change the electromagnetic field simulations from the calculations made when designing an empty system.

He discussed a closed system (i.e., a TEM cell), an open system used for in vivo work, and the requirements for their design and characterization. The goal in designing an accurate TEM cell is the reduction of reflection by using the time domain reflectometry technique. This technique determines the impedance through the transmission line system of a TEM cell. Dr. Martens pointed out that SAR peaks occur at the edge of the septum, which is important to consider when designing the placement of cell cultures; however, even the empty area above the septum does not have completely uniform electric fields. To illustrate that point, he described the results of quantifying the exposure of animal phantoms placed above and below the septum in a TEM cell. The results of that characterization show differences in SAR distribution between the two animals based on their placement in the cell.

Using numerical modeling, Dr. Martens reported in detail the results of field polarization and distribution inside an in vitro TEM cell system. Reviewing an open in vivo system that exposes animals nose-first toward an antenna, he described the methods by which the system developers modeled the antenna and the animals to quantify the exposure fields. He also reported the use of a nonperturbing temperature probe to further verify exposure in animals. Dr. Martens concluded his presentation by stressing the importance of appropriate characterization of exposure systems to accurately interpret biological effects.

Safety guidelines for wireless communication instruments are based on the specific absorption rate (SAR) of radiofrequency (RF) radiation, which is measured in W/kg. The two primary methods to measure the output of wireless communication instruments and the resulting SAR levels in the exposed tissues are either analytically or experimentally based. The analytical dosimetry uses numerical modeling methods such as the finite-difference time-domain (FD-TD). These models calculate the specific absorption rate distributions for the coupling of RF devices, such as cellular phones, to biological bodies. The experimental method uses E-field sensors embedded in a phantom head filled with tissue-simulating gels. Each method has its strengths and weaknesses. The FD-TD method models the head's tissue properties with high resolution, converting MRI scans of the body into complex models of the human head with all of its tissues like bone, cartilage, brain matter, etc. The disadvantage is that accurately modeling the communication device being tested it is difficult. On the other hand, the experimental method uses the actual telephone to test output. The downside is that the head model is crude compared with the computer model method. Validations of both methods are ongoing.

Dr. Om Gandhi's presentation dealt with numerical and experimental dosimetry related to the assessment of risk caused by using hand-held cellular phones. In the first part of his presentation, Gandhi focused on numerical dosimetry by illustrating the different numerical methods used internationally. From the analysis, the finite-difference time-domain (FD-TD) method emerged as more advantageous than the other methods considered for the study of bioelectromagnetic problems. Gandhi emphasized that the FD-TD method allows the use of heterogeneous phantom models without the loss of simplicity. It allows the evaluation of both the specific absorption rate (SAR) distribution and the radiation pattern of the antenna and needs the least computer memory of all the numerical methods. Gandhi discussed four near-field tests that have been used to validate the University of Utah's FD-TD cellular telephone code. They obtained these tests from published data that considered simple phantom models (as a layered half-space, box, and sphere) and simple electromagnetic source models (dipole antenna, infinitesimal dipole). He showed good agreement between simulations made at the University of Utah and the published data.

The last validation, which is currently under development at the University of Utah, is between the FD-TD code and data obtained with measurements on an actual cellular phone. With reference to the measurements, Gandhi reviewed the international work done with particular attention on the phantoms used. These phantoms typically contain about four different tissues (e.g., skull, brain, ears, eyes). Gandhi outlined recent results in this field related mainly to the development of new, smaller-sized E-field probes to measure higher frequency fields and to the characterization of phantoms with new dielectric tissue properties that are emerging from Dr. Camelia Gabriel's work. Gandhi considered the correct characterization of the human phantom as an important detail in numerical dosimetry. To illustrate this point, he showed a short videotape where differences in the absorption of the electromagnetic field were found by varying the head dimensions when modeling a 5-year-old child, a 10-year-old child, and an adult. The tape clearly showed that in the model of the 5-year-old child, absorption is much deeper than absorption in the 10-year-old model or the adult model. Gandhi's group is still investigating the reason for such a difference. Finally, in his concluding remarks, Gandhi expressed concern over the lack of an internationally accepted testing procedure for wireless devices to assess their compliance with existing standards.

Dr. Kuster's presentation focused on the issue of compliance testing on hand-held communications equipment. He described the key requirements needed for good testing procedures, then focused attention on the uncertainties of such procedures with respect to the experimental approach.

Kuster identified the sources of uncertainty related to a testing procedure in modeling a group of users, modeling the actual telephones, and the variations of measurements. Concerning uncertainties of measurement, Kuster analyzed the experimental apparatus developed at the Swiss Federal Institute of Technology, Zürich (ETH) to measure spatial-peak SAR in shell phantoms. He concluded the analysis with an estimate of the error of less than plus or minus 20%. With reference to the experimental uncertainties in modeling cellular phones, Kuster noted that they are reduced to zero because actual cellular phones are used in the measurements.

The biggest question related to the experimental testing procedure at ETH is whether a homogeneous shell phantom can accurately represent a human being. To answer this question, Kuster studied the exposure on three experimental (physical) phantoms and three numerical phantoms, with differing numbers of tissues, sizes, and geometries. Small differences were found in the absorption when he compared his shell phantoms with the physical phantoms, while larger differences were found with the numerical analysis. Kuster explained these differences as related to the varying thickness of the skin and bone used in the numerical models.

Kuster showed that they almost completely eliminated the differences when the comparison was made on the SAR values as averaged over 1 gram or 10 grams as required by the safety standards. He stated that the differences between the two types (experimental and numerical) of models are all within 10% for SAR averaged over 10 grams and within 25% for SAR averaged over 1 gram. Kuster concluded that the homogeneous phantom represents the worst-case absorption without excessive error in the SAR evaluation, while allowing for a reduction in the number of tests necessary to comply with industry standards. The measurement technique developed at ETH also satisfies other testing requirements: the ability to test randomly selected devices, a higher degree of reproducibility and reliability, and time efficiency. Finally, the measurement procedure developed at ETH is simple enough to be used without specialists. Kuster stated that it takes about two days of intensive training for an engineer to use it properly.

Scientific Discussion

Dr. Michael Schuller (Maannesmann Mobilfunk) asked Dr. Martens if he calculated the influence of the biological structure on the electromagnetic field for different structures. His presentation covered TEM cells, but Dr. Schuller thought that for narrow-band signals, like GSM, a waveguide is a good alternative.

Dr. Luc Martens replied that he did not cover the waveguides because of time limitations.

Dr. Schuller did not think that higher order modes were a problem in waveguides, and that the ability to expose several samples at once was a benefit.

Dr. Dina Simunic (Tu Graz, Institute of Biomedical Engineering) first posed a question to Dr. Chou. She asked that since the issue of thermoregulation is clearly very complex, how does he estimate the error resulting from extrapolating exposure from animals to humans?

Dr. C. K. Chou pointed out that the ANSI/IEEE standard does not differentiate between thermal and nonthermal effects. The standard is based on a whole-body exposure of about 4 W/kg, to which they then apply a safety factor to extrapolate to humans. The resulting ANSI standard of 0.4 W/kg does not consider the difference between thermal and nonthermal, as long as there is an effect.

Dr. Simunic replied that she thinks you can not calculate SAR up to 4 W/kg; you can only calculate the temperature rise. She asked if he could estimate this error.

Dr. Chou said that the temperature is just a by-product of the SAR absorption. Those in the field have debated whether the effect is thermal or nonthermal for a long time. He described working in Dr. Guy's laboratory where they never referred to thermal or nonthermal effects, just high-level or low-level effects. Even a small amount of power resulting in a very small temperature rise can still be a thermal effect. He used the example of a study on microwave pulses which involved a very small amount of energy. He said you could hear the pulses, but you could not measure any temperature rise. It was, however, a thermal effect. He pointed out that Dr. Ken Foster did an analysis using thermal expansion to explain the phenomenon. They tried to isolate the temperature and understand how the microwaves interacted with biological tissue. Dr. Chou concluded with the statement that extrapolation is why we want to use SAR as a quantifying unit; it does not matter if it is a thermal or nonthermal effect.

Dr. Simunic thanked Dr. Chou and asked Dr. Gabriel what she thought about homogenizing brain tissues since she showed significant differences [in dielectric properties] between grey and white matter.

Dr. Camelia Gabriel agreed that there are differences between grey and white matter, but thinks that homogenizing the brain tissues is satisfactory for estimating the value inside the brain using macroscopic dosimetry. If we wanted to study dosimetry at the molecular level, then we would have to consider the different parts.

Bernhard Eicher (Swiss Telecom PTT) asked Luc Martens if in his time domain reflectometry measurement of the TEM cell, could he clearly see the transitions between the coaxial and the conical section and between the conical section and the straight section? He said that it is well known that discontinuity produces high SAR levels. He wanted to know how far they extended into the parallel section of the cell, and could they meet in the central region to produce field distortions?

Dr. Martens thought that was difficult to answer, but that Mr. Eicher was right, that at those transitions, higher-order modes are excited. A system should be designed so that the structure is as far as possible from this discontinuity. Also, you must compare the structure length with the frequency before you put the structure to the test, then you really excite the TEM mode. He added that the second effect is that if the discontinuity is large, you could produce standing waves. In his study, he expanded the vertical axis of the figure to clearly see the discontinuities, but if you look at the values in the figure, there is not much of a discontinuity effect. The percentage of reflection is small.

Dr. Mays Swicord (Motorola) asked Dr. Gabriel to expand on her thoughts concerning microdosimetry. He said that it seemed obvious to him that a large molecule will relax very rapidly, so that any thermal responses would not affect function any more than raising the temperature of the surrounding environment. However, one might consider some large structure, like the cell membrane, which might have an elevated temperature compared with the surrounding environment, causing functional effects. He asked Dr. Gabriel to comment.

Dr. Gabriel replied that she was not referring to the effect on the molecule or whether that effect was significant or not significant. She was pointing out the preferential rate at which the two molecules absorb energy. Even a simple binary system with one macromolecule and water will have a preferential rate—or could have—if all our assumptions are correct. We should have a preferential deposition of the energy in the water system. The repercussions of this uneven distribution of energy at the molecular level have to be looked into for each system.

Dr. Martin Meltz (University of Texas Health Sciences Center at San Antonio) wanted to express a concern and ask a question of Luc Martens. He said he was concerned about using the exposure agent under study (microwaves) to control temperature during a study of their effects. He was not sure if he could tell if an effect was due to the on-and-off switching of the microwaves or a continuous exposure. Normally, in cell biology, he said they did studies where they keep the temperature at $37\,^{\circ}$C as a starting point, and then do the exposure to the reagent: ultraviolet, ionizing radiation, x-rays, or microwaves. He asked for anyone's response and expressed his concern for this approach.

Dr. Martens replied that they have found that with the tube inside the waveguide system, you could have a temperature rise, but not see it because of cooling through the tube. For example, if you are measuring both the E-field and the temperature, then you can find that in some cases the temperature is not changing, though the fields are large enough. He suggested that it could be a way to distinguish between thermal and nonthermal effects. The problem is that the cooling through the wall may bring the temperature up to a constant level.

Dr. Meltz said that if someone does a study using far-field microwave exposures, basing them on an SAR in the most uniform area, and they see no effect, should they not be more comfortable if they detected E-field hot spots—not necessarily thermal hot spots—in the flask? He continued that this was not if there *is* an effect detected. If there is an effect, you clearly have to go back and look at the E-field hot spots.

Nevertheless, if you have an absence of an effect reported under those conditions, it should give you an even greater level of confidence.

Dr. Chou agreed, if you do not believe in the window effect. But if your SAR indicator is low because you are measuring in the middle, you missed the hot spot. If you do not see any effect measuring the whole system, based on the ordinary threshold effect, then it should be safe. However, if there is a power window, that is another story.

Dr. Bill Guy (Wireless Technology Research) responded by saying that near the edges, you have a very high gradient. You would not know whether it was a gradient effect, or just a standard SAR effect.

Dr. Meltz clarified that he was talking about an absence of an effect. He was arguing that when there is no effect, you can still be comfortable using far-field exposure when you learn that there are E-field hot spots in the types of tissue culture vessels used. If there is an effect, he said he would be the first to say that you have to be concerned about E-field hot spots. It is only if there is an absence of an effect that it provides an additional margin of confidence in the original SAR used, since the SAR at the sides have to be even higher. He asked people to remember that we are looking at all the cells in a given container, not just the cells in the middle. He summarized his points by saying he felt the need to defend the issue of Dr. Martens not including far-field microwave exposures as a way of doing these types of studies.

Dr. Don McRee (WTR Director of Extramural Research) asked Luc Martens how well he thought Dr. Balzano's head-first exposure system simulates the exposure to the head from cellular telephones, referring to thermographic charts that Dr. Martens had shown.

Dr. Martens said that his laboratory did not do that characterization; he just used it as an example of an open system with an antenna.

Dr. McRee asked if he knew the SAR patterns for the system, and Dr. Martens told him that Niels Kuster might be better to answer the question.

Dr. Niels Kuster replied that since the rats are exposed in the close near field of a dipole antenna, the SAR is induced by the H-field. Therefore, the induced SAR pattern is comparable to that of an eddy current pattern. You find high SAR levels at the upper part of the skull and low SAR levels at the bottom. In this respect, it reflects the actual absorption from a mobile phone fairly well, high absorption close to the surface and low absorption in the rest of the brain.

Dr. Guy asked what the ratio would be between whole-body average SAR and the peak SAR.

Dr. Kuster said that the average absorbed in the brain is about three times higher than the average absorbed by the whole body.

After thanking the presenters, Dr. Guy closed the session with some comments. He said that he sees very precise approaches being taken with certification issues, where we are talking about fractions of SAR either below the perceived standard coming up on the 1.6 W/kg and the fractions of SAR above it. There is tremendous precision available to detect whether you are above or below a certain level.

He added that if we look at the different exposure systems presented, they represent the types of exposures that led to the present standards, which are essentially based on whole-body exposure with estimated hot spots that are 20 times higher. Though he could not speak for European, Australian, or New Zealand standards, that is the basis of the IEEE and NCRP standards.

He continued to say that these hot spots result from a situation that starts with whole-body loading, then adds hot spots on top of the whole-body loading, and that is essentially where the 8 W/kg comes from; a whole-body average of 0.4 times the highest SAR level of 20 is 8 W/kg. This number was reduced further when the different standard-setting organizations decided to add an extra safety factor for differentiating between general population exposures and uncontrolled exposures. Part of the reduction of one-fifth occurred because occupational exposures generally last for 40 hours a week, whereas the general population exposure could be 24 hours a day (e.g., someone living near an FM radio station). A good part of the rationale for that one-fifth reduction comes from the increased potential exposure for the general population. Also, the NCRP and the IEEE/ANSI have a specific statement that says that the person who has control over his or her use of the radiofrequency device automatically falls under the occupational exposure. Dr. Guy noted on the other hand, there is a need for caution because that 8 W/kg hot spot probably never occurred in the heads of animals exposed for the development of the standard. Those hot spots occur in places like the ankle, the tail, etc. Overall, the head exposures were lower than what the peak exposures are over the rest of the body.

He feels that the present database does not support an exposure situation which results in extremely low whole-body averages with a peak SAR in the brain area. This is why having a head-only exposure system is essential. If your exposure is not in the head, but you try to produce peak SARs above what you would consider safe in the head, the rest of the body will get even higher SARs, and you then run into a thermal loading problem.

Dr. Guy concluded by saying in certification we are getting ahead of a good standard that would provide some assurance of safety from highly localized head exposures. He feels that an important parameter will be the ratio between the peak SAR in the head to the whole-body exposure that is close to what would exist for a human.

Dr. Guy asked for any additional questions.

Dr. Alessandro Chiabrera (University of Genoa) returned to the previous question asking Dr. Chou, Dr. Gabriel, and Dr. Martens what they thought about the possibility of using a statistical characterization of the dielectric properties of biological material. He noted that this new method has nothing to do with the kind of errors mentioned in the session because it is a completely different mathematical approach.

Dr. Martens replied that if a statistical characterization of a biological system were used in simulations, it would take too much time using today's computers. He considered the possibility that statistical distributions could be directly implemented in more analytical modeling such as Method of Moment, but with other numerical techniques, it would take weeks to simulate one single problem.

Dr. Sheldon Wolff (University of California)reiterated that it is not the SAR which is important to the dose, but the amount of energy that is absorbed. A high peak SAR for one second does not have the same biological effect as a high SAR over a longer period of time. If there are rest periods throughout the exposure, the organism will time have to cool before any biological effects are observed.

Dr. Meltz emphasized that before invoking a need for a recovery period, you have to show an effect exists to recover from at a given SAR. A high SAR for a short time or continuous exposure at lower SARs have the same average but different effects. He returned to a statement made by Dr. Chiabrera, saying that, as a biologist, he would like to know SAR even within the diameter of a single cell, so he did not think a statistical approach to measurement was useful.

Dr. Joe Wiart (CNET France Telecom) asked Dr. Gandhi to comment on the new Perfectly Matched Layer (PML) absorbing condition, with particular reference to this condition's influence on the FD-TD resolution of near-field problems.

Dr. Om Gandhi replied that they have used all three absorbing boundary conditions at one time or another, but that for near-field problems, PML does not seem to have a major advantage because most of the energy is absorbed close to the source, and very little is left to reach the boundaries. He did not see much advantage in PML or Berenger's boundary conditions for cellular telephone dosimetry problems.

Dr. Quirino Balzano (Motorola) asked Dr. Gandhi if he could explain the higher SAR that he found in the model of a 5-year-old child at 900 MHZ, since they used a similar model in their experimental set up and did not find any increase.

Dr. Gandhi replied that at this time they do not understand the reason behind the higher SAR found in the 5-year-old child head model other than more in-depth penetration. In order to understand this deeper penetration, they are studying the coupling of the electromagnetic field with different sized spheres, which is an easier problem to tackle. In his closing remarks, Dr. Balzano suggested that Dr. Gandhi first investigate the problem experimentally.

Dr. Martens (University of Gent) noted that defining canonical cases for the certification of numerical methods is important. With reference to this, he showed slides on the work done in the COST 244 project. In this project, the researchers defined a canonical problem made with simple phantoms (cube and sphere), and simple antennas (dipole and monopole on a conducting box) and calculated various results (e.g., SAR in particular points, radiation patterns, etc.). Martens presented some results showing large variations from one group to another.

Dr. Gandhi replied that he was unable to comment because he had looked at data from a limited number of COST 244 participants, who had given him detailed SAR distributions. He noted that those groups were, by coincidence, fairly experienced in using numerical electromagnetic techniques. He found a decent comparison of the SAR distribution data from those three or four groups. Dr. Gandhi suggested that perhaps Dr. Martens was comparing the newly formed groups in the field, who may not have known how to do the problem correctly.

Dr. Kuster added that a high level of expertise is required to perform accurate computations—even for simple problems—and that many groups were relatively new in the field, which could explain the large differences in results.

Mr. Thomas Schmid (ETH Zürich) noted that Dr. Gandhi had shown simulations using both homogeneous and heterogeneous phantoms. He asked Dr. Gandhi to confirm that the homogeneous phantom can be a good approximation for the worst-case model.

Dr. Gandhi replied that all the cases he showed were used to validate their FD-TD code, and that these validations will continue, with three or four additional comparisons with published data.

Mr. Eicher noted that Gandhi's presentation suggested that a longer antenna could be better. He asked if this was also true for the so-called worst case condition where the antenna touches the head. Moreover, he asked if there were any data on the uncertainties of modeling the variations of output from an actual handset antenna approaching the head, since Dr. Gandhi used only one number in his simulations.

Dr. Gandhi replied that they modeled the phone straight up and down and at a 33° tilt, which corresponds to the actual position of the phone. They have not modeled the antenna touching the head. He added that more analysis needs to be done in order to answer the question on actual versus idealized radiating devices.

Dr. Masao Taki (Tokyo Metropolitan University) showed transparencies on the calculations he performed using FD-TD. He showed large differences in the SAR values obtained when modeling a dipole or a monopole antenna as the electromagnetic source, when changing the position of the phone, and when using homogenous or heterogenous head models. In particular, his peak SAR results obtained with a homogeneous model were higher than those obtained with a heterogeneous model. However, he noted that they obtained the highest SAR with a heterogeneous model and a monopole antenna and that it was located in the cheek. He speculated that air in the oral cavity caused the result. He noted that unless this air cavity is taken into consideration, estimating SAR in a phantom could be inaccurate and that this could generate some problems in Kuster's method.

Dr. Wolff asked how safety limits could be set with the scarcity of information on biological effects, and why use SAR, which is the rate at which the human body absorbs electromagnetic energy instead of the amount of energy absorbed? He felt that the latter is more representative of the electromagnetic hazard.

Dr. Gandhi noted that, unfortunately, health agencies must enforce already existing safety limits, which use SAR.

Dr. Chiabrera noted that a big problem in dosimetry studies is the difficulty in correctly characterizing each cell of the biologic system, both from a geometrical and from an electrical point of view. He asked whether they felt it was time to change the approach used in dosimetric analyses. He suggested that statistical distributions be used to characterize the system with respect to the electromagnetic field emitted from the phone, the dielectric properties of the biologic material, and the geometry of the head.

Dr. Gandhi reiterated his answer to the preceding question. He noted that the safety guidelines are in terms of SAR and, therefore, to certify hand-held devices the SAR must be determined.

Dr. Chiabrera noted that to link different research areas, studies on the interaction mechanisms need to include not only the SAR distribution, but E-field distribution as well.

Dr. Kenneth R. Foster (University of Pennsylvania), noted that measuring SAR from a near-field exposure is difficult because the SAR is highly variable depending on the location of the antenna, etc. He asked if they could suggest a method in which engineering constraints could be more precisely specified to avoid this tremendous variability.

Dr. Kuster replied that a CENELEC working group is attempting to define the different positions of phone use (i.e., the angles of the phones with respect to the axis of the head).

Dr. Bill Guy summarized the session noting that the presentations had shown the very precise approach being taken toward certification, looking at a fraction of SAR above and below the standard. However, the exposure systems presented represent the types of exposures on which the current standards are based (i.e., whole body with estimated hot spots). The present database does not support an extremely low whole-body average with peak SAR in the head, which is why a head-only exposure system is important in this research.

APPENDIX D-2

EPIDEMIOLOGY

Rebecca A. Steffens and Mirka Zago

Summary

The epidemiology section of the State of the Science Colloquium took place on the second day and began with a one-hour invited paper by Dr. Kenneth Rothman, of Epidemiology Resources Inc. (ERI). Dr. Rothman's paper, entitled, "State of the Science in RF Epidemiology," first described the history of the cellular telephone, the rapid growth in the number of subscribers since its introduction, and issues raised as to the possibility of subsequent health effects. These issues have implications for health professionals, industry, and the legal profession.

Next, Dr. Rothman explored how epidemiology can make a significant contribution to the field of radiofrequency (RF) exposure research. He first described past research, the current state of research, and what the future holds. Initially, Dr. Rothman outlined basic concepts integral to the science of epidemiology such as the definition of causation and sufficient cause. Cause in epidemiology usually refers to one component of an entire causal mechanism that, when combined with other factors such as time (or a long induction period), leads to a particular disease. He referred to examples such as smoking and lung cancer and diethyl stilbestrol (DES) exposure of pregnant women and adenocarcinoma of the vagina in their daughters. Both instances are nice models for an exposure occurring at a certain point in time and health effects appearing much later. Another basic concept in epidemiology is that when studying the effects of environmental agents epidemiologists rely on "non-experimental" or "observational" studies. This means that controlling for outside factors that differ between the two groups being studied and that may affect the study results, commonly known as confounders, must be controlled for in the data handling or analysis stage of the study.

Dr. Rothman went on to explain that results from epidemiological studies are expressed in a variety of ways. Some common measures of effect are mortality rates, risk and odds ratios, and their appropriate confidence intervals. He emphasized that clear progress has been made in studying exposures such as cigarette smoking, but that there is more difficulty in studying effects that are either non-existent or subtle. This difficulty was encountered earlier in the study of electromagnetic fields (EMFs). There is debate as to whether results from RF studies will show similar inconsistencies; however, Dr. Rothman felt this would not be the case. Epidemiology, he said, can provide clearer answers about the potential health effects of cellular telephone use much more quickly than EMF studies were able to do in terms of EMF exposure. Next, he summarized the major epidemiologically relevant differences between EMF exposure and RF exposure from cellular telephones. The primary difference is total body exposure versus localized head-only exposure. He also emphasized that while EMF exposure is increasing, RF exposure is showing explosive or exponential growth. This would most likely result in any health effects, if they exist, eventually showing up in health registry statistics due to this dramatic time trend. Dr. Rothman further elaborated on other sources of possible RF exposure for the population in addition to that from cellular telephones. Next, focusing on specific aspects of RF epidemiology studies, Dr. Rothman discussed markers of RF exposure that could be or are already being used in epidemiologic studies. These include occupational exposure, residential exposure, telephone company billing records, and self-reports. Other important markers are type of telephone; level of cellular power output, for which geographic location may be a surrogate; and laterality of exposure or which side of the head the user most often holds the phone against, for which handedness may be a surrogate measure. Dr. Rothman also mentioned metal implants, jewelry, and eyeglasses as possible important factors to consider.

Following this, Dr. Rothman then summarized results from several published epidemiologic studies on RF exposure. Within this context he discussed the "healthy worker" effect and how this may impact studies of various occupational groups. He also pointed out the overall difficulty of controlling for any particular confounding factors that might affect the results, and the important distinction between mobile (car or bag) phones and hand held portable telephones in terms of RF exposure. With car and bag phones the antenna is not in the handset and therefore there is little or no direct exposure to the head. Dr. Rothman turned next to two studies being conducted by ERI, as part of the WTR program. First, a preliminary survey of a group of phone users from a particular carrier was used to assess the correlation between the individual using the phone and the actual account holder. In addition, this survey was used to explore the question of laterality and its relationship to handedness. Next, Dr. Rothman discussed the large mortality surveillance study also being conducted by ERI based entirely on telephone user records. The goal of this large cohort study will be to evaluate the risk of death particularly from brain cancer of cellular telephone users. Phone records provide information on amount of use (number of calls, minutes of use, and start of service date), type of telephone, and unique identifying information. This unique identifier allows linkage with mortality data in order to evaluate overall death as well as specific causes of death. Dr. Rothman mentioned that at some point a prospective cohort of users will be assembled and contacted directly using questionnaires in order to evaluate not only phone use but other lifestyle factors as well. This will allow better control of confounding and provide long-term follow-up of any health outcomes. Finally, Dr. Rothman described two case-control studies of RF exposure and brain cancer currently being conducted: one by the National Cancer Institute, and the other by the American Health Foundation, of which the latter study is being partially funded under the WTR program.

After Dr. Rothman's invited paper were three 20-minute invited panel responses. These were made by Dr. Robert Morgan of Environmental Health Strategies, Inc., Dr. John Goldsmith, of the Ben Gurion University of the Negev, and Dr. Ernst Wynder of the American Health Foundation. Dr. Goldsmith spoke to the state of the art guidelines for RF epidemiology. Dr. Goldsmith separated his presentation into three topics. First was the existing state of public health and scientifically-based regulations. Second was the critique of two key studies as examples of how we can update our epidemiologic input to improve the understanding of this problem. The third topic was to discuss innovative ways to address the issues encountered in RF epidemiology and present some concepts of epidemiologic monitoring that may apply. Dr. Goldsmith elaborated on the importance of narrowing the gap between the three major scientific disciplines: exposure estimation, experimental sciences such as toxicology, and population-based scientific disciplines such as epidemiology in response to the study of possible health effects of RF exposure from cellular telephones. Up to this point standards in regard to RF, radar, and microwave exposure have been derived from military studies with little or no epidemiologic input. Therefore, these regulations may not apply to RF exposure from cellular telephones. Dr. Goldsmith went on to critique several of these studies, highlighting several inconsistencies in the data and their interpretation. He emphasized that scientists must not be distracted from epidemiologic studies by inferences drawn from toxicology, physics, or existing regulatory standards. He further emphasized that exposure estimation is difficult and one should start with semi-quantitative indices and focus on population-based studies. There is always a need to study high-risk groups, with that risk being identified by other exposures, inherent attributes, or health history. Finally, Dr. Goldsmith discussed results of a study of Moscow embassy staff. This study showed no excess of cancer mortality when compared with other Eastern European embassies; however, when site-specific cancers were examined there were some excesses seen. Dr. Goldsmith addressed several other studies and finished by advising that scientists involved in RF epidemiologic studies not limit their outcomes to cancer, consider epidemiological monitoring, and assume that the future of epidemiology is on the line.

Following Dr. Goldsmith was Dr. Ernst Wynder of the American Health Foundation. Dr. Wynder's presentation focused on the epidemiology of small effects or weak associations. He began by describing disease prevention as the most important method for treating diseases that are largely not treatable. One of these is brain cancer. He further stated that most cancers are related to metabolic overload. Smoking, drinking, eating, and sexual behavior have all been associated with certain types of cancers. Dr. Wynder referred to his own study published in 1950 indicating smoking as a cause of lung cancer. This study was an example of how significant data speak for themselves. However, with weak associations (OR <3 or 2) there are three major problems: case-control selection and bias, confounders, and subgroup analysis. Dr.

Wynder described a hospital-based case-control study, partially funded by WTR, on brain cancer and cellular phones that is currently underway at the American Health Foundation. As discussed earlier, this study will face similar problems as other studies of weak associations. One of these problems is confounding. Dr. Wynder used the study of cigarette smoking as an example where numerous confounders are found. Increased alcohol intake, increased fat intake and other nutritional deficiencies are all characteristics of smokers and are also associated with certain cancers. Therefore, these may confound the outcome of a case-control study, especially a study involving weak associations. Next, Dr. Wynder explored a type of bias found in case-control studies which he has termed the "wish bias." This is the unconscious, inaccurate reporting of behaviors or results due to persons wishing for a certain outcome, and is prevalent in self-reported data. The investigator in industry may hope the product is not harmful and therefore wish for a negative outcome whereas an investigator in academia may wish for a positive outcome which is more likely to be published and attract funding. For subjects participating in the study, the wish bias is apparent in the underreporting of negative behaviors and the overreporting of healthy behaviors, and this differs depending on whether the subject is a case or a control. Finally, Dr. Wynder approached a new topic area relevant to the cellular telephone and brain cancer issue. This is the negative placebo or nocebo effect in relation to a specific exposure. This effect implies that a suggestion of harm or pain from a specific exposure made to a group of subjects will result in many of the subjects experiencing that outcome even if the exposure is really harmless. A few early studies have suggested that the nocebo effect differs by personality type; if secondary gain in the form of monetary compensation is involved, the subject is more likely to claim damage from the exposure. Dr. Wynder summarized his presentation by emphasizing the importance of applying Bradford Hill's, "Criteria of Judgement," to all epidemiologic studies, but especially those of weak associations before anyone has the right to claim causation. These criteria include:

1.   strength of the association;
2.   consistency within the study and between studies;
3.   specificity;
4.   temporality;
5.   dose response;
6.   biological plausibility.

For cellular telephones and brain cancer the biologic plausibility exists; however, the next steps are to address the remaining criteria. Finally, in addition to the epidemiology of cellular telephone exposure, factors contributing to the mortality and morbidity of brain cancer must be thoroughly examined in both the United States and other parts of the world. This is necessary in order to fully evaluate RF exposure from cellular telephones and the contributing environmental effects on the subsequent development of brain cancer in the population.

The final speaker of the morning was Dr. Robert Morgan of Environmental Health Strategies, Inc. Dr. Morgan first commented on issues discussed by the previous speakers. He discussed the issue of latency and induction time for a specific disease and the difficulty epidemiological studies have in determining either of these. He suggested that, perhaps, epidemiologists need to spend more time differentiating between a cause and a risk factor. In terms of RF epidemiology, the field is being driven more by a public health imperative than a biologic imperative, meaning primarily that with a rapidly expanding technology there is a need and desire to know whether or not there is any health effect, regardless of the lack of biologic evidence at the time. Dr. Morgan emphasized that this problem of changing technology combined with the problem of latency which is probably around ten years for almost any type of malignancy will have an effect on the results of any epidemiological study in this field. He continued describing that epidemiologists in the past saw relative risks of 10 or 20, but now have the statistical tools to detect relative risks of 1.2 to 1.5. This makes it increasingly difficult to separate a true risk from possible confounders and that this is something of which epidemiologists must always be aware and carefully address in their research and subsequent publications. He also said this same caution should apply to using old data to try and find answers to current problems.

Next, Dr. Morgan addressed the topic of occupational studies. Pointing out that the workplace is the sentinel for the community, meaning that people manufacturing or designing certain equipment or materials are exposed to a certain substance or level of energy at higher levels than the general population. This leads to both advantages and disadvantages inherent in occupational studies. As advantages, Dr. Morgan lists primarily that occupational studies deal with a defined population and that employment and health records are fairly readily available for this same population. Exposure estimates are sometimes available, but this is true in more semi-quantitative terms such as job title, and length of employment. Occupational studies can also be of either cohort and/or case-control study designs. Some disadvantages include restricted sample size, leading to more confounding and decreased statistical power. Dr. Morgan also discussed the issue of ascertainment bias. For example, a person that is considered affluent, employed or adequately insured may be more likely to seek health care and thus be diagnosed with the disease in question at a higher rate than a person without these characteristics. Next, he discusses the "healthy worker effect" which is a bias common in occupational studies arising from the fact that persons who work and are able to work tend to be healthier than the general population. Finally, Dr. Morgan discusses the factors involved in using occupational studies as an approach to studying the possible health effects of RF exposure. The primary issues include the probability of exposure (dose, intensity, and duration) based on job title, and the need for good demographic data such as social security numbers. When conducting a cohort study there is the advantage of looking for multiple outcomes since cohort studies select their population based on exposure and then follow them over time for a disease outcome. This can also be a disadvantage because you are being given data for which you had no prior hypotheses which can create a multiple comparison problem in a statistical analysis. Cohort studies in many cases can also provide the appropriate latency period: for example, a company in the telephone or radio business since the 1940's will have valuable long term data on their workers. This occupational cohort can also be a very good source of cases and controls for case-control studies. Because these people have a high probability of exposure your statistical power increases and you can get better data than by interviewing people in the general population. Some confounders can be controlled for but not others. For example, smoking history is rarely available in occupational studies. In conclusion, Dr. Morgan emphasized that no one type of study is without certain limitations and that in anticipation of results, scientists must look forward to their studies being interpreted and misinterpreted by various people in various ways. However, Dr. Morgan asserts that epidemiology will provide the definitive answer as to whether RF affects human health, but not to expect these answers too quickly.

Scientific Discussion

Dr. Niels Kuster:
I have a question to all four of you. In what year will we be able to say that the odds ratio of brain cancer among mobile phone users is lower than two?

Dr. Rothman:
We should be able to say that within one or two years. But the trick is to understand what that means. Let us assume we had data showing that there was no effect. After a short time we will be able to produce that data. But what it will refer to will be a short length of follow-up from initial exposure. And we will not be able to estimate what the effect is for long-term follow-up or for the long-term effects of early exposure, because we have to wait for that to occur.

Dr. Kuster:
I put the question wrongly. In which year do you think you are able to state that the brain cancer risk of mobile phone is lower than a factor of 2?

Dr. Rothman:
We can say that it is shortly, but only for the short term. If you want to know what the risk is 20 years after sustained exposure, you'll have to wait 20 years after sustained exposure to find out.

Dr. Wynder:
From our case control studies, we will be able to tell within two years what the odds ratio is. I disagree with the *Science* article that an odds ratio of 1.8 can be significant if it meets all the criteria of judgment that I have indicated. There I believe the *Science* article made a grievous error. But what I also said, the lower the odds ratio, the more likely you are to make one or several of the mistakes that I have listed. But a case control study historically will be able to give much data long before the cohort studies are completed. One of the major advantages of the cohort studies is that they give you an actual absolute risk.

Dr. Goldsmith:
I differ slightly with some of my colleagues in epidemiology on the emphasis I put on

odds ratios. I want to make this point because it is likely to be troublesome, particularly for a relatively infrequent disease. To take the odds ratio alone, or even the 95 percent probability limit, without looking at the probability that such an odds ratio could occur for random reasons, or without looking to see how small a number of cases you are examining, is a rather risky business. In many circumstances, we have expected numbers that are less than 1 with only 4 possible outcomes: 0,1,2, or 3. The ability to draw a fine judgment based on odds ratios...when you have, for example, an expected number of .2, you have 0, 5, 10, and 15. Those odds ratios are not meaningful as such. If we're using odds ratios as the criteria of success of an epidemiologic program, they are not an adequate one in and of themselves.

Dr. Morgan:

If the odds ratio or the Standardized Mortality Ratio is not elevated enough to become statistically significant, the argument will be made that you haven't followed the cohort long enough. At what point is long enough? If you have to wait 30 or 35 years, then the study is obsolete by the time it's finished because the technology you measured is no longer in use. I think the case control studies under way...you're not going to have an answer to this question that anyone is going to be happy with for many years, if at all.

Dr. John Vena:

With regard to the cohort study design, I think that given the unique characteristics of the exposure to cellular phones, it's the only way to get the answer. The discussion about the issues of exposure time and mechanisms and latency, I think the cohort design will give us answers in a relatively short period of time because of the issue of "Is the exposure really promotional in nature, or are we talking about an initiator?" If they are promotional in nature, then the cohort design is ideal to study this and find an answer within a short period of time. The studies we've done have indicated that brain cancer latency for some occupational exposures is around 20 years. They aren't as long as some of the other solid tumors. If they are promotional in nature, like some of the other EMF exposures have been considered, then I think the answers will come sooner than 20 years. My other comment is that with the changing exposure nature of the cellular phone technology, the only way we can be sure of someone's exposures and the changing nature of that exposure is through the cohort design. The cohort design is ideal to ask the right questions and to come up with some of the right answers. Regarding the studies that are being proposed, why omit the commercial users? What proportion of the users are commercial accounts? What proportion of the business phones or commercial users would be sole users? I think they could be a unique group, as in the meter readers we heard about in the study in Sweden. By omitting them, we might be missing an important group.

Dr. Rothman:

In response to the question about omitting business accounts and focusing on consumer accounts, we expect to enroll millions of people in our study and follow them for a long period of time. Size is not going to be a problem, but validity is. What an epidemiologist facing this research question has to bear in mind is that if you end up finding no effect, then the most serious criticisms that you have to be able to deal with are have you successfully dealt with those issues that would have led to exposure misclassification that could be explaining a lack of an effect even if there were one? So misclassification is our primary preoccupation. Our concern with the business accounts is that we have learned that for many of such accounts, it's difficult to get the linkage information that we need, the Social Security information accurately, to link with mortality records. Sometimes the Social Security number that is obtained for such accounts may relate to a purchasing person in the company, and somebody else may be the user. We also think that, though many business phones may be used by one individual, they're more likely to be passed around and used by various employees in the company than is a private consumer telephone. Because of these uncertainties and others that we had about business telephones, we just opted to exclude those, because we still had sufficient numbers of people from the various companies that we intend to enroll to have a good-sized cohort with less misclassification from the remainder. So it was really the validity issue with respect to being able to interpret the possible results if we found nothing that prompted this exclusion.

Dr. Morgan:

I tend to agree with your concern about the commercial users. I think the commercial users may have been among the earliest users, because business was quick to adopt the new technology. I also agree with your comment that the cohorts may well give an answer earlier—our cohort is supposed to be finished in six or seven months—of people who were employed in the industry. We'll see how it comes out with 133,000 people. It's a relatively large cohort. In spite of my own optimism about the set of studies that I am undertaking, I think we have to still put a lot of caveats that this is an issue which is not going to be decided very quickly.

Dr. Vena:

I think the other issue is the outcomes of study. If we just concentrate solely on brain cancer, we would be missing an opportunity to look at their potential effects that could be related to the use of technology and how they might interact with other psychosocial factors. It's going to be tough. As Dr. Wynder discussed, if we're going to outcomes that aren't going to be quantified through cancer registries and the like, or definitive diagnosis, we're going to more morbidity outcomes, like headaches or skin rashes or neurological-type conditions. Then they'll be much more difficult to validate the outcome as well.

Dr. Goldsmith:

I was about to say the same thing. It seems to me that if we focus on outcomes that are solely restricted to cancer, we're not using the biologic experience that we ought to be able to use in a cohort study. There hasn't been any paper, as for as I know, on neurologic findings, particularly peripheral neurologic findings associated with cellular telephone use. I inquired of a colleague in neurology and he said, "Yes, we get an occasional case of persons with numbness or tingling in the distribution of the trigeminal nerve, which supplies the face, that is associated with cellular telephone use. It's just that nobody has written it up. We haven't organized our information." I think there are a number of malignant outcomes to which a good deal more attention should be paid. If we fail to do that, we're failing to use the cohort system adequately.

Dr. Wynder:

As to the last question, there are so many of us here interested in brain cancer, and there's clearly more to brain cancer than cellular telephones. It seems to me if we already go through the trouble of doing large case-control studies, what are some of the other variables that relate to the etiology of cancer of the brain? By and large, we are relatively ignorant. There's one age group that occurred before 20, one that's later on in life. This being the "Age of the Brain," I would suggest that all of us give some more broader thought about the etiology of brain cancer. Most of our discoveries in epidemiology have been linked to epithelial cancers. By and large, we have never done very well with types like cancer of the brain, but this is a great, great challenge. The final point I want to make, and a point that was made on the piece that we heard about headaches—the brain is a remarkable thing, how it influences the body. Let me just give you one example. Some years ago I was swimming in the Dead Sea. And I looked at my toe, and I found what seemed to me a melanoma. Now the worst thing in terms of a negative perceiver would be a doctor. Because when I went to medical school, we always had five students, whatever the disease symptoms were, they thought they had the disease. So for months I was really concerned about my toe. I felt pain in my groin. I felt pain in my head. I thought I had terminal melanoma. Now I can tell you next when I swim in the Dead Sea, I will be much happier. The point I am making is that you have certain symptoms that you may think relate to a disease, or you read in *The New York Times* that A may cause B, it has a dramatic effect. And the final point I really want to make—when I talked about secondary gain—I attended a colleague control council meeting last week in Orlando. A fellow from Pepsi Cola brought the history of fraud of the American people because somebody found a needle in a single can. We are told there were 150 reports about people finding a needle--this a disgrace to the American people as such. But what brought it about were the media, with one report after the other. Pretty soon all kinds of fraudulent people said, "We found a needle in the can." And so it is with symptomatology. The more we hear in the papers that something relates to a symptom, like headaches, the more of us will get it. When we are discussing next week is the mechanism whereby we believe the brain influences the body in all types of things, including pain, nausea, dizziness, insomnia, irritability, and as some study suggested, divorce rate.

Dr. Rothman:

I described, in my talk, the ERI mortality study, which is a purely record-based study linking phone records with death certificates. It's obvious that in a record-based study like that, you cannot study headache or skin rash or other symptoms of problems that do not get reported on death certificates, do not even lead to death. On the other hand, I also described a study that we are planning in which cellular telephone users are going to be identified and are going to be followed by regular contact through mail questionnaires periodically. In that cohort study, which hasn't yet started, we hope to look at a large variety of outcomes, including all of the outcomes that have been recently discussed. So it's obviously a question of study design. If you've got death records and death certificates as your measurement of outcome, you're not going to look at skin rash. But in the studies we are planning with direct contact with the cellular phone users, we do not expect to be measuring a wide variety of outcomes.

Dr. Matthew Meltz:

To start with, Dr. Wynder, you made a very direct statement that you saw "biological plausibility." I need to understand what that means to you. And I'd like to ask if the other epidemiologists are also coming from that same belief, that there is biological plausibility, as compared to hypothetical plausibility?

Dr. Wynder:

When I said "the biological plausibility," I wasn't discussing degrees, from a hundred to one. Maybe it's only one. But at least you hold the cellular telephone to the ear. As we showed yesterday, there are certainly some effects on the brain. And in general, I would like to think it is more hypothetically possible then biologically plausible. But it's not entirely so far out of range that you wouldn't begin to think about it. A final point in regard to that: I have always felt that carcinogenesis primarily relates to metabolic overload. As far as minimal exposures are concerned, including to cellular telephones, we have the anatomic and the physiologic and the metabolic capacity to deal with small amounts of whatever the toxic elements are. This includes things like dioxin and environmental tobacco smoke and other things. So it always comes down to dose. When I said "biologically plausible," I really meant that hypothetically it's plausible. I think I stand corrected on that point.

Dr. Asher Sheppard:

The question I had goes to the larger issue of exposure assessment. It seems to me that the importance of business accounts was that they would represent the different part of the exposure distribution. In order to validate my assumption and other assumptions about what kind of exposures are going on, how do you look at the issue of exposure assessment here? In particular, Dr. Rothman, I was struck by the comment about the difference you believe between the EMF magnetic fields, power frequencies, and the exposures from cellular telephones, as to the ability to get good exposure assessment. I wonder what the basis for that trust is?

Dr. Rothman

Let me just repeat the obvious, which is that for EMF exposure, you're not going to learn much about an individual's exposure without a detailed examination of the individual's habits and circumstances, and probably site measurements of field strength. But we do have surrogates for RF exposure from cellular telephones. We have billing records that tell us how long a person has been on the phone, or at least how long the phone has been used. By our survey data, we can infer that we have a fairly good surrogate for actual individual exposure. As I have pointed out, there are very many other elements to the ultimate question of exposure if you're talking about it in terms of, say, SAR to specific tissues. There is the power output of the telephone. There is the presence or absence of metal eyeglasses. There is the side of the head. There are quite a number of other factors involved. We believe we're going to have large enough data in our record-based cohort study so that we're going to be able to single out a large number of individuals at the high end of the exposure distribution. Even though there are going to be various factors that are still uncertain in defining whether or not these people had sustained high exposure, in general, we can segregate people with low-level exposure from people with comparatively high exposure. Now, what we're calling "high exposure" may not correspond to what you might think of as high exposure in biological terms or in terms that you can generate in the laboratory for animal exposure. The point is, in terms of consumer use, we can find people who are heavy users, whose account and whose reports make it clear that these are the people at the top of the distribution. And we'll be able to look at the outcome rates in such people. So that's not the basis for my optimism. There is nothing comparable that you could do in terms of EMF exposure without an entirely different approach to exposure assessment.

Dr. Morgan:

I think there's a danger that we will move from issues of exposure, in terms of dose to body tissues, to the consideration of whether people are "exposed" or "unexposed." If we look at what has happened before in issues like asbestos, where the first studies were done on people who were exposed over many years to very high doses—and there has been a willingness to extrapolate downwards from those high doses to bystanders who have had little or no true dose when you come to exposure—and with the proliferation of devices that emit radio frequency energy, you're going to get people who claim to be exposed or who know they're exposed who, in fact, have had very little doses. And I think there we start to get closer to the EMF issue, where people will claim or think they've had, or epidemiologists will assume that there has, in fact, been continuous exposure, not the intermittent exposure through use. So, something we must be concerned about in the future is the indiscriminate assignment of exposure categories without a lot of thought.

Dr. Sheldon Wolff:

I have one question for Ken Rothman and one perhaps for Dr. Wynder. I was struck by your slide showing that the use of phones is going up exponentially. And that stopped in '94. We're two years beyond that, and this is just going to keep climbing. If we're going to have a 20-year, perhaps, latency period, where do we really get our control population? Because it seems to me the people that you're considering to be unexposed right now are going to be recruited into the users and would no longer be valuable as controls. The other question I had, again came from a slide of yours showing that the median use or length of a telephone call was two minutes, median number of calls was eight per week. So now you begin to wonder, because Dr. Gandhi has told me that at high SARs, it takes about six minutes before an effect is seen. The effects are transitory, so that once you stop the exposure, the animals, and then people, sort of return to normal. This makes me want to raise the question: Is there really a biological plausibility thing that we're really dealing with—is it a real problem that we're dealing with? With such short exposures, could they really cause the kinds of effects that seem to be driving this whole problem?

Dr. Rothman:

First, there may be a misunderstanding of what we're using for our comparison group. Let me clarify it. In our mortality-based cohort study—and probably in the population-based cohort study that we're talking about—the essential comparison is people using portable handheld telephones. That is, a comparison of their experience with the experience of people using mobile telephones, car telephones. So as long as technology expands, as long as there are people in both of these groups, the comparisons are internal among the cellular telephone customers. Some customers get no exposure because they use a car phone. And some customers get exposure because they're using a handheld telephone and placing the antenna next to their head. We don't envision that there will be a problem running out of comparison people, because the comparison group are all cellular telephone customers. The problem could come if there were a dramatic shift in the technology so that everybody started using handheld telephones and there were very few people using car phones. So far, we don't have that problem. But then, that would be something that we would get concerned about as time goes by. For now, there is no issue with respect to comparison groups. In fact, there's a very nice balance in terms of numbers in the two groups that we're looking at.

Dr. Wolff:

But don't you think that some of the people who are now perhaps using mobile phones will be converted to what may be the more convenient handheld phones as the technology changes or as time goes on, so that suddenly one group is being changed and being recruited into another group? And you're not going to see the results for another 20 years.

Dr. Rothman:

Yes, it's certainly possible that as time goes on, that people that have not been exposed to the exposure that we're studying, which is basically the handheld portable telephone, will become exposed. As an analogy, imagine that you're studying the effects of cigarette-smoking, and you're comparing that, as an exposure, to the effects of chewing gum. Well, it may be that people who chew gum later in life would take up cigarette-smoking, and then they become smokers. So you don't count them as a non-smoker if they start smoking. And the same would occur in our studies. We can get information, ideally, on what kind of instrument a person is using and when the person starts using that, and we treat the data accordingly. This is not a new issue for epidemiologists. The only trick here is to get the information. And we certainly will know how to deal with it. Now your question was about biological plausibility. If I remember, you said that it looks like at the median level of use, that we are talking about exposures that are considerably below the levels that seem to cause measurable laboratory-measured effects. That may well be the case. But our focus of course is not going to be on people who are using the median level of use. So we hope to look at the most extreme contrast that we can. This is something that having a very large study enables us to do with a little more flexibility than we could in a small study. We can still get sizable numbers of people in the very high exposed categories and measure the effects of extreme use. Now let's just suppose that in those highest categories we still are dealing with levels of exposure below those that Dr. Gandhi was talking about as being of concern. Does it make sense to do a study like this? You have to ask that from various points of view. From the point of view of some biologists, it might not. But I have talked to other biologists who say that even at that level there are changes in cell membranes and gap junction openings that are shut off, and the conduction of possible harmful agents that accumulate between one cell and another, so some people claim that there is still some biological concern. But even if you don't accept that point of view, from the point of view of the industry, it still seems to be worthwhile to study the effect of the highest level of consumer exposure that is experienced in order to provide reassuring information that can reassure the very wide customer base that the industry is privileged to have and a customer base that is continually expanding. So, from the industry point of view, it would make sense to study it, even though the laboratory information and the biological information weren't there. Even if that were true, that they weren't there to support it, there wold still be motivation to study it. From the epidemiologic point of view, it follows that if this is the pattern of use that people have, then it makes some sense to study what is the effect of this particular pattern. For those reasons, it is still a sensible idea, I believe, to go ahead and measure what we can about people who are in that current distribution of use. The problem that Bob Morgan referred to earlier is one that we're very preoccupied with, and that is that we're talking about doing long-term studies over years, or even decades, about a technology that's changing month by month. This is a real challenge, and it's something we have to consider. Ultimately, that may cloud the interpretation of our study results since we can't predict how the future of this technology is going to change. We do know though that we have a lot of users right now using a certain kind of technology. What we're doing is the only thing that could be done under the circumstances, study what people are doing.

Dr. Goldsmith:

First, I want to speak to the problem of biologic plausibility. It is one of the criteria that we have held improves in trying to evaluate whether an association is likely to be viewed as the causal mechanism. But the point I tried to make in my first slide is that epidemiologic study must never, never be deferred or evaded because the end point that has been suggested and that you are looking for is not biologically plausible. A very high proportion of the known human carcinogens were discovered first by epidemiologic studies, and only later were biologic mechanisms found that were relevant. So it's a very important question, but it must not be used to defer our work. I wanted to make another comment about the problem of comparing exposures. An unwritten assumption in the statistical and epidemiologic logic, when one is comparing a high-exposure group and a low-exposure group—or even more gradations—is that the other risk factors are identical, that you're not confounding the exposure with something else. And in order to do that, you must know something about the risk factors. We know a little bit about the risk factors for brain cancer. In a number of studies, it seems to have been somewhat higher in chemists than other occupations. And in the petrochemical industry, there is some suggestive evidence that the risk ratios are not very high, although the probabilities are such as to make it statistically significant. We also know that brain cancer has been associated with ELF, and that's a relatively new finding. So we have to be very careful when we compare populations that we've chosen for contrasting exposure, to make sure we've balanced them or adjusted for or taken into account the other risk factors.

Dr. Wynder:

Relative to plausibility, *The Lancet* in 1950, when we first reported our first study on lung cancer and smoking, wondered what the biological plausibility was. In other words, we have not always been brightest. And obviously this one is more difficult. One of the questioners listed the points of initiation, promotion, and progression—where is it that possibly cellular telephones come in, if anywhere? Certainly since the cellular telephone has been around only for a few years, you wouldn't imagine there was initiation, because you would know it takes 20 or 30 years for cancer to develop. So it would be more likely progression and promotion. I probably don't think that is quite likely, though hypothetically, everything is likely. The final point I want to make relating to epidemiology—I always do something that I call the epidemiology control. To what extent do the cellular telephone users differ from anyone else? Do they smoke less? Do they eat differently? Certainly as I walk along the streets of Rome and I see someone in Piazza Novona while I look at the statue and he talks on the cellular telephone, we are different. And so we've got to look at some other variables. I think it is crucial to this debate, in the final analysis, what will establish whether something causes or does not cause is the science of epidemiology. I may not have a clue on how it happens. In all of our dietary work, we're never precisely sure of the relative role of fiber and diet and fat, but we know epidemiology works. And it may take years or centuries, if ever, until we understand the intricacy whereby certain factors initiate, promote, or progress cancer.

Dr. Rothman:

Just a quick follow-up comment. Several speakers recently have questioned whether cellular telephone users, or the ones with high exposure, differ from people who don't use cellular telephones. I just want to remind people I showed a graph today which was preliminary results from our record-based mortality study. In that graph, we looked at mortality rates for portable phone users and compared that with mobile phone users. The question about whether cellular telephone users differ from people who don't use cellular telephones is of no interest to us in our study, because we are not comparing cellular telephone users with people who don't have cellular telephones. We are comparing one type of user with another type of user. And we do think cellular telephone users differ from people who don't use the telephone, and we think that they differ in ways that might affect brain cancer. But we don't think that those differences will apply, because we don't think that they occur among cellular telephone users with respect to the type of phone they use.

Mr. Bill Moyer:

I wanted to ask the panel to give us some insight as to what examples there are from the history of epidemiology, where correlation factors as low as 1.2 to 1.5, basically a small number, have actually led to uncovering causes that resulted in real-world health problems? I was wondering historically if other sources, particularly if there were industrial sources involved, would give the industry some insight as to what we might expect as we go through the process.

Dr. Goldsmith:

How large an increase in the probability of cancer would you expect to have to find before you change your behavior about some practice that you're using, how you drive your car, how you eat? I think if we put that kind of question to most people, something like ten percent increase is about all they really want to be passive about. When it gets a bit more than that, they get rather interested. Although we're talking about a small number, we're talking about numbers which take large populations and which are difficult to interpret. The acceptability of small proportional increases in serious disease by the public is not very great. I think they want us not to have any increase at all, if possible, and to that end, we have to devote considerable effort.

Dr. Morgan:

There are two kinds of answer to the question. The first is the scientific issue. And remember that the acceptance or rejection of the hypothesis is really a subjective phenomenon, where you see sufficient data to say that "I believe there's an association that's causal," or not. There's no magic statistics. Where you set that level will vary by individual background, training, bias, whatever. The other issue, which may be more important, is the regulatory issue. Whereas the scientist is generally trained to avoid Type 1 error, we don't want to accept a false association. The regulator, on the other hand, by nature tries to avoid a Type 2 error, in the thought that they're trying to be protective and will accept an association that maybe the scientist doesn't. And I think it's one of the reasons why scientists and regulators argue and why you can't really be both. So that your question in many ways is unanswerable—that if someone says, "You found a relative risk of 1.3, does that mean it's causal," I may or may not think it's causal. But it's perhaps more important what somebody else thinks of it and how they will interpret it. I can't think at the moment of any risk of 1.3 that has been translated into public health policy, except perhaps less than 1.3, which is the kind of thing you're seeing with breast implants. And yet there was FDA action in the absence of any association. So that regulators and industry people, or whatever, will take action even though there isn't necessarily statistical significance and even though there isn't necessarily a strong effect. But that's not a scientific question, I don't think.

Dr. Wynder:

Where they have taken action is on the environmental tobacco smoke, which is about 1.3. I happen to believe the causation has not been established, but tobacco is such an enemy of the people that anything goes. In terms of alcohol and breast cancer, they hover around 1.3. Dr. Willard believes it's causative. I have some doubt. Perhaps the best example wold be people who have serum cholesterol levels of about 160, which we believe are quite normal. But I would estimate there's probably a risk of about 30 percent over those who have 140. For some of the major causes of death, like cholesterol and other heart disease, we probably can do what you say. But for most other things, where the only evidence we have is 1.2 or 1.3, taking that out of some studies, it's probably not likely that this is causative. But our willingness, as a society, to act on it depends on how strong or how weak the enemy is for our government.

Dr. Goldsmith:
I just want to say, in passing, I think that many clinical decisions in medicine are made with much lower probabilities.

Dr. Rothman:
I think I can cite an example of relative risk 1.2 in which regulatory action has been taken, and that's with regard to air pollution effects, where the highest relative risks are about 1.2, not an area without debate, but still an area where there are small effects and in which there is regulatory action. I just want to make one final comment on this though. Epidemiology is sometimes criticized as being a scientific area where it is really difficult or impossible to infer whether or not effects in the area that you've outlined are actually causal or not. And it's a reasonable criticism to a point. But in response and in defense, I like to point out that it's true that in epidemiology we have this area where it is difficult to make certain inferences. More difficult. But in fact, epidemiology is the only hope of making inference about effects that are as small as these. In other sciences, such as in toxicology, there is absolutely no hope of studying enough subjects to make good inferences about effects that are as small as the ones that you have raised. Epidemiology, like any science, would have its gray zones where there are levels of difficult-to-detect effects. But in epidemiology, these effects are smaller than in any other area of investigation.

INTERFERENCE WITH MEDICAL DEVICES

Gretchen K. Findlay and Andrea Donato

Session One Summary

As mobile communications devices have proliferated, concern has been raised about the potential for medical equipment to malfunction due to interference from mobile phones in the vicinity of a hospital or other medical care facility. The papers presented in this section provide a good overview of the myriad of issues that are present when assessing and dealing with the potential for interference between medical equipment and communications instruments. The papers present research results, discuss governing standards, and offer recommendations for managing the problem.

Dr. Ken Joyner gave the invited paper regarding the state of the science in wireless instrument medical equipment interference. Dr. Joyner is Manager of the Electromagnetic Compatibility Section at Telstra Research Laboratories in Clayton, Victoria, Australia.

Dr. Joyner began his presentation by pointing out that the effects of electromagnetic interference (EMI) on medical electrical equipment are of concern because of potential interference with the safe operation of life-support and other critical care equipment. He stated that EMI is not a new phenomenon and is not only caused by wireless or radiated communication instruments, but by a variety of sources. The problem of EMI between medical devices and cellular instruments has two major components. First, hospital equipment is particularly susceptible to EMI. Second, as mobile communication devices proliferate, the number of situations where medical electrical equipment might be exposed to relatively high electromagnetic fields increases.

Before describing a number of studies in which he has been involved, Dr. Joyner first familiarized the attendees with the communication technologies available in Australia and included in his studies. The two mobile telephone systems in use in

Australia are the Advanced Mobile Phone System (AMPS), which is an analog system, and the Global System for Mobile Communications (GSM), which is a digital system. He compared the power, modulations, and field strengths of these systems.

In the first study, AMPS and GSM phones were placed near 15 pieces of in-service medical electrical equipment to detect any abnormal behavior due to EMI. Three pieces of equipment were affected by AMPS and eight by GSM. He stated that the following symptoms were observed: false error conditions and shut down, changes in pump infusion rates, blanking of oscilloscopes, and vulnerability in monitors with long leads and radio transmission. Findings from the study indicated that although all items met the 1979 U.S. Food and Drug Administration voluntary standard of 7 V/m, many were susceptible to the phones. These findings prompted the Australian Therapeutic Goods Administration to make policy recommendations to hospitals.

A more recent study aimed at evaluating the performance of a number of currently available drug infusion pumps and syringe drivers when subjected to electromagnetic fields from AMPS and GSM handsets. The devices were graded according to the following performance classifications: 1. No EMI—normal operation; 2. Permanent failure, but fail safe (defined as appropriate device warning and shut down); 3. Intermittent EMI, with reversion to normal operation when EMI source is removed; and 4. Subtle but permanent failure, and unit does not fail safe. Eight of the 17 devices tested so far have exhibited a category 2 failure; none of the devices have failed without appropriate warning to the operator.

In addition to in-service medical devices in hospital settings, Dr. Joyner discussed ongoing research with hearing aids and cardiac pacemakers. Based on the findings of a preliminary study confirming that GSM phones caused EMI in various types of hearing aids, a collaborative joint investigation has begun. Involved parties include Telstra Research Laboratories, the National Acoustics Laboratories, the Spectrum Management Authority, AUSTEL (the Australian Telecommunications Industry Regulator), Mobile Service Providers, representatives from the hearing aid industry, and consumer groups, including hearing aid user organizations. The group had defined a series of goals for the study, including: assessing the degree of EMI caused by GSM phones in a wide range of hearing aids; assessing the effectiveness of various treatments and design modifications to hearing aids to reduce interference; developing a reliable and practical measurement system; and developing hearing aid standards for immunity to digital mobile interference. Dr. Joyner also described a pacemaker study which tested 25 patients with a GSM mobile telephone and simulated signals; results included occasional inhibition of output and oversensing. The consulting cardiologist concluded that no consistent, clinically significant abnormalities existed.

Next, Dr. Joyner provided an overview of current international standards for medical electrical equipment and hearing aids. He discussed the International Electrotechnical Commission's recommended standard of 3 V/m for both categories and raised questions regarding its adequacy.

In conclusion, Dr. Joyner offered four strategies to manage EMI issues with medical electrical equipment in the hospital setting. First, he recommended a mobile communications management strategy, which included utilizing controlled communications services in the medical industry. Second, he recommended an education strategy aimed to make personnel in the medical industry more aware of

EMI. Next, a prevention strategy, in which biomedical engineers identify and control sensitive medical equipment, was recommended. Lastly, Dr. Joyner recommended a new EMI standards strategy in which medical equipment requires new immunity levels defined by risk categories:

- High Risk: Life support devices, key resuscitation devices, and other devices whose failure or misuse is reasonably likely to seriously injure patients or staff.

- Medium Risk: Devices whose failure or misuse would have a significant impact on patient care, but would not be likely to cause direct serious injury.

- Low Risk: Devices whose failure or misuse is unlikely to result in serious consequences. This category would also encompass an "Annoying" classification.

He recommended that medical equipment placed in a medium or high risk category should have a minimum level of immunity of no less than 10 V/m.

The invited panel response was given by Dr. Bernard Segal, a member of the McGill Biomedical Group on Electromagnetic Compatibility. His presentation covered a discussion of studies of electromagnetic environments, ad hoc equipment testing, and recommendations to minimize risk. Dr. Segal is an Electrical Engineer at McGill University and Director of Research in Otolaryngology at the SMBD Jewish General Hospital in Montreal, Quebec, Canada.

Dr. Segal stressed the importance of understanding the electromagnetic environment. He described studies conducted by the McGill group including free-space propagation predictions, measurements of fields of fixed sources, and measurements of fields of portable sources. He explained that to estimate the risk of interference in a given device, the electromagnetic environment must exceed the equipment immunity. To assess the equipment's immunity, Dr. Segal suggested ad hoc testing.

He described a series of ad hoc tests conducted by McGill. He tested a series of common communication devices with medical equipment under realistic conditions in a hospital setting. He tested typical orientations, cables, rooms, and operational modes looking for serious, repeatable malfunctions. Walkie talkies were the most powerful sources tested and were found to cause the most interference. Testing using cellular phones produced many fewer device malfunctions, and testing with a very low power source (10 mW) produced no malfunctions.

Finally, Dr. Segal presented recommendations for minimizing risks of EMI malfunctions. During the next five to ten years, he recommended requiring management of radiofrequency (RF) sources and medical devices in the hospital environment, education of hospital personnel and phone users, and ad hoc estimation of immunity of existing medical equipment inventory. During the next 10 to 20 years, he suggested implementing better equipment designs and increased standards.

Session One Scientific Discussion

Dr. Bernard Eicher, Swiss Telecom, PTT:

This is not a very suitable way to do it because there are people that are very suspicious when you put the base station just on a hospital because they feel that they get even more ill when the base station is on the hospital. Okay, then, now my question. I feel there is an inherent communication problem in how we deal with the fact that one part of the engineers are making standards for, let's say, 3 V/m for interference of electronic equipment. And the other part of the engineers are producing devices which, by definition, conflict with exactly that standard. How do we deal with that?

Dr. Joyner:

First of all, a comment about sitting base stations on hospitals. I guess we do things differently in the southern hemisphere. We have a lot of base stations on hospitals. But we have a sitting criteria that says that field strength in hospital wards must not exceed 1 V/m. So although we put the base stations on top of the hospitals, we limit the field strengths in the hospitals to no more than 1 V/m.

Dr. Peter Excell, Bradford University, United Kingdom:

Well, it's a variation on the same theme as the other questioners, but I put my perspective to it. In the U.K., vehicle electronic systems are required to be immune to 50 V/m. But the manufacturers realize that it isn't good enough. They are testing to 200 V/m. Is an anti-lock braking system or a fuel injection system more important than a medical system? I'm saying this as a devil's advocate. You repeatedly refer to the question—the instruction that the hand-held phones must not be, in quotes, used in the hospital. The general public does not realize that these things radiate even when they're not talking into them. Usage is not clear enough. There is a long track record of established skills in the military industry that is transported now into the automotive industry, plus security industries. We can make that immune to 200 V/m and more. Three volts per meter seems incredibly low to me. So I would suggest that in the medium to long term, high immunity or bullet proofing, as you put it, is the real way to go. And in the short term, I would suggest that something like an alarm that goes off like a siren when it detects a field strength is an idea. One possible problem that occurs to me, that makes this different from, say, a military equipment is that there may be an inherent problem in shielding. The flying leaves that are attached to the heart muscle may be inherently antenna like in their behavior. Is that so? Is there a way around it?

Dr. Joyner:

One has to ask the question what is a reasonable level of immunity. And I guess if you want to regulate and make every piece of medical equipment immune to 100 V/m, the cost is going to go up initially. I think one has to be reasonable about this and say that some level between 3 V/m and higher would be a reasonable level. I feel quite comfortable, personally, with 10 V/m, with restrictions in hospitals for patient and visitor use of mobiles. But you have to realize that clinicians and health keepers now need mobility in the hospital environment. And if the equipment had reasonable immunity, you could have the two criteria met in that equipment wouldn't malfunction and that clinicians would have access to mobile communications, which is essential in modern day patient care. So I don't think that bullet proofing medical equipment to a 100 V/m would be a reasonable thing to request. That's my opinion.

Dr. Segal:

I'd like to say that I would very much like to see equipment at 100 V/m. I would be quite happy to see equipment at 20 V/m. The problem is, we can wish for standards. We have to be able to have standards that the medical device industry can produce. There is a major problem with standards, with regard to patient applied parts. When you have a medical device that is attached to a patient, whether that be through wires or through fluid lines, particularly when a patient is connected to several medical devices—if you look at a patient in an intensive care unit, you can count ten antennas radiating from that patient. And the biggest antenna is the patient himself. And the medical device manufacturers quite rightly claim that how can I design a piece of equipment if I don't know what is attached to it. And this is where the FD-TD technique might help us in trying to understand what the fields are like in this sort of complex environment. But I'm also assured by medical device manufacturers that it is possible to design equipment that will be able to do this. You have a design problem in the medical device industry that you both have to prevent very low leakage currents from going into the medical device for safety reasons. And you have the high frequency requirements. And these are often conflicting requirements. But I am told that it is possible to do. It's going to take time. It's going to take research.

Dr. Quirino Balzano, Motorola:

The question is directed to all of you, essentially. What I have seen this afternoon, that everybody is ready to ban the radio, but nobody seems to say, hey, this lousy medical equipment that interferes so easily, why are we not going to fix that? You cannot take that much—it cannot take that much of an effort to actually substantially improve the existing equipment that is out there. Can you give me an idea if that is feasible or not, please?

Dr. Joyner:

In day two, one of my slides did put an onus on the bioengineers to identify this sensitive equipment and formulate specific controls. Now those specific controls do include hardening of that equipment. But it often is not that easy with some of the older equipment to actually do. And sometimes the bioengineers don't have the skills to actually do that.

Dr. Balzano:

I wouldn't leave it to the bioengineers. There is such a thing as an EMC engineer. That's who we leave it to.

Dr. Joyner:

I work for the Telco, not the hospital. Again, it's a cost item, too. Some equipment is really expensive.

Dr. Balzano:
Another cost is that doctors not have access to medical communication in case of emergency? And that might be pretty high also.

Dr. Joyner:
Well, we have hardened some equipment so that it does perform much better. But, I mean, there is an enormous amount of equipment out there. It is a huge task.

Session Two Summary

For the past year and a half, the potential for cellular phones to interfere with implanted devices such as pacemakers has received considerable attention from the media, researchers, and the government. On October 5, 1994, a congressional hearing was held by the U.S. House of Representatives' Subcommittee on Information, Justice, Transportation, and Agriculture to uncover what was known of the interaction. At that time, it was concluded that further research was necessary and interdisciplinary cooperation was required. Although there have not been any clinical reports of a pacemaker malfunctioning due to interference from a communications device to date, there is a growing body of experimental evidence suggesting that the interaction does exist and could pose a serious public health problem. The papers presented in this session represent the majority of the body of knowledge in this area. The following papers present the state of the science on the issue from the interdisciplinary viewpoint of clinicians and biomedical engineers, and cover topics such as clinical and in vitro research, clinical significance, risk management, and mechanisms of the interaction.

Dr. David Hayes gave the invited paper regarding the state of the science in wireless instrument pacemaker and defibrillator interference. Dr. Hayes is director of the Pacing Laboratory and a cardiologist at the Mayo Clinic in Rochester, Minnesota, USA.

Dr. Hayes began his presentation by stressing that he was speaking as a clinician and did not assume expertise in physics, engineering, or epidemiology. For the benefit of the attendees, he provided background on the structure and operation of a pacemaker. He discussed polarity, including descriptions of bipolar and unipolar configurations, single and dual chamber pacing, sensitivity, and pacing abnormalities or interference types. He defined and displayed example tracings of inhibition, noise reversion, inappropriate tracking, crosstalk/safety pacing, and undersensing. He concluded this background with a discussion of the NBG code and the concept of pacemaker dependency.

Following this foundation, Dr. Hayes continued with a thorough review of the literature. He reviewed the findings reported by Barbaro, Eicher, Joyner, Strandberg, Irnich, Carrillo, and Grimm. He also briefly reviewed the results and methodology of his own preliminary research. Dr. Hayes offered the following summary of the studies to date. There is some trend toward phones of higher power resulting in more EMI, but no definitive answers have been reached. The greatest risk of EMI occurs when the antenna of the phone is in close proximity to the pacemaker. It is too early to say if any public safety risk exists. No definitive conclusions can be drawn; however, it appears that many pacemakers will display some form of EMI in response to digital cellular phones. It is not yet clear if pacemakers of a specific manufacturer or specific pacemaker models from a given manufacturer are more susceptible to cellular phone interactions. Dr. Hayes stressed that based on the current state of the science, further research is clearly necessary.

A unique concept Dr. Hayes presented was the importance of the clinical significance of EMI. Clinical significance is the health impact on a patient, and it is the key to understanding the public health risk of the interference issue. To determine the clinical significance of EMI, Dr. Hayes suggested that it is necessary to draw from in vitro and in vivo studies. He described a classification scheme of clinical significance developed by himself, colleagues, and WTR. Possible pacemaker responses were divided into the following categories: Class I, definitely clinically significant; Class II, probably clinically significant; and Class III, probably not clinically significant. He proposed that such a classification scheme should be considered when reporting results from studies of pacemaker EMI.

Dr. Hayes concluded his discussion of pacemakers with a description of the investigative approach he was undertaking in coordination with WTR. This approach includes three phases. Phase I is to conduct clinical studies to assess if and how implanted devices interact in vivo. Phase II is to assess the clinical and public health significance of EMI. Phase III is risk management research and making recommendations for corrective intervention as necessary. The in vivo protocol includes three clinical centers testing more than 1000 pacemaker patients. While the patient is electrocardiographically recorded, a series of currently available (AMPS, U.S. Digital Cellular, and MIRS) and soon to be available (CDMA and PCS-1900) U.S. phone technologies are tested in normal talking position and in sequenced movements over the pacemaker. The phones are operated in the test mode at maximum average power; U.S. Digital Cellular is also tested in actual transmission.

Lastly, Dr. Hayes briefly touched on the state of the science of interference research with implantable cardioverter defibrillators (ICDs). He stated that EMI could potentially result in failure of the ICD to detect a lethal rhythm disturbance and also potentially result in the delivery of unnecessary shocks in the presence of normal heart rhythm. He reported that there is no significant information regarding ICD susceptibility to EMI generated by wireless technology and that pilot studies are underway.

As the first panel response, Dr. Vincenzo Barbaro presented his own results and observations on cellular phone interference with pacemakers. Dr. Barbaro is Research Director of the Diagnostics and Function Monitoring Unit of the Laboratory of Biomedical Engineering at the Istituto Superiore di Sanita (ISS), Rome, Italy.

Dr. Barbaro explained that his team had started to investigate electromagnetic compatibility issues regarding wireless hand-held phones and pacemakers in response to a request from the Italian Minister of Health. He also explained the structure of the ISS. He then gave a description of the methodology and results of the study conducted. He described the phone technologies tested, and, in particular, the observations conducted with two analog and two digital models. The digital models

392

worked with the European standard GSM, the analog with the TACS standard. The in vitro trials were conducted using a Plexiglas box filled with saline solution. Dr. Barbaro's results showed that the electromagnetic field radiated by GSM and TACS phones interfered with a number of pacemaker models tested. Dr. Barbaro showed three typical effects induced by GSM phones: pulse inhibition, asynchronous pacing, and synchronization with the interfering signal. He said that the effects persisted as long as the interfering signal was on. Pulse inhibition and undersensing phenomena were detected with the TACS phones. The worst case of pulse inhibition observed consisted of the skipping of three non-consecutive beats. Undersensing and oversensing phenomena persisted while the TACS signal was on.

Pulse inhibition and/or synchronization were also observed when the connection had not succeeded. Even if there is no ringing, both TACS and GSM phones emit a series of random bursts. Dr. Barbaro reported that when GSM phones were tested, 20 seconds of pulse inhibition was observed during the phase. Upon testing TACS phones, pacemakers skipped a maximum of three beats. Dr. Barbaro said that since no permanent malfunctioning was observed, the team was encouraged to assess the validity of the experimental model with an ad hoc series of in vivo trials. Inhibition, synchronization, and asynchronous pacing phenomena were detected in vivo as well, in good agreement with in vitro results.

Further in vivo trials were conducted to verify the effect induced by GSM phones on a wider population of 101 informed, pacemaker-implanted patients; TACS observations were carried out on 15 patients. Dr. Barbaro reported that GSM interference was detected in 26 of the 101 patients; TACS-induced effects were observed in 3 of the 15 implanted patients. Dr. Barbaro concluded his presentation by describing the issues that require further studies. He stated that he strongly believed in the usefulness of in vitro trials because they allow the investigators to conduct tests in a controlled and repeatable manner.

Dr. Jiri Silny followed with the second invited panel response, focusing on the mechanisms of interaction between electromagnetic fields from cellular technologies and pacemakers in in vitro results. Dr. Silny is a Professor for Biomedical Measurements at the Aachen University of Technology and head of the Department for Biophysical Measurement at the Helmholtz-Institute for Biomedical Engineering in Aachen, Germany.

After a short introduction, Dr. Silny reported results from his own research experience. He explained how the input electronic circuits of the pacemaker might react to the application of a strong outside signal. The amplifier and band-pass filter of the pacemaker are designed for processing of the intracardial signal—which has only low frequency components ranging between 10 and 120 Hz—so he hypothesized that the semiconductor circuits work nonlinearly, causing the demodulation of the microwave signal in the input stage of the pacemaker. These new signal components are then filtered and processed in the same manner as the intracardial signal and can induce pacemaker malfunctioning.

Dr. Silny showed the signal emitted by a GSM cellular phone during the dialing, listening, and talking phases after demodulation and low pass filtering at a cut frequency of 1 MHZ, and after demodulation and band-pass filtering in the first electronic stage of the pacemaker. He showed the dominant frequency patterns of the

GSM signal during three phases. The band-pass filtered GSM signal forms a saw-tooth signal with a strong amplitude of 2 Hz and a weak 8 Hz component during the dialing and listening phases; during the talking phase, 217 Hz and 8 Hz are predominant.

Dr. Silny also described the experimental setup of bench tests that he had conducted. A 900 MHZ signal with an amplitude of up to 30 V simulates the signal emitted by an 8 W handset in the three phases, and can be directly injected into the input stage of a pacemaker. With 13 unipolar pacemakers, he found that interference thresholds varied widely in the 90 to 15,000 mV range. The lowest interference threshold recorded for pacing inhibition was found during the listening and dialing phases, whereas switching to fixed rate mode during the talking phase was associated with a higher interference threshold.

The behavior of the same unipolar pacemaker models was also studied in a tank model of the thorax filled with saline solution. The model was exposed to an electromagnetic field up to 100 W. Dr. Silny said that his results showed that the maximal transmission of the electromagnetic field from the phone antenna to the pacemaker input occurs when the portable phone lays directly over the case of the pacemaker with the antenna oriented in the direction of the lead. He also reported measured or calculated values of the emitted power needed to obtain the same effect observed with bench tests. He showed that the calculated transmission loss factor between the near electromagnetic field of the antenna and the voltage at the input of the pacemaker varies between 15 and 35. He concluded that the threshold of interference depends strongly upon several factors such as lead configuration, location of the pacemaker, characteristics of the single pacemaker, and position of the phone antenna with respect to the pacemaker.

Lastly, Dr. Silny reported that preliminary investigations in vivo on those pacemakers that had shown high sensitivity to interference in vitro seemed to suggest that the interference thresholds of the pacemakers had been underestimated.

The third panel response was provided by Dr. Roger Carrillo, a cardiovascular and thoracic surgeon at Mt. Sinai Medical Center in Miami Beach, Florida, USA. Dr. Carrillo has been involved in research into interference in pacemakers for more than three years. Dr. Carrillo focused his presentation on the mechanisms of the interaction, drawing on both the in vitro and in vivo studies he has conducted.

Dr. Carrillo first reviewed the results of his clinical work. He reported completing 211 tests on 65 patients, using 10 portable and transportable cellular phones of both analog and digital technologies. Phones were held to the ear and with the antenna in the proximity of the pacemaker. Interference was detected in 21 of the 65 patients.

Based on the preliminary observations of his studies, Dr. Carrillo described certain variables responsible for the EMI. First, Dr. Carrillo reported that the power of the cellular phone was correlated with the incidence of interference. Modulation was also involved, as all of the digital TDMA phones tested were able to produce interference, but the analog phones did not. He reported that antennas differ in their electromagnetic configuration, and that the magnetic field is responsible for producing more interference when compared with the electric field of the antenna. Therefore, he reported that antenna configurations may be the cause of some variability. In addition, he stated that the orientation of the antenna over the pacemaker had a significant effect on the incidence of interference. The epoxy header of the pacemaker is the most susceptible to interference. Dr. Carrillo suggested that the connecters and feed-through of the epoxy header would be capable of carrying the energy inside the sensing circuitry of the pacemaker. Dr. Carrillo also stated that the particular angles of the magnetic field vector over this location will produce more EMI. Lastly, he identified distance as a factor, and stated that laboratory studies have shown interference over a distance range of 0.8 to 12.9 centimeters.

Dr. Carrillo also discussed variables associated with the pacemaker. He identified the depth of the implantation, sensitivity, and sensing electronics as factors in susceptibility to EMI. He reported that some pacemaker models were resistant and some susceptible to interference. In a further investigation of pacemakers from a single manufacturer, he identified a feed-through filter that was the source of resistance, and he suggested that the presence of this filter might be a reliable and efficient solution to the interference problem.

Dr. Carrillo concluded with the recommendation that pacemaker patients should not use digital cellular phones in proximity to their pulse generator and that further tests should be done to clarify the importance of the variables and make risk management recommendations.

Session Two Scientific Discussion

Dr. Hank Grant, Center for the Study of Wireless Electromagnetic Compatibility:
I don't have a question, but I would like to explain the in vitro study that is currently underway at our center (the Center for the Study of Wireless Electromagnetic Compatibility). Our testing is currently 90 percent complete, and I would like to present the preliminary results of our pacemaker-cellular phone interaction study.

The objective of our study is to investigate the interaction between cellular phones and pacemakers. The scope of the study is that we are using pacemakers from five major pacemaker companies and TDMA, GSM, MIRS, PCS, CDMA, and analog phones. Our main focus is on United States technology.

MIRS and TDMA testing is 95 percent complete. GSM and CDMA are being initiated and will be completed by October. Our testing will include high frequency (1900) PCS testing. We will also add defibrillators in the next phase of testing.

We are testing pacemakers from the following companies: Medtronic, CPI, Pacesetter, Intermedics, and Telectronics. We are using eight to ten devices from each company.

The TDMA phones we are testing are from the following manufacturers: Nokia, Ericsson, Motorola, and AT&T. The MIRS phone we are testing is from Motorola. The GSM phone we are testing is from Ericsson; others manufacturers will be added in the future. The CDMA phone we are testing is from Qualcomm.

We used a technique similar to others. We used a torso-simulator that is similar to others. We placed the pacemaker in saline solution and then interjected heart beat wave forms. We then monitored the action of the pacemaker.

Another important part of our study is the simulation on both technology sides. We indicate ability to test with simulated phone signals, but we have a base station simulator for each technology and use standard phones available. Most technologies are not widely available in the United States so the base station allows us to test particular devices and also put phones in variety of modes and test things like ring and registration modes. We did find some interaction between phones and pacemakers.

As I said the study was large. Initially, the study was developed through an industry advisory board in conjunction with us. The board had members from phone technology companies, pacemaker companies, and government groups like the U.S. Food and Drug Administration. The first cut in experiment landed 90 million data points, and we did preliminary studies to cut that number down to 75,000 points and 500 test runs. Still a large study, but something more manageable.

A slide showed the following information:

- Phone/Phone Mode Combinations
  Maximum = 1 MIRS + (4 modes x 4 TDMA) = 17
  Realistic = 1 MIRS + (2 modes x ~2 TDMA) = ~5

- Maximum Number of Test Points:
  = 30 pacers x 177, 600 points x 17 phone modes
  = 90,576,000 points

- Estimated Realistic Number of Test Points
  = (67 MIRS + 218 TDMA) x (30/17) x ~150
  = ~75,000 points from ~500 test runs

Three hundred seven of 500 estimated runs are complete; approximately 61 percent. 80 of 307 runs had some interaction; 26 percent. Most of the interaction was with MIRS and TDMA technology. 31 of 217 TDMA runs had some interaction; 14 percent. 15 of 123 TDMA had ringing-interaction; 12 percent. 16 of 94 TDMA had talkback-interaction; 17 percent. This was the main type of interaction found. We are testing for 12 different types of interaction modes which are mutually exclusive. We will be providing a large published report that will be available to you sometime in January. It will have all the data from our studies.

The major conclusions that we found were that there was no instance of pacemaker reprogramming, and no instance of permanent inhibition. We plan to complete testing in the next couple of months. In the future, we will do more PCS work, and look at implantable defibrillators.

Mr. Norbert Leitgeb, Institute for Biomedical Engineering, Graz University of Technology:
I missed the possible risk...the fibrillation risk? From a theoretical point of view, the switching from the normal mode to asynchronous mode is combined with a certain risk of fibrillation. Could you exclude this risk?

Dr. Hayes:

You could not completely exclude the risk, but the risk would be indefinitely small. Yes, it is possible but extraordinarily rare. But if it does occur it is extremely serious and lethal.

Dr. Carrillo:

I agree with David. When patients come in for normal pacemaker follow-up we put a magnet on top of pacemaker to bring it into asynchronous mode. So this is part of routine follow-up. When a database of Veteran's Administration Hospitals where more than 40,000 patients follow-up has been done in asynchronous mode, there have been no reports of ventricular fibrillation. So this shows how rare of a phenomenon this could be.

Mr. Leitgeb:

It was very important to me to hear that interaction mode changes during active and passive phase of a conversation, so the active phase...the device is asynchronous mode and in listening may be triggering or inhibition. So the device switches from one interference to another one. This is bad and good news. The good news in not to be a possible risk is that in inhibitory pacemakers the time interval of continuous inhibition is small. The bad news is constant switching may increase fibrillation.

Dr. Silny:

The question is if it is possible that in talking phase you have a fixed rate mode and in listening phase you have inhibition or asynchronous. The signals after depolarization or filtering are very slow, so in very sensitive patients you may have only synchronous sometimes and then the normal behavior.

Dr. Carrillo:

Our experience with GSM phones on transmitting or talking mode have shown inhibition on American pacemakers. We are trying to find out exactly why. Filters are different pacemaker company to pacemaker company, that's one variability. Two, there is a DTX mode with 4 Hz, that's another because of inhibition and there are other factors that we are looking at. But we have seen inhibition in talking mode with GSM phones.

Dr. Eicher:

I have two comments for Dr. Hayes. You showed studies already done on a slide. The study by Naegeli and Eicher is the same study. One was presented by cardiologists and one was by engineers. The cardiologists piled up all trials in respect to any setting of pacemakers to get 600 experiments and very few errors. But like all other studies, 7 of 39 produced errors. The other comment is to question if the 2 Hz signal in the GSM is the most sensitive signal to a pacemaker. We found in the laboratory that this is completely pacemaker-dependent. We tried to use 8 Hz, 2 Hz, and 217 Hz and depending on the pacemaker it is more or less sensitive so this is not a general statement.

Dr. Silny:

To his second comment, it is true that could be possible, but in the signal in cell phones we only have 2, 8, 217 Hz. That means after filtering you see very high amplitude after 2 Hz, low amplitude at 8 Hz. You have interference at these frequencies. Eight Hz is also very important but the amplitude of 8 Hz is much lower as the number of bursts is also lower.

Dr. Eicher:

That is absolutely clear. But this is not a question. It is just a finding in experiments that it is dependent on a pacemaker if it reacts with 2, 8, 217 Hz. It is a very strange finding but you can do it in the laboratory.

APPENDIX D-4

BIOLOGICAL RESPONSES: GENETIC EFFECTS

Graham Hook and Micaela Liberti

Summary

An evaluation of potential genotoxicity is the initial stage of a regulatory assessment of potential toxicity, is an important tool in the evaluation of mechanisms of action of toxic substances, and is directly relevant to the evaluation of carcinogenic potential. Standardized tests for genotoxicity have been available for more than 20 years. Since the introduction of standardized test batteries thousands of chemicals have been tested using standardized tests. Much is now known about the chemicals that illicit genotoxic responses in these tests. In addition each of the standardized tests for genotoxicity is now well characterized. For these reasons standardized batteries of tests for genotoxicity are currently used as a first screen in the testing of virtually all newly developed compounds. In addition standardized test batteries or variants of individual tests are part of many research projects aimed at understanding the underlying mechanism of action of chemical and physical agents. In this regard the study of potential biological effects of radiofrequency radiation is no exception.

In the first presentation of this session Dr. David Brusick presented a preliminary review of the available literature related to the evaluation of potential genotoxic hazards associated with exposure to radiofrequency radiation. Simply stated genotoxicity is the alteration of the normal structure of the genome in such a way as to represent a potential hazard to the cell or organism being tested. Dr. Brusick divided genotoxic hazards into three groups: DNA disruption, recombination, and other (dominant lethal test, etc.). Using a database of over 100 studies compiled and reviewed as part of the efforts of an Expert Panel established by Wireless Technology Research, Dr. Brusick compared the results of these studies with what would be expected by chance. Dr. Brusick referred to this method of analysis as a macro-view. Using the macro-view allows for the identification of important endpoints when faced with a large database.

To identify potentially significant endpoints the frequency of positive results were compared to the expected frequency of positives based on chance alone. The frequency of expected positive results was calculated based on Dr. Brusick's experience with these endpoints and published information. Based on this analysis Dr. Brusick concluded that there was no evidence for base pair substitutions (point mutagens) or recombinogenic effects from radiofrequency radiation. However, there was some evidence for the induction of large rearrangements (chromosome aberrations and dominant lethal mutations). The significance of these results to the question of potential effects from radiofrequency radiation from wireless communication devices was limited due to the small number of studies at relevant frequencies.

The three presentations which directly followed Dr. Brusick's focussed on what future studies need to be done to fill in the gaps identified by Dr. Brusick. Dr. Verschaeve presented work from his laboratory which demonstrated the importance of looking at potential synergistic action of radiofrequency radiation with known genotoxic agents. Dr. Martin Meltz presented an overview of the extensive research program on radiofrequency radiation he and his colleagues have conducted for the Air Force. Finally Dr. Roti Roti of the Washington University described the types of tests, and the rationale for their selection, his group was going to conduct as part of a Motorola-sponsored project. Of particular interest were Dr. Roti Roti's plans to try to confirm the studies of Drs. Lai and Singh using the COMET assay. The final presentation was given by Dr. Sheldon Wolff, a renowned expert in the field of radiation biology and genotoxicity. Dr. Wolff's presentation focussed on the rationale for conducting genotoxicity tests given that it is generally agreed that radiofrequency radiation lacks the energy to directly affect DNA. In addition Dr. Wolff pointed out many of the pitfalls that should be avoided in designing and analysing these tests based on his experience with ionizing radiation.

Scientific Discussion

The presentations were followed by a unique question and answer period moderated by the session chairman Dr. Gary Williams of the American Health Foundation. Dr. Williams started the session by asking each of the speakers to comment on what they had heard from the other speakers. This part of the session was especially informative and gave the speakers the opportunity to rebut points made by other speakers and to expand upon important points from their own presentations. Dr. Verschaeve used his time to reemphasize the importance of developing new methodologies for evaluating radiofrequency radiation given its physical characteristics and unique exposure scenarios. In particular Dr. Verschaeve reiterated his call for further studies to evaluate synergistic effects and to identify potentially sensitive human populations. In contrast to the other speakers Dr. Meltz took the position that sufficient information exists to conclude that radiofrequency radiation does not directly induce DNA damage. Dr. Meltz agreed with Dr. Verschaeve that further work on potential synergistic effects needs to be done. Dr. Roti Roti emphasized the need to develop a focussed program since a shot gun methodology will always find some positive effects, which may just be sporadic or false positives.

The session ended with questions and comments from the audience. Dr. Om Gandhi commented on the relationship of SAR to the development of safety guidelines. Dr. Andrew Sivak and Dr. Mary Beth Jacobs (U.S. FDA) asked for clarification of the mechanism of synergism and the types of databases used by Dr. Brusick to develop his frequencies of expected positives respectively. Two questions were raised concerning the paper published by Drs. Lai and Singh showing increased DNA damage in rat brain cells following whole body exposure to 2450 MHZ radiofrequency radiation. Dr. Jacobs asked the panel whether they were aware of the status of an international validation study of the COMET assay used by Drs. Lai and Singh. Drs. Brusick and Verschaeve answered for the panel. The validation effort had been initiated by Dr. Raymond Tice of Integrated Laboratory Systems. Although the effort had not yet begun Dr. Verschaeve stated that he felt several groups in Great Britain would start shortly. Dr. Thomas Tenforde (Battelle Pacific) asked Dr. Roti Roti to comment on the results presented in the Lai/Singh paper. An extensive discussion of this paper followed including a description of the methodology and a discussion of possible indirect mechanisms which could produce the reported effect.

In keeping with the mandate of the colloquium the session on Biological Responses - Genotoxicity covered the state of the science to date. The session was ably chaired by Dr. Williams who summed up the session reiterating the aspects of genetic effects that make them a valuable area of research. Genetic effects are causally related to both reproductive toxicity and carcinogenicity. Most chemical and physical carcinogens are genotoxic. If radiofrequency radiation is a carcinogen then genetic effects are a "plausible biological mechanism."

BIOLOGICAL RESPONSES: CARCINOGENIC AND OTHER

Kelly G. Sund and Francesca Apollonio

Summary

Session Chair Professor Guglielmo D'Inzeo of the University "La Sapienza" of Rome opened the session by showing a diagram of the many levels at which bioelectromagnetic interaction can be considered. Central in the diagram was the progression from electromagnetic fields interacting with molecular processes at the atomic level, to possible microscopic polarization and subsequent function alteration at the cellular level, to possible macroscopic polarization and subsequent communication alteration at the tissue level, to possible heating and subsequent function alteration at the organ level, to possible thermoregulation and either disease or therapeutic consequences at the level of the total body. The mechanisms session was organized so that the speakers followed a similar progression from the molecular level to that of potential effects on humans due, for example, to mobile communications. Professor D'Inzeo then introduced Dr. Alessandro Chiabrera of the University of Genoa to give his invited paper on the state of the science in recent advances in mechanisms potentially related to radiofrequencies.

Dr. Chiabrera began his talk by stressing that he would only focus on modeling the first interaction step, at a molecular level. The complexity of, and limited knowledge about, the sequence of many steps after that caused him to infer that no conclusions about either therapeutic or adverse health consequences could be suggested based on the first interaction step.

This first interaction step considered by Dr. Chiabrera concerned ion-protein systems, which would be relevant to either the binding of ligand ions to cellular receptor proteins or the transport of messenger ions through cellular channels. He noted that there are two established models for examining such ion-protein systems: the Langevin-Lorentz (classical) approach, which studies how the displacement of a messenger ion could be affected by an electromagnetic field, and the Zeeman-Stark (quantum mechanical) approach, which focuses on how the reduced density operator of a messenger ion is affected by an electromagnetic field. Although neither model provides a good approximation of reality, Dr. Chiabrera stressed that it is possible to write state equations describing the dynamic evolution of the ion and protein system using either model. He explored the possibility of radiofrequency electromagnetic fields changing the ion dynamics inside a protein crevice or a protein channel so that the probability of the ion being bound to the protein or the ion transit time would be altered. Dr. Chiabrera focused mainly on ligand-receptor interactions.

According to Dr. Chiabrera, the ion is usually attracted to the protein by an endogenous field. He reported that the predictions obtained from the Protein Data Bank of the endogenous force typically experienced by the ion can be too high because the presence of the ion is not considered. For this reason, one must add to the field reported in the data bank the reaction field of the protein due to the displacement of the protein charges induced by the approaching ion. The resulting reaction field lowers the actual endogenous field, so that effects of low-intensity electromagnetic exposure become possible.

Dr. Chiabrera discussed the theory that the collision of water molecules would prevent effects from being seen after exposure to low-levels of exogenous radiofrequency electromagnetic fields. He stated that, to the contrary, high and spatially nonuniform endogenous fields would decrease the number of water molecules in the protein cavity by up to several orders of magnitude, so that they would not interfere with the effects of exposure to the low-intensity radiofrequency electromagnetic field.

Dr. Chiabrera did agree that low-level exposures would have negligible effects if the ion-protein system were at thermodynamic equilibrium, due to the thermal "noise" in the system. He noted, however, that living cells are not at thermodynamic equilibrium due to their basal metabolism. Dr. Chiabrera then went on to update the Langevin-Lorentz and Zeeman-Stark models to include this basal metabolism, which could lead to possible signal "amplification." He theorized that, under the right conditions, the exogenous energy from a low-intensity radiofrequency electromagnetic field, plus the endogenous energy from cellular basal metabolism, could interact through the nonlinear characteristic of the endogenous force to give an ion enough energy to escape being bound to its protein. Dr. Chiabrera also discussed the possibility of radiofrequency down-conversion, due to the aforementioned nonlinearity, and the consequent demodulation of a modulated radiofrequency carrier.

Dr. Chiabrera discussed the problem that often arises in assessing electromagnetic interaction, namely, how the power added to the system by the exposure, which can be slight in comparison to thermal energy, can give an effect. He said that what seems to be accepted at the moment are different aspects:

- the basal metabolism processes fueling the cell are the source of steady power that can sustain signal amplification through the nonlinearities of the state equations for the ion-protein system;

- the nonlinearities are also responsible for possible demodulation of radiofrequency signals down-converted to direct current or low frequency ranges;

- cooperativity and synchronization are potential enhancers of cell sensitivity to electromagnetic exposure; and

- thermal noise must always be considered in any theoretical attempt to evaluate potential electromagnetic bioeffects.

Dr. Chiabrera then discussed new numerical results from his laboratory, which he considered to be the first theoretical proof of a mechanism for a low-intensity radiofrequency field having an effect on an elementary biological process. He and his colleagues planned to reconfirm the results and then present them at the annual meetings of the European Bioelectromagnetics Association in February 1996 and the Bioelectromagnetics Society in June 1996. As Dr. Chiabrera described the preliminary results, starting at thermodynamic equilibrium (which would not occur in a living cell), a calcium ion was not bound to the receptor protein. No effects were seen, he reported, upon application of 915 MHZ to this system in thermodynamic equilibrium. Dr. Chiabrera continued that, upon adding in the force from basal metabolism, which was enough to keep the ion bound, an exogenous sinusoidal radiofrequency electromagnetic field gave an effect above 1% at 1 mW/cm^2. Changing the exposure conditions, he stated, resulted in an effect above 10% at 10 mW/cm^2. Thus, Dr. Chiabrera concluded that it is the basal metabolism which would allow a radiofrequency electromagnetic field to have an effect, via the nonlinearity of the protein's endogenous force.

In closing, Dr. Chiabrera noted again that "as far as in vivo experiments and epidemiological studies are concerned, any theoretical attempt to predict biological effects would be premature because of the highly complex (cascade, feedback, and feedforward aspects) processes and of the gaps in the related knowledge. The biophysical basis presented in this paper can provide only some guidelines for the specification of [electromagnetic] exposure parameters that are scientifically reasonable and practically affordable."

Professor D'Inzeo resumed his place at the podium and displayed his schematic to refresh the memories of the participants on the progression of the session; he then introduced Dr. Asher Sheppard of Asher Sheppard Consulting to give the first invited response.

Dr. Sheppard devoted his talk to addressing the question of where microwave energy absorbed by biological objects goes on the microscopic and molecular levels. He categorized the possible loss mechanisms into ohmic losses by ionic currents, as well as dielectric losses in cells, proteins (not only through forces on polar groups, but also through bound water and rotationally free groups), and water. Dr. Sheppard stated that this last mechanism provides the major contribution to heating at 1-20 GHz and posed the question of whether it provided the major contribution to biological responses.

He showed H.P. Schwan's categories of energy dispersion, namely: biological cells composed of water, membrane, and protein; bare cells consisting of water and membrane; solutions of water and protein; and just water.

Dr. Sheppard suggested a definition of a "nonthermal experimental condition" as one where there is so little energy input that, even if there were no way to remove heat, there would be no significant effect on temperature (in vitro and in vivo) or thermoregulation (in vivo). He said "athermal conditions" occur in vitro when the temperature would be changed if there were no way to compensate for the energy input, but by removing enough heat the temperature is held constant (and at a normal value). "Thermal conditions" were said to occur when heat input is sufficient to cause a significant rise in temperature (in vitro and in vivo).

Dr. Sheppard discussed the equation for reaction rate. He cited authors who found that the transference of energy by structural water and/or the absorption of microwave photons may affect protein structure.

In conclusion, Dr. Sheppard stated that at about 1 GHz absorbed energy goes into free water and bound water and then is rapidly transferred by collisions to proteins, lipids, and both microscopic and macroscopic structures.

Professor D'Inzeo then returned to the podium to show the progression of the session through his diagram, and introduced Dr. Bernard Veyret of Universite Bordeaux for his invited response.

Dr. Veyret began his talk by comparing and contrasting biointeraction (which he defined as the values of electric and magnetic fields inside organisms), bioeffects (changes in biochemical and physiological parameters in cells or systems due to biointeraction), and health consequences (hazardous or beneficial changes in health status because of bioeffects).

He noted that microwave biointeractions are typically thought to involve bulk water, although the heating of bulk water is unlikely at the low powers of mobile telephones. Since modulation by extremely low frequency fields has been cited as the cause of specific bioeffects, Dr. Veyret recommended conducting experiments on the same biological model with both extremely low frequency fields and radiofrequency fields modulated by extremely low frequencies. He predicted that such an approach would provide insight on demodulation mechanisms.

In terms of bioeffects, Dr. Veyret agreed with Dr. Sheppard's definitions of nonthermal (which he called specific), athermal, and thermal effects. He raised the questions of whether possible effects from mobile telephones would be nonthermal/specific or athermal, and what organ systems would be targeted.

Dr. Veyret mentioned recently completed or ongoing areas of bioeffects research in Europe: genetics, behavior, cell proliferation, cancer, blood-brain barrier, nervous system, and neuroendocrine system. He noted that some of these studies were conducted on humans. Dr. Veyret summed up the European work by stating that many studies were negative, but that some were positive and needed to be repeated. On the whole, he concluded that the European research suggested possible effects on the nervous system and endocrine system.

In conclusion, Dr. Veyret noted that mechanisms of specific effects were not yet known either for extremely low frequency fields or for microwave fields. He cautioned that possible interactive mechanisms should be studied, since, for example, some effects of extremely low frequency fields were only seen in his laboratory following preparation of cells in a particular fashion.

Professor D'Inzeo then revisited the progression of the session by use of his schematic and introduced Dr. Thomas Tenforde of Battelle Pacific Northwest Laboratories to give his invited response.

Due to time constraints, Dr. Tenforde termed his presentation merely a comment on the scientific literature relating to electromagnetic fields and cancer. To review the multistage model of carcinogenesis developed from skin-painting studies, he showed a diagram including the stages of initiation, promotion (with stage I being early events and stage II described as conversion), and tumor progression. Since an earlier session that day covered initiation, Dr. Tenforde did not include that topic in his remarks.

Dr. Tenforde first discussed results obtained in vitro that he considered relevant to promotion and progression. He categorized these results as variable, and suggested that more study was needed in three areas. The first of these was the reported decrease in protein kinase activity in response to extremely low frequency fields and radiofrequency fields modulated by extremely low frequencies. The second was the conflicting data on the possible increased expression of certain oncogenes following exposure to extremely low frequency fields. The third concerned the elevated cytoplasmic activity of ornithine decarboxylase seen with extremely low frequency fields and radiofrequency fields modulated by extremely low frequencies, which could be interpreted as evidence of tumor promotion (although less than that seen with the chemical promoter phorbol ester 12-ortho-tetradecanoylphorbol-13-acetate, or TPA) were it not for the absence of increased synthesis of ornithine decarboxylase and/or DNA.

Dr. Tenforde also discussed data obtained in vivo, which he said showed no convincing evidence of tumor promotion except for perhaps the effects of extremely low frequency fields on rat mammary tumors as reported by Beniashvili et al. (1991) and replicated by another laboratory. Dr. Tenforde presented the hypothesis that melatonin production at night could be suppressed by extremely low frequency fields, with four consequences: increased concentration of estrogen and subsequent promotion of breast tumor cell growth; decreased immune system response to tumor-specific antigens; reduced oncostatic effects of melatonin on estrogen-receptor-positive breast tumor cells; and reduced scavenging of free radicals that damage DNA.

Dr. Tenforde concluded his talk by calling for a broad range of carcinogenesis studies.

Professor D'Inzeo returned to the podium and illustrated how the session was covering the various levels of biological responses. He then introduced Dr. Andrew Sivak, a consultant, to give the final invited response to Dr. Chiabrera's paper.

Dr. Sivak prefaced his remarks by stressing his public health orientation, particularly in terms of cancer, which he said was typically studied by epidemiology studies, animal bioassays, and mechanistic studies. Dr. Sivak noted that there were not yet any published epidemiology studies on the wavelengths relevant to wireless communication instruments, although some studies, such as those funded by Wireless Technology Research, LLC, were underway.

As for animal bioassays, Dr. Sivak cited three that had been completed on carcinogenesis, two that were done on other endpoints, and two more that were underway. None of the three finished carcinogenesis bioassays, he reported, showed any significant increase in a particular target site, although one saw an overall increase and one saw an overall decrease in cancer. One of the other chronic bioassays mentioned by Dr. Sivak reported no difference in survival following exposure to 800 MHZ, but no pathology was done in that study. The other chronic bioassay he discussed showed no change in life span following exposure to 2450 MHZ at 2 W/kg for an hour a day for two years, but a 30% decrease in life span when the exposure was increased to 6.8 W/kg. Dr. Sivak pointed out that the exposure in these studies was many times that to which humans using wireless communication devices are exposed.

Dr. Sivak discussed four types of mechanistic studies. He stated that none of the handful of studies on inducing cell proliferation showed an effect from microwave exposure, that the studies on the enhancement of tumor cell growth had no increase in the number of dead animals, and that the one in vitro study on calcium transport reported no effect.

The fourth type of study mentioned by Dr. Sivak, tumor promotion, was the focus of an expert panel assembled by Wireless Technology Research, LLC. Dr. Sivak explained the charge to this panel, which he chaired, as evaluating in vitro and in vivo studies involving radiofrequency radiation, determining the relevance of animal promotion models to humans, and examining possible mechanisms of tumor promotion by radiofrequency radiation. He relayed the panel's conclusions that there was no in vitro or in vivo evidence that radiofrequency radiation acted as a tumor promoter, that direct inferences from experimental tumor promotion studies to humans could not be supported, and that there were not enough data to suggest a mechanism by which radiofrequency radiation could act as a tumor promoter.

Dr. Sivak concluded his remarks with his opinion that scientific data do not dictate a significant concern about carcinogenesis due to exposure to radiofrequency radiation from wireless communication instruments, but that other health effects including neuroendocrine ones should be considered. He wished that the database on biological effects would be as extensive as that for some chemicals, and called for biologically-based regulatory standards.

Scientific Discussion

After the break, the session resumed with a question and answer period. Dr. Sivak began by clarifying that his concluding statement was not meant as an attack on regulators, whom he recognized as working diligently to create standards.

Dr. Quirino Balzano of Motorola next asked Dr. Chiabrera for his values of the metabolic field and its force. In his answer, Dr. Chiabrera noted that a metabolic field force of 2×10^{-17} N seemed to show an appreciable (above ten percent) effect at 10 mW/cm^2. Dr. Balzano then suggested that Dr. Chiabrera incorporate statistical fluctuations of the metabolic force. Dr. Balzano also questioned Dr. Veyret's suggestion that research on extremely low frequency fields could be relevant to radiofrequency fields, since the mechanisms involved might be completely different. Dr. Veyret countered that extremely low frequency field research could be relevant if the same bio-effect was being reported.

Dr. Mary Elizabeth Jacobs of the Food and Drug Administration then asked Dr. Sivak why he recommended studying neuroendocrine effects. Dr. Sivak replied that this was a likely hypothesis following from application of electromagnetic fields to the brain, and that it seemed to have some support from the European research.

An epidemiologist, Dr. John Vena of the State University of New York at

Buffalo, asked the entire panel how their mechanistic perspective would direct epidemiology studies. Dr. Chiabrera believed it worthwhile to consider concurrent exposures to power lines and to report the actual earth's magnetic fields, because radiofrequency demodulation may occur. Dr. Sheppard did not consider the mechanistic work far enough advanced to guide epidemiology, but noted that the work of Dr. Henry Lai at the University of Washington on rats suggested studying behavioral effects correlated with the acetylcholine neurotransmitter. Dr. Veyret recommended studying persons with a history of neurologic disorders. Dr. Tenforde cautioned against trying to incorporate biomarkers of radiofrequency radiation exposure in epidemiology studies at this point, due both to their expense and to their current lack of correlation with any health effects. Dr. Sivak observed that politics appeared to dictate an examination of cancer, but repeated that the state of the science did not yet support any direction for epidemiologic research.

Dr. Arthur W. Guy of Wireless Technology Research, LLC questioned the modulation and magnetic field focus of Dr. Chiabrera's model, suggesting that the electric field component of any demodulated extremely low frequencies associated with his model would produce effects far outweighing those of any demodulated extremely low frequency magnetic field component. In other words, with perfect 100 percent demodulation of the one milliwatt per square centimeter fields in the tissue of his model, the electric field strength would be far above the thresholds of action potential stimulation and cardiac fibrillation, while the magnetic field flux density would be a weak five milligauss. The demodulation would have to be less than 2.5 percent to prevent action potential stimulation, which would limit the magnetic field strength to an innocuous 0.125 milligauss or less, far below any threshold of observed effects. Dr. Chiabrera clarified that his effect was just seen at the carrier radiofrequency of a transverse electromagnetic sinusoidal wave, so that both the pertinent electric and magnetic field components were considered.

Dr. Martin Meltz of the University of Texas Health Science Center at San Antonio took issue with Dr. Veyret's call for consideration of extremely low frequency research, stating instead that researchers in that field should observe researchers in the radiofrequency field, and that both fields could learn lessons in designing studies from those who work on chemical exposures. Dr. Meltz also observed that the public seemed to experience considerable confusion about the difference between extremely low frequencies and radiofrequencies already, and did not want to add to that. Dr. Veyret responded that, looking outside bioelectromagnetics, there were lessons to be learned from extremely low frequency work in terms of coordinating research.

In his closing remarks for the session, Professor D'Inzeo summed up the session's progression through his diagram of the many levels at which bioelectromagnetic interaction can be considered. He noted that the end effects could be either harmful or beneficial. He then showed a second diagram showing how advances in cell biology, membrane biophysics, biochemistry, and quantum and classical studies can all affect each other. Professor D'Inzeo ended by concluding that much work remains to be done before arriving at any conclusions in this field.

COLLOQUIUM SUMMATION

George L. Carlo and Susan E. Hersemann

Dr. George Carlo, Chairman of Wireless Technology Research, LLC, began his observations and perspectives on the colloquium by thanking the staff and all the participants for their hard work over three long days. He believed that the colloquium had been successful in moving the scientific and public health aspects of these issues forward, and that the ambitious goals of the meeting had been met.

Dr. Carlo explained that his own interest in wireless communication instruments comes from a public health perspective. He noted that this approach is quite straightforward and in some ways much simpler than some of the discussions held over the last several days. The public health approach seeks an answer to the question, "Is there a problem that requires intervention, and if so, when and how do we intervene?" A public health approach is distinguished from hypothesis testing, such as seeking to establish the safety of a device or a product prior to marketing, or to be absolutely sure that there is no risk. The public health approach has to do with enough evidence to require intervention.

Dr. Carlo returned to the four questions he had posed at the beginning of the colloquium. First, how should the abundant existing scientific information generally applicable to biological effects of radio frequency radiation be applied to this new question of low-power, head-concentrated emissions from cellular telephones? Dr. Carlo felt that the colloquium had been enlightening with regard to this question. Many existing data are relevant and useful. We are not in the position of knowing nothing; we know a great deal. Although there have not been numerous studies done directly on cellular telephones, some judgments can be made. Most significantly, from the perspective of public health protection, we have not seen anything which indicates an immediate need for intervention with regard to direct biological effects.

Second, what safety standards should apply to new generations of wireless technology, and how can compliance be measured? Dr. Carlo believed that discussions at the colloquium illustrated that, with respect to safety standards, regulation may be leading the science. There was a sense of frustration among the biologists that there may not be enough biological basis to support guidelines for near-field, low-power exposures in the low SAR range. At the same time, significant strides have been made in characterizing output from wireless instruments. While the advances in measurement are encouraging, comfort can not be taken blindly just because a number can be measured. Dr. Carlo cited an example from the area of environmental exposures to illustrate this point. In the early 1960s, dioxin was measured in parts per million. As measurement science progressed, dioxin could be measured in parts per billion, parts per trillion, and beyond. The ability to measure dioxin far outstripped the ability to interpret that data in the context of biology and public health.

In Dr. Carlo's perspective, standards should be biologically-based. If they are not, the science base needed to support them must developed without letting political pressures drive premature, speculative regulatory decisions. Dr. Carlo mentioned the assertions of some that regulatory needs are having an impact on the direction of the science. Science-first thinking requires that science should lead to regulatory decisions, not the other way around.

Third, do we have the scientific tools necessary to study near-field, low-power exposures with a reasonable degree of scientific certainty? He related that he was encouraged that the scientific community had taken up the challenge to modify existing tools for application to the specific problems of wireless instruments' biological effects. He gave the examples of new, head-only exposure systems and measuring heat distributions in TEM cells in an effort to interpret those studies better.

Dr. Carlo related that even with such progress, however, the rapidity of technological evolution is outstripping the usefulness of our standard tools and approaches for testing products in the pre-market arena and monitoring them in the post-market environment. A new paradigm is needed. In this vein, Dr. Carlo was encouraged by the epidemiology reports detailing new ways of identifying cohorts and study procedures for post-market surveillance. He considered the move toward new and creative ways of monitoring users of the products through post-market surveillance to be very important given the fact that it is impossible to predict what the technology might be next month, let alone what the health effects of that technology may be.

Finally, how do we address biological effects that are indirect, such as those that might follow from interference between digital signals and cardiac pacemakers or defibrillators? Dr. Carlo believed that the pacemaker research to date was a tribute to the timely, constructive, and integrated response of the medical, scientific, industrial, and regulatory communities. The problem was little more than a year old, yet tremendous steps forward had been made. He praised the response as a model for other areas.

Dr. Carlo closed by challenging the participants to utilize the knowledge gained at the colloquium in their research and in their thinking, and to continue to interact with each other, the WTR, and the ICWCHR on this important public health issue.

Several other speakers offered comments during the summation session. Thomas Damboldt of Deutsche Telekom expressed support for the public health approach, but confessed uncertainty as to whether research would address the concerns of the public. He indicated that direction on the type of studies needed and some standardized guidelines for exposure characterization would be welcome. He suggested that ICWCHR might take the lead in developing this information. Tom Lukish of the

Cellular Telecommunications Industry Association communicated the industry's commitment to the research program and their confidence in the tremendous scientific power being brought to bear on the issue. He discussed the rapid proliferation of cellular technology in the US and highlighted the safety features of cellular telephones, such as the ability to make emergency calls.

Questions regarding Italian exposure limits and siting of base stations were posed by Francesco de Lorenzo of Radio Ouda Rossa, and prompted reflections from Dr. Paolo Vecchia of the Istituto Superiore di Sanità, Dr. Paolo Bernardi of the University "La Sapienza" of Rome, and Dr. Gary Williams of the American Health Foundation on the issues of risk perception among members of the public and risk communication by scientists. Dr. Martin Meltz of the University of Texas Health Science Center at San Antonio concluded the session by challenging reporters to research their topics thoroughly, and challenging the public to demand such thoroughness.

Keyword Index